Infection in the Immunocompromised Host

T0177474

Oxford Specialist Handbooks published and forthcoming

Oxford Specialist Handbooks in Infectious Diseases

Infection in the Immunocompromised Host

Simon M. Fox

Locum Consultant in Infectious
Diseases, Sheffield Teaching
Hospitals NHS Foundation Trust;
and Oxford Centre for
Tropical Medicine,
University of Oxford, UK

Angela M. Minassian

Chief Investigator on Clinical
Vaccine Trials; and Honorary
Consultant, Jenner Institute,
University of Oxford; and Heart of
England NHS Trust, UK

Thomas Rawlinson

The Jenner Institute, University of
Oxford, Wellcome Trust Research
Training Fellow, UK

Brian J. Angus

Associate Professor and
Reader in Infectious Diseases,
Director Oxford Centre for
Tropical Medicine, University of
Oxford, UK

OXFORD
UNIVERSITY PRESS

OXFORD
UNIVERSITY PRESS

Great Clarendon Street, Oxford, OX2 6DP,
United Kingdom

Oxford University Press is a department of the University of Oxford.
It furthers the University's objective of excellence in research, scholarship,
and education by publishing worldwide. Oxford is a registered trade mark of
Oxford University Press in the UK and in certain other countries

© Oxford University Press 2019

The moral rights of the authors have been asserted

Impression: 1

Published in the United States of America by Oxford University Press
198 Madison Avenue, New York, NY 10016, United States of America

British Library Cataloguing in Publication Data
Data available

Library of Congress Control Number: 2018945626

ISBN 978–0–19–878998–7

Printed and bound in China by
C&C Offset Printing Co., Ltd.

Contents

Symbols and abbreviations

➔	cross-reference
~	approximately
↑	increased
↓	decreased
→	leading to
↔	normal
♨	website
ADCC	antibody-dependent cellular cytotoxicity
AFB	acid-fast bacilli
aGvHD	acute graft-versus-host disease
AHSCT	allogeneic haematopoietic stem cell transplantation
ALT	alanine aminotransferase
AML	acute myeloid leukaemia
ARDS	acute respiratory distress syndrome
ARV	antiretroviral
ASA	aminosalicylic acid
ATG	anti-thymocyte globulin
BAL	bronchoalveolar lavage
BCG	Bacillus Calmette–Guérin
BD-glucan	1,3-beta-D-glucan
BHIVA	British HIV Association
BIS	British Infection Society
CDAD	*Clostridium difficile*-associated diarrhoea
CDI	*Clostridium difficile* infection
CGD	chronic granulomatous disease
cGvHD	chronic graft-versus-host disease
CID	combined immunodeficiency
CML	chronic myeloid leukaemia
CMV	cytomegalovirus
CNS	central nervous system
COPD	chronic obstructive pulmonary disease
CPE	carbapenemase-producing Enterobacteriaceae
CSF	cerebrospinal fluid
CT	computed tomography
CVID	common variable immunodeficiency disorder
EBV	Epstein–Barr virus
ECG	electrocardiogram

EDTA	ethylenediamine tetraacetic acid
EIA	enzyme immunoassay
ELISA	enzyme-linked immunosorbent assay
ESBL	extended-spectrum beta-lactamase
ESCMID	European Society of Clinical Microbiology and Infectious Diseases
G6PD	glucose-6-phosphate dehydrogenase
G-CSF	granulocyte colony stimulating factor
GI	gastrointestinal
GM-CSF	granulocyte-macrophage colony-stimulating factor
GvHD	graft-versus-host disease
HAART	highly active antiretroviral therapy
HACEK	*Haemophilus parainfluenzae, Aggregatibacter actinomycetemcomitans, Cardiobacterium hominis, Eikenella corrodens,* and *Kingella kingae*
HAV	hepatitis A virus
HBcAb	hepatitis B core antibody
HBsAG	hepatitis B surface antigen
HBV	hepatitis B virus
HCV	hepatitis C virus
HDV	hepatitis D virus
HEV	hepatitis E virus
HHV	human herpesvirus
HIES	hyper IgE syndrome
HIV	human immunodeficiency virus
HLA	human leucocyte antigen
HPV	human papillomavirus
HSCT	haematopoietic stem cell transplantation
HSV	herpes simplex virus
HTLV	human T-cell lymphotropic virus
ICU	intensive care unit
IFA	immunofluorescence assay
IFN	interferon
Ig	immunoglobulin
IGRA	interferon-gamma release assay
IL	interleukin
IRIS	immune reconstitution inflammatory syndrome
IUIS	International Union of Immunological Societies
IV	intravenous
IVIG	intravenous immunoglobulin
JEV	Japanese encephalitis virus

KS	Kaposi's sarcoma
LCMV	lymphocytic choriomeningitis virus
LFT	liver function test
LTBI	latent tuberculosis infection
MAC	*Mycobacterium avium* complex
MAI	*Mycobacterium avium–intracellulare* infection
MDR	multidrug-resistant
MERS	Middle East respiratory syndrome
MHC	major histocompatibility complex
MIC	minimum inhibitory concentration
MMF	mycophenolate mofetil
MMR	measles, mumps, and rubella
MRI	magnetic resonance imaging
MRSA	methicillin-resistant *Staphylococcus aureus*
MSSA	methicillin-sensitive *Staphylococcus aureus*
MTB	*Mycobacterium tuberculosis*
MTBC	*Mycobacterium tuberculosis* complex
mTOR	mammalian target of rapamycin
NAAT	nucleic acid amplification test
NAT	nucleic acid testing
NHL	non-Hodgkin lymphoma
NICE	National Institute for Health and Care Excellence
NNRTI	non-nucleoside reverse-transcriptase inhibitor
NRTI	nucleoside reverse transcriptase inhibitor
NTM	non-tuberculous mycobacteria
NtRTI	nucleotide reverse transcriptase inhibitor
NTS	non-typhoidal *Salmonella*
OGD	oesophagogastroduodenoscopy
PAMP	pathogen-associated molecular pattern
PCP	*Pneumocystis* pneumonia
PCR	polymerase chain reaction
PHE	Public Health England
PI	protease inhibitor
PID	primary immunodeficiency disorder
PML	progressive multifocal leucoencephalopathy
PRR	pattern-recognition receptor
PTLD	post-transplant lymphoproliferative disorder
qPCR	quantitative polymerase chain reaction
R-CHOP	rituximab + cyclophosphamide, doxorubicin, vincristine, and prednisolone

RPR	rapid plasma reagin
RSV	respiratory syncytial virus
SARS	severe acute respiratory syndrome
SBP	spontaneous bacterial peritonitis
SCID	severe combined immunodeficiency
SIRS	systemic inflammatory response syndrome
SLE	systemic lupus erythematosus
SMX	sulfamethoxazole
SOT	solid organ transplant
STD	sexually transmitted disease
TMP	trimethoprim
TNF	tumour necrosis factor
TRIM	transfusion-related immunomodulation
TST	tuberculin skin test
UCB	umbilical cord blood
UK	United Kingdom
UNAIDS	Joint United Nations Programme on HIV and AIDS
US	United States
VISA	vancomycin-intermediate *Staphylococcus aureus*
VRE	vancomycin-resistant enterococci
VRSA	vancomycin-resistant *Staphylococcus aureus*
VZV	varicella zoster virus
XDR	extensively drug-resistant

Section 1

Background

Introduction

Introduction

The term 'immunocompromised host' defines individuals with either non-specific (e.g. skin and mucous membrane, phagocytic activity, complement) or specific (humoral or cellular immunity) dysfunction of defence mechanisms, or a combination of these. The alteration of these defence mechanisms may be a consequence of underlying disease (e.g. tumours, HIV infection), the effects of medical therapies (e.g. chemotherapy, steroids, immunosuppressants, radiation), or primary genetic defects.

In recent decades, the population of immunocompromised patients has steadily increased, largely due to the combination of advances in medical therapies and the human immunodeficiency virus (HIV) pandemic. The extended use of high-dose chemotherapy in the treatment of malignancies, as well as autologous or allogeneic transplantation of bone marrow or peripheral blood stem cells, has offered new therapeutic options, but has also increased the number of patients at risk of opportunistic infection. Similarly, increasing numbers of solid organ transplants with the corresponding need for anti-rejection immunosuppression along with an expanding number of patients taking corticosteroids or other immunosuppressive drugs make the immunocompromised host an increasingly common entity.

The advent of highly active antiretroviral therapy (HAART) in the treatment of HIV has markedly reduced immunosuppression and opportunistic infections in patients with access to these drugs. Unfortunately, many patients (particularly in resource-limited settings) are still unable to benefit from these drugs and continue to present with infections related to immunocompromise.

Key principles

- It is essential to recognize and consider the roles played by the underlying illness of the host, the state of the host immune system, and the drugs administered, in the aetiology of infection—both in diagnosis and therapy.
- Common and uncommon pathogens are both important in the immunocompromised host, making for an extensive list of differential diagnoses and a challenge in establishing an early accurate diagnosis.
- Several non-infectious pathologies may mimic clinical syndromes of infection. Failure to recognize this possibility can result in unnecessary invasive and non-invasive diagnostic procedures and administration of potentially toxic medications, detrimental to the health of an already fragile host.
- The urgency of establishing an accurate diagnosis needs to be weighed against the risks associated with the diagnostic procedures, some of which may be invasive. In critically ill patients or patients in whom invasive procedures may be precluded, empiricism may be the most appropriate or only choice. While recognizing that antimicrobial resistance is widespread in wards housing compromised hosts, broad-spectrum empiric therapy may often be the most prudent strategy. Under such circumstances, the duration of empiric therapy needs to be constantly evaluated and the antimicrobial spectrum narrowed as soon as possible.
- Timing of appropriate intervention, based on sound clinical judgement, is crucial for a good outcome—not too early, but not too late.

Chapter 2

The immune system

Introduction

This introduction to the immune system provides just a brief overview of the fundamental processes that constitute innate and adaptive immune mechanisms. In reality, our understanding of this intricate apparatus is still evolving at the molecular, cellular, and systems levels. Such a complex system might be expected to incorporate some redundancy and the spectrum of immunodeficient states in which the host is unable to effectively combat pathogens and cancer underlies the fine tuning.

Host defence

Colonization versus infection

Colonization would not typically be expected to harm or cause signs and symptoms, and therefore does not usually need treatment. From birth, large areas of the human body surface are colonized with microorganisms—including the skin and the mucous membranes of the oropharynx, nasopharynx, intestinal tract, and genital tract. The human microbiota is in fact estimated to consist of 10–100 trillion microbial cells, primarily bacteria in the gut, with the so-called human microbiome consisting of the genes these cells harbour. Importantly, these 'normal' or commensal microbes help to prevent colonization of an individual by more dangerous pathogens which could lead to infection. A carrier is colonized with a microorganism and may transmit to other people. This status can persist for long periods of time, and may be influenced or altered by the immune response to the organism, local competition from other microorganisms, and the use of antimicrobials.

Infection is when a disease-causing microorganism(s) is present and causing damage to body tissues, which typically induces inflammation during the acute stage. However, the difference between infection and colonization is almost always related to circumstances. Colonizing organisms can become pathogenic under certain conditions, and even highly virulent organisms require the right circumstances to invade and cause successful infection of the host.

Distinguishing colonization from infection is an important factor in making a correct diagnosis for many conditions and is especially problematic in the immunocompromised host.

Physical barriers

Infectious complications occurring in the compromised host are a direct result of faulty defence and often there is a clear relationship between specific predisposing factors (e.g. changes in the skin and mucosal barriers, neutropenia, humoral or cellular immunity deficiency) and the predominant pathogen(s).

The outer defence system includes physical barriers (the skin, cilia, mucosa of the buccal and nasal cavities, genitourinary and the gastrointestinal tracts) and chemical barriers (tears, mucus, stomach acid, urine flow). Opportunistic pathogens can enter the host by taking advantage of physical injury or breaches in these barriers, while other pathogens have evolved mechanisms to cross host barriers.

The skin is a common site of contact with many pathogens. The presence of specific immune cells and production of antimicrobial molecules plays a very important role in cutaneous defences. The skin also provides structures such as hair follicles and sebaceous, eccrine, and apocrine glands that constitute discrete niches for microbes, with variable environmental pressures including humidity, temperature, pH, and the composition of antimicrobial peptides and lipids. Although most pathogens are unable to cross the skin barrier, they can access underlying tissue via cuts, injury, lesions, insect bites, or medically inserted devices.

Mucosae are composed of three layers: an epithelium, connective tissue called lamina propria, and a thin layer of smooth muscle. Epithelia are in

contact with the extracellular environment, and are covered by a protective mucus layer composed mainly of mucin glycoproteins, digestive enzymes, antimicrobial peptides, and immunoglobulins. Some pathogens have
evolved mechanisms to breach the mucus layer in order to reach epithelial
cells, including production of proteases, flagella-based motility, or resistance
to antimicrobial molecules.

Innate humoral and cellular defence mechanisms

Following a breach of these physical barriers, the host immune system
forms the second line of defence, seeking to contain and ultimately destroy the invading pathogen through a variety of cellular and humoral means.

In the early stages of infection, defences are often termed 'innate' or
'non-specific' to contrast with the subsequent 'adaptive' response mediated by the expansion of specific B and T lymphocytes that also provide long-lasting immunological memory. The innate immune system is an
evolutionarily older defensive strategy, and the dominant system found in
less complex species. As the first responder, this system seeks to contain,
engulf, and destroy pathogens. It initiates inflammation, signals through
the secretion of soluble immune molecules, and directs any ensuing adaptive response. As a pathogen may be extracellular or intracellular, the immune system has established mechanisms to respond accordingly. Innate
pathogen recognition mechanisms are central to this process, with an array
of different pattern-recognition receptors (PRRs) on cells of the immune
system able to detect evolutionarily conserved pathogen-associated molecular patterns (PAMPs) comprising protein-, sugar-, lipid-, or nucleic acid-
based molecules that differ from the host but are frequently expressed by
foreign microorganisms. These families of PRRs include the Toll-like receptors (TLRs) and C-type lectins on the cell surface, and cytosolic PRRs such
as nucleotide-binding oligomerization domain (NOD) proteins and the
caspase recruitment domain (CARD) helicases.

The 'innate' cells of the immune system are detailed in Table 2.1.

The binding of PRRs with PAMPs triggers the release of cytokines, most
notably interleukins and interferons. These are chemical messengers that
signal the presence of pathogens and regulate gene expression, cell differentiation, proliferation, activation, and apoptosis. The first soluble signals
are cytokines and chemokines leading to a pro-inflammatory response. This
is characterized clinically by localized redness, swelling, heat, and pain—a
dynamic tissue response mechanism that has evolved as an initial defence
against pathogens. The outcome of pathogen-driven inflammation is destruction of the pathogen whenever possible, or its containment when destruction is not achievable. Vasodilation and increased vascular permeability
are key components of tissue inflammation, allowing for the movement of
plasma proteins and immunoglobulins into the tissue. Subsequently, the cellular components, which normally reside in blood, are enabled to move into
the inflamed tissue via extravasation and a chemokine gradient towards the
site of infection. Depending on the cell type and invading pathogen, these
cells may phagocytose or degranulate.

Within the humoral system, an array of soluble complement proteins
is abundant in the plasma and functions to destroy extracellular pathogens. Complement proteins bind to the surfaces of microorganisms in a

Table 2.1 The characteristics and location of cells involved in the innate immune system

Cell type	Characteristics	Location	Image
Mast cell	Dilates blood vessels and induces inflammation through release of histamines and heparin. Recruits macrophages and neutrophils. Involved in wound healing and defence against pathogens but can also be responsible for allergic reactions	Connective tissues, mucous membranes	
Macrophage	Phagocytic cell that consumes foreign pathogens and cancer cells. Stimulates response of other immune cells	Migrates from blood vessels into tissues	
Natural killer cell	Kills tumour cells and virus-infected cells	Circulates in blood and migrates into tissues	
Dendritic cell	Presents antigens on its surface thereby triggering adaptive immunity	Present in epithelial tissue, including skin, lung, and tissues of the digestive tract. Migrates to lymph nodes upon activation	

(Continued)

Table 2.1 Contd.

Cell type	Characteristics	Location	Image
Monocyte	Differentiates into macrophages and dendritic cells in response to inflammation	Stored in spleen, moves through blood vessels to infected tissues	
Neutrophil	First responder at the site of infection or trauma, this abundant phagocytic cell represents 50–60% of all leucocytes. Releases toxins that kill or inhibit bacteria and fungi and recruits other immune cells to the site of infection	Migrates from blood vessels into tissues	
Basophil	Responsible for defence against parasites. Releases histamines that cause inflammation and may be responsible for allergic reactions	Circulates in blood and migrates to tissues	
Eosinophil	Releases toxins that kill bacteria and parasites but also causes tissue damage	Circulates in blood and migrates to tissues	

specific and regulated sequence according to three different pathways (Fig 2.1). Activation leads to opsonization and phagocytosis by C3b deposition, bacterial lysis by C5b–9 membrane attack complex (MAC) formation, and inflammation by the recruitment of immune cells, endothelial and epithelial cell activation, and platelet activation.

Adaptive humoral and cellular defence mechanisms

Acquired immunity is triggered in vertebrates when a pathogen evades the innate immune system thus generating a threshold level of antigen. An antigen is defined as a substance within the body that is capable of eliciting an immune response (traditionally an antibody response).

Key to the initiation of this response is the processing and presentation of the antigen by a professional antigen-presenting cell (APC), which specializes in presenting antigens to T cells. Protein antigen internalization may occur either by phagocytosis (macrophages and dendritic cells) or by receptor-mediated endocytosis (B cells). Proteins that are internalized by the endocytic pathways are degraded into short peptides by lysosomal enzymes and presented back on the cell surface bound to major histocompatibility complex (MHC) class II molecules (the exogenous antigen-presenting pathway). Similarly, protein antigens can also be transferred to the cytosol for 'cross presentation' by the endogenous antigen processing pathway. In this case or following direct cellular infection by a pathogen, short peptides (nine to ten amino acids long) are generated by proteasomal degradation of cytosolic proteins. These are subsequently translocated into the endoplasmic reticulum, via the TAP transporter, to meet MHC class I molecules held in close proximity to the transporter by a network of chaperone proteins. Once a peptide is loaded onto the MHC class I molecule, the complex leaves the endoplasmic reticulum through the secretory pathway to reach the cell surface. Generic MHC molecules are known as human leucocyte antigen (HLA) molecules in humans (and H-2 molecules in mice, a species widely used for immunology research).

Professional APCs also possess a wealth of PRRs whose ligation not only activates the APC, but also induces the secretion of cytokines in a manner dependent on the combination of PRRs that are activated. The ensuing cytokine milieu is tailored to instruct the adaptive system about the nature of the response required to eliminate a particular class of pathogen. Once activated, dendritic cells migrate from the periphery to the secondary lymphoid system bearing peptide antigen in the context of relevant MHC molecules, and present their findings to naïve T lymphocytes. Linear peptide epitopes are recognized in the context of a MHC molecule by the T-cell receptor and CD4 or CD8 co-receptor, and in conjunction with a panel of co-stimulatory molecules and cytokines upregulated by the activated dendritic cell, activate the naïve T cell. This cell will undergo rapid clonal expansion into an armed effector T-cell population that migrates into the periphery. Following expansion, this population contracts to form circulating effector memory (T_{EM}) and central memory (T_{CM}) T-cell populations.

CD4+ T cells
CD4+ T cells recognize peptides presented in the context of MHC class II molecules on the surface of APCs. Many different types of CD4+ T cell have

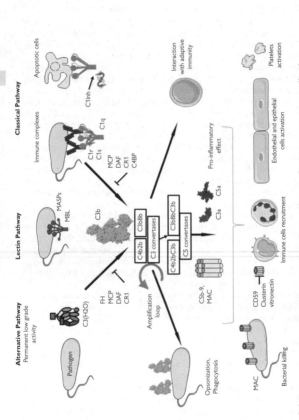

Fig 2.1 The complement system. Reproduced from Merle, NS. et al. Complement system part II: role in immunity. *Frontiers in Immunology.* 6(257). Available at: https://doi.org/10.3389/fimmu.2015.00257. Copyright © 2015 Merle et al. Open Access.

now been characterized and are defined in terms of their functional roles, phenotypic markers, and cytokine profile (2.2).

CD4$^+$ T cells show remarkable plasticity and are able to differentiate into many different subsets based on the soluble molecules secreted during priming of the subsets by APCs (e.g. interleukin (IL)-12 for T-helper 1 cells). The different subsets can be distinguished by the transcription factors that regulate and maintain their lineage-specific effector functions (e.g. T-bet for T-helper 1 cells). The molecules secreted by these subsets (e.g. interferon (IFN)-γ for Th1 cells) are finely tuned to control the pathogen that mediated the release of the specific molecules by the APC during activation of the naïve (Th0) cells into the various subsets.

IL-12 secretion by macrophages and dendritic cells, and IFNγ secretion from natural killer (NK) cells, promote the induction of CD4$^+$ Th1-type responses. CD4$^+$ Th1 cells are required to provide help for CD8$^+$ T-cell responses, but can also act as effectors by themselves as part of a protective immune response. Th1 cells also secrete many effector cytokines, most importantly IFNγ and tumour necrosis factor (TNF)-α, which mediate pro-inflammatory responses and activate cellular arms of the immune response.

Th2 cells predominantly secrete IL-4, IL-5, and IL-13, which are required in the production of protective immune responses to extracellular pathogens. Specialized T follicular helper cells provide essential help for antibody production by B cells within germinal centres of the secondary lymphoid tissues. Regulatory T cells (formerly known as suppressor T cells), are defined by the expression of CD4, high levels of CD25, and the forkhead transcription factor FoxP3. They produce anti-inflammatory cytokines such as IL-10 and transforming growth factor (TGF)-β, thus exerting an immunosuppressive effect to down-regulate and control an immune response. Traditionally associated with the maintenance of self-tolerance, these cells are also induced by infection, whereby they may prevent immunopathology, or down-regulate protective Th1-type responses leading to persistent infection.

CD8$^+$ T cells

CD8$^+$ cytotoxic T lymphocytes play a crucial role in protection from intracellular pathogens. These cells recognize peptides presented in the context of MHC class I molecules, expressed by all nucleated cells. If the MHC class I-peptide complex is recognized by the T-cell receptor of a circulating CD8$^+$ cytotoxic T lymphocyte then apoptosis is initiated, in a utilitarian fashion. This occurs by the polarized secretion of cytotoxic effector proteins (perforin and granzymes) or alternatively by the Fas–FasL interaction. Secretion of IFNγ by CD8$^+$ T cells contributes to defence in several ways. These include the direct inhibition of viral replication, up-regulation of MHC class I and class II molecule expression along with other vital components of the endogenous antigen processing pathway, macrophage recruitment and activation, the further induction of cytokines such as IL-12 and TNFα from APCs (which up-regulate IFNγ production by T cells and NK cells in a positive feedback loop), the stimulation of inducible nitric oxide synthase to generate nitric oxide, and activation of the tryptophan-catabolizing enzyme (indoleamine 2,3-dioxygenase), to effectively starve intracellular pathogens of this essential amino acid.

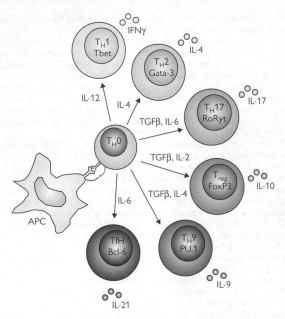

Fig 2.2 CD4+ T-helper cell subset differentiation. Reproduced from Russ, B.E. et al. T cell immunity as a tool for studying epigenetic regulation of cellular differentiation. *Frontiers in Genetics.* 2013. 4(218). doi: 10.3389/fgene.2013.00218. Frontiers Media S.A. Open Access.

B cells and antibodies

B cells bind and internalize circulating antigen as APCs via their specific B-cell receptor or membrane immunoglobulin. Unlike the T-cell receptor, the B-cell receptor can recognize linear or conformational epitopes of proteins. The internalized antigen is processed by the exogenous pathway, and linear peptide epitopes presented on MHC class II molecules to await CD4+ T follicular helper cell recognition. Clustering of the membrane immunoglobulin and concomitant ligation of CD40 on the B-cell surface by CD40 ligand (CD40L/CD154), expressed by activated CD4+ T follicular helper cells, activates the B cell to undergo clonal expansion. Activated B cells secrete an initial burst of immunoglobulin (Ig)-M, before undergoing isotype switching of their constant Fc region to IgG, IgE, or IgA (dependent on the instructive cytokine profile and CD4+ T follicular helper cell). These isotypes define the effector function of the antibody (Table 2.2). Short-lived plasma cells migrate to the periphery to secrete antigen-specific antibody, whilst others remain in the B cell follicles and germinal centres of the secondary lymphoid

Table 2.2 Human antibody isotypes

Class	IgG₁	IgG₂	IgG₃	IgG₄	IgM	IgA	IgD	IgE
CDC	++	+	+++	−	+	+	−	−
ADCP	++	±	++	+	−	+	−	−
ADCC	++	−	++	−	−	−	−	−
Serum conc. (mg/mL)	13.5				1.5	3.5	Traces	0.0.5
Half-life (days)	23				5	6	3	2
Secreted form	Monomer				Pentamer	Dimer	−	Monomer
Binding sites	2				10	4	2	2
M.W. (Da)	150,000				900,000	385,000	180,000	200,000
% in plasma	75–85%				5–10%	10–15%	0.001%	0.001%

ADCC, antibody-dependent cellular cytotoxicity; ADCP, antibody-dependent cellular phagocytosis; CDC, complement-dependent cytotoxicity; M.W., molecular weight.
Reproduced courtesy of Carlo Pifferi. Available at: ⅋ http://www.glycopedia.eu/Humoral-adaptive-immune-responses

tissues to undergo antigen-driven affinity maturation and somatic hyper-mutation of the specific immunoglobulin. Long-lived plasma cells are finally generated that move into the bone marrow to secrete high-affinity antibody over many years. Memory B cells remain behind as sensitized precursors, ready for immediate proliferation upon antigen re-exposure. It is the development of these long-lived memory B- and T-cell populations that enables the immune system to respond more rapidly and effectively to a pathogen upon secondary encounter.

Section 2

Clinical approach

Primary immunodeficiency

Introduction

Primary immunodeficiency disorders (PIDs) consist of a group of genetically determined conditions that result in a spectrum of immunodeficiency, autoimmunity, and malignancy. This can range from the complete absence of a functioning immune system to very specific defects in the immune response. While the more severe forms usually present in childhood, PIDs can present at any age. There are now in excess of 300 PIDs recognized, and the number is expanding every year. While individual conditions are rare, as a combined group primary immunodeficiency is not a rare occurrence with an estimated 1:2000 to 1:10,000 individuals affected.

Although the majority of individuals with known PIDs are managed in specialist centres, there is often a significant delay in diagnosis due to a lack of awareness in non-specialists. Early diagnosis is important in order to reduce end-organ damage and to facilitate genetic counselling if necessary.

The International Union of Immunological Societies (IUIS) has categorized PIDs into nine groups based on phenotypic features.[1] These categories are based on the predominant defect in immune response such as cellular immunity or humoral immunity, innate or acquired, and immune regulation.

IUIS categories of PID

- *Immunodeficiencies affecting cellular and humoral immunity* (~15% of all PIDs): severe combined immunodeficiency (SCID) and the less severe combined immunodeficiency (CID).
- *CID with associated or syndromic features*: generally associated with T-cell immunodeficiency (e.g. DiGeorge syndrome).
- *Predominantly antibody deficiencies* (~65% of all PIDs): the most common group. Includes the often asymptomatic selective IgA deficiency which has a prevalence of 1:500.
- *Diseases of immune dysregulation*: e.g. haemophagocytic lymphohistiocytosis.
- *Congenital defects of phagocyte number, function, or both* (~10% of all PIDs).
- *Defects in intrinsic and innate immunity.*
- *Autoinflammatory disorders.*
- *Complement deficiencies.*
- *Phenocopies of PID.*

Pathogenesis, clinical features, and laboratory features are summarized in Table 3.1.

Table 3.1 Summary of International Union of Immunological Societies classification of primary immunodeficiency disorders (April 2014)

Category and representative diseases	Pathogenesis	Clinical features	Laboratory features	Treatment
Combined immunodeficiencies (~15% of all PIDs)				
Severe combined immunodeficiency (SCID)	>13 genetic defects causing the absence of B and T lymphocyte function; XL and AR defects	1:65,000; presents in early childhood; severe overwhelming infections	↓ lymphocytes on FBC, abnormal lymphocyte subsets, ↓ immunoglobulins	Isolation measures, augmented nutrition, antimicrobial treatment/prophylaxis, avoidance of live vaccines, immunoglobulin therapy, definitive treatment is with haematopoietic stem cell transplantation
Combined immunodeficiency (CID)	Heterogeneous group of generally less severe conditions with impairment of cellular and humoral immunity (e.g. Omenn syndrome)	Recurrent infection often with autoimmune features and failure to thrive	Usually normal lymphocyte count on FBC, lymphocyte subsets may be abnormal, can also present with neutropenia, ↓ platelets, haemolytic anaemia	As for SCID depending on severity and complications
Combined immunodeficiencies associated with syndromic features				
Wiskott–Aldrich syndrome	Mutations in WAS gene affecting stem cell derivatives. XL	1:100,000 to 1:1,000,000; triad of recurrent infection, bleeding due to thrombocytopenia and eczema. Also have ↑ risk of autoimmune disease and haematological malignancy	↓ platelets on FBC, abnormally small platelets on blood film. Sequencing of WAS gene	Frequent antimicrobial therapy/prophylactic antimicrobials, avoidance of live vaccines. Platelet transfusions for active bleeding. Immunoglobulin therapy, definitive treatment with haematopoietic stem cell transplantation (gene therapy under development)

(Continued)

Table 3.1 Contd.

Category and representative diseases	Pathogenesis	Clinical features	Laboratory features	Treatment
DiGeorge syndrome	Deletion on chromosome 22 (22q11.2) (90%) causing abnormal development and migration of thymic cells and other developmental abnormalities. Majority de novo or AD	1:4000; phenotypic variability; absent or hypoplastic thymus (↓ T cells), absent parathyroid glands (↓ Ca²⁺), cardiac abnormalities, facial abnormalities	↓ serum calcium, may have ↓ lymphocytes (T cells); significant phenotypic variability. Genetic analysis (FISH)	Antimicrobial therapy/prophylaxis, avoidance of live vaccines. More severe cases may need haematopoietic stem cell transplantation/thymus transplantation. Specific management for cardiac/parathyroid abnormalities
Ataxia–telangiectasia	Mutations in ATM gene causing DNA repair defects causing selective IgA deficiency or hypogammaglobulinaemia and T-cell dysfunction. AR	1:250,000; ataxia, telangiectasia, recurrent pulmonary infections, dysphagia, lymphoreticular malignancies	Usually have ↓ immunoglobulins, may have ↓ lymphocytes, ↑ αFP, ↑ CA 125, radiosensitivity. Genetic analysis	Antimicrobial therapy/prophylaxis, avoidance of live vaccines. Avoid unnecessary X-rays/radiation. Immunoglobulin therapy. Feeding gastrostomy
Predominantly antibody deficiencies(~65% of all PIDs)				
Selective IgA deficiency	Unknown, variable inheritance	~1:500; often asymptomatic, recurrent sinopulmonary infection	↓ IgA	Antimicrobial therapy/prophylaxis
Common variable immunodeficiency (CVID)	Mostly unknown, variable inheritance	1:25,000 to 1:50,000; variable phenotype, predominantly recurrent sinopulmonary infection	↓ IgG and IgA ± IgM	Antimicrobial therapy/prophylaxis, immunoglobulin therapy
X-linked agammaglobulinaemia (XLA) (Bruton's disease)	Mutations in BTK gene; a cytoplasmic tyrosine kinase. XL	1:70,000 to 1:400,000; recurrent and severe infections (mostly sinopulmonary)	↓ immunoglobulins	Antimicrobial therapy/prophylaxis, immunoglobulin therapy

Diseases of immune dysregulation			
Haemophagocytic lymphohistiocytosis (HLH)	Several mutations for proteins affecting the cell membrane, AR	↓ NK activity, cytopenias, ↑ ferritin, abnormal liver function tests	1:50,000; fever, hepatosplenomegaly, cytopenias, albinism, rash, morbilliform eruptions	Antimicrobial therapy/ prophylaxis, immunoglobulin therapy, haematopoietic stem cell transplantation
Autoimmune lymphoproliferative syndrome (ALPS)	Germinal mutations for cell-surface apoptosis receptors (FAS) and intracellular apoptosis pathways, defective lymphocyte apoptosis, variable inheritance	↑ double-negative T cells (CD4−/CD8−), cytopenias	Splenomegaly, adenopathies, autoimmune cytopenias, ↑ risk of haematological malignancy	Aimed at autoimmune and lymphoproliferative manifestations; corticosteroids, sirolimus mycophenolate, rituximab
Congenital defects of phagocyte number, function, or both (~10% of all PIDs)			
Chronic granulomatous disease	Mutations affecting electron transport proteins causing defective oxygen free radical production in NK and macrophage cells. AR and XL	↓ neutrophil and macrophage function—neutrophil oxidative burst activity (dihydrorhodamine 123 assay)	1:200,000; early-onset severe and recurrent infections (skin, pulmonary, GI tract), including fungal infection. Progressive granulomata formation in the respiratory, urinary, and GI tract. Particularly susceptible to Staphylococcus aureus, Burkholderia cepacia, Serratia marcescens, Nocardia, and Aspergillus spp.	Antimicrobial therapy/prophylaxis, interferon gamma, haematopoietic stem cell transplantation

(Continued)

Table 3.1 Contd.

Category and representative diseases	Pathogenesis	Clinical features	Laboratory features	Treatment
Leucocyte adhesion deficiency	Mutations or deficiency of leucocyte adhesion proteins (e.g. CD18) causing defective leucocyte adherence and chemotaxis. AR	Recurrent infection; in particular, skin infection/ulcers without pus or inflammation. Periodontitis	Leucocytosis, immunophenotyping, genetic testing	Antimicrobial therapy/prophylaxis, haematopoietic stem cell transplantation
Defects in innate immunity				
NEMO deficiency	Mutations in *NEMO* gene, a modulator of expression of NF-kappa B family of transcription factors. XL	1:250,000; ectodermal dysplasia (thickened skin, conical teeth, absence of sweat glands, and thin, sparse hair with recurrent infection). Particularly susceptible to pyogenic organisms (staphylococci/streptococci) and mycobacteria	May have ↓ immunoglobulins, genetic testing	Antimicrobial therapy/prophylaxis, immunoglobulin therapy, avoidance of live vaccines (particularly BCG). haematopoietic stem cell transplantation
Auto-inflammatory disorders				
Familial Mediterranean fever	Mutations in *MEFV* gene, involved in modulation of the inflammatory response. AR	~1:500 in the highest-risk populations; people of Mediterranean origin (particularly Armenian, Jewish). Much lower incidence in other populations. Paroxysmal attacks of fever, polyserositis, abdominal pain, chest pain, arthritis, and erythema (erysipelas-like). Secondary amyloidosis	↑ neutrophils, and CRP/ESR. Episodic proteinuria/haematuria. Genetic testing.	Acute attacks treated with analgesia and supportive measures. Colchicine is effective as a continuous prophylactic therapy at reducing severity and frequency of attacks.

Complement deficiencies

C2 deficiency	C2 mutations causing defective classical complement pathway. AR	~1:20,000 in Caucasians. Recurrent sinopulmonary infection. Particularly susceptible to encapsulated organisms. Associated with systemic lupus erythematosus	May have positive ANA (speckled) and positive anti Ro (SS-A). Complement function tests; absent CH50 haemolytic activity	Antimicrobial therapy/ prophylaxis, immunoglobulin therapy, rituximab
C1 inhibitor deficiency (hereditary angio-oedema (HAE))	Deficiency (type 1) or dysfunction (type 2) of C1 inhibitor. Causes excessive bradykinin production and other inflammatory effects. AD	1:50,000; recurrent angio-oedema without urticaria or pruritus. Often presents with paroxysmal abdominal pain and recurrent laryngeal oedema	↓ C4 levels (natural substrate to C1 esterase). C1-INH antigenic levels and C1-INH functional levels	Acute attacks may require advanced airway management. Human plasma derived or recombinant C1 inhibitor concentrate

Phenocopies of PID

Autoimmune lymphoproliferative syndrome (ALPS—somatic FAS mutations)	Somatic mutation of the FAS gene, TNFRSF6, causing defective lymphocyte apoptosis	Splenomegaly, lymphadenopathy, cytopenias	↑ double-negative T cells (CD4−/CD8−), cytopenias	Aimed at autoimmune and lymphoproliferative manifestations; corticosteroids, sirolimus mycophenolate, rituximab
Pulmonary alveolar proteinosis	Auto antibodies to GM-CSF	Diffuse lung disease caused by periodic acid-Schiff-positive lipoproteinaceous material causing progressive dyspnoea and intercurrent infections with opportunistic pathogens (Nocardia, mycobacteria, fungi). Association with cryptococcal meningitis	Characteristic radiographic findings, BAL, and histology. Autoantibodies to GM-CSF.	Treatment of intercurrent infection, 'whole lung lavage', subcutaneous or inhaled GM-CSF

Table 3.1 Contd.

Category and representative diseases	Pathogenesis	Clinical features	Laboratory features	Treatment
Acquired angio-oedema	Auto antibodies to C1 inhibitor	Recurrent angio-oedema without urticaria or pruritus. Often presents with paroxysmal abdominal pain and recurrent laryngeal oedema. Presents in the fourth decade of life or later. Often associated with haematological malignancy (non-Hodgkin's lymphoma)	Autoantibodies against C1 inhibitor protein, ↓ C4, C1-INH	Acute attacks may require advanced airway management. Human plasma derived or recombinant C1 inhibitor concentrate

AD, autosomal dominant; αFP, alpha-fetoprotein; ANA, antinuclear antibody; AR, autosomal recessive; BAL, bronchoalveolar lavage; CA, cancer antigen; CRP, C-reactive protein; ESR, erythrocyte sedimentation rate; FBC, full blood count; FISH, fluorescent in situ hybridization; GI, gastrointestinal; GM-CSF, granulocyte-macrophage colony-stimulating factor; INH, inhibitor; NF, nuclear factor; XL, X-linked.

Presenting features

Infections are the most common presentation of PIDs; these may be recurrent, chronic, unusually severe, or infections with opportunistic/unusual pathogens. While severe forms of PID are usually diagnosed in early childhood, the less severe forms may not come to medical attention until adulthood and require a high index of suspicion on the part of the clinician.

The following should prompt the consideration of PID:
- Recurrent ear, sinus, or pulmonary infections.
- Failure to thrive in children or weight loss in adults.
- Recurrent abscesses, thrush, or persistent fungal infection.
- Recurrent viral infections (e.g. cold sores, warts).
- Unusual pathogens (e.g. *Pneumocystis jirovecii*).
- Family history of primary immunodeficiency.
- End-organ damage (e.g. bronchiectasis).
- Chronic diarrhoea.

Common presenting syndromes

Sinopulmonary infection

Usually due to immunoglobulin deficiencies (e.g. IgA deficiency) and common variable immunodeficiency disorder (CVID). Immunoglobulin deficiency results in particular susceptibility to encapsulated bacteria such as *Streptococcus pneumoniae* and *Haemophilus influenzae*. As sinopulmonary infections are common, a 'rule of thumb' for gauging abnormality would be more than four new ear infections or more than two pneumonias in 1 year in a child, and more than two new ear infections or one pneumonia per year for >1 year in adults.[2]

Skin disease

Chronic or persistent mucocutaneous candidiasis is a strong indication of immunodeficiency, as are recurrent or unusually deep skin abscesses. Classic PIDs presenting like this are hyper IgE syndrome (HIES) and chronic granulomatous disease (CGD), alongside combined immunodeficiencies such as SCID.

Gastrointestinal disease

Chronic diarrhoea and malabsorption are common presenting features of antibody deficiency, in particular, CVID and IgA deficiency. Typical gastrointestinal infections include *Campylobacter jejuni*, *Salmonella* spp., *Yersinia enterocolitica*, and *Clostridium difficile* as well as parasites and protozoa such as *Giardia lamblia*. There is a strong association with autoimmunity such as inflammatory bowel disease and coeliac-like disease.

Broad and profound susceptibility to infection

Usually presents within the first few months of life with multiple severe infections (pulmonary, gastrointestinal, skin), growth failure, and mycobacterial disease following Bacillus Calmette–Guérin (BCG) vaccination (e.g. SCID).

Autoimmune disease

There are strong associations between PIDs and autoimmune conditions such as autoimmune haemolytic anaemia, idiopathic thrombocytopenia, pernicious anaemia, inflammatory bowel disease, primary biliary cirrhosis, autoimmune hepatitis, rheumatoid disease, thyroiditis, alopecia, erythroderma, and uveitis.

Malignancy

PIDs are strongly associated with lymphoproliferative disorders, particularly those that are due to immune dysregulation and T-cell deficiency.

Investigation of primary immunodeficiency

Most PIDs can be diagnosed with standard laboratory tests. It is important that, before suspecting a primary immunodeficiency in patients presenting with recurrent, severe, or unusual infections, the much more common acquired and non-immune-mediated causes are excluded. Chief among these are HIV infection, medical comorbidity, and immunosuppressant drugs.

Specific features of the history and examination may suggest a likely diagnosis. This may include the age of the patient, sites of infection, causative organisms, syndromic features, and associated autoimmunity/malignancy.

Useful screening tests
- Full blood count with differential.
- Serum immunoglobulins (IgG, IgM, IgA, IgE).

The majority of common/important PIDs will show some abnormality on these tests.

More specific tests
These include the following:
- *Antibody deficiencies*: specific antibody titres against vaccinated antigens (protein: tetanus, diphtheria; or polysaccharide: pneumococcus). Genetic analysis.
- *Combined deficiencies*: lymphocyte subsets (T, B, and natural killer (NK) cells), *in vitro* functional assays of T and B cells, protein expression analysis.
- *Complement deficiencies*: complement protein function (CH50 and AH50). Measurement of individual complement proteins. Genetic analysis.
- *Phagocyte function*: measurement of phagocyte oxidase activity (chemotaxis and bacterial killing). Genetic analysis.

Management of primary immunodeficiency

Management of all but the least severe PIDs should be by specialist centres.

Goals of treatment

- Prevent recurrent infection.
- Reduce severity of infections.
- Minimize end-organ damage.
- Treat concomitant autoimmunity/malignancy.
- Correct the underlying defect if possible.

Therapeutic options

- Early antimicrobial therapy.
- Prophylactic antimicrobial therapy.
- Immunoglobulin replacement (intravenous or subcutaneous).
- Haematopoietic stem cell transplantation.
- Gene therapy.
- Given the genetic nature of these conditions, genetic counselling may be appropriate.

Acknowledgement

This chapter was kindly reviewed by Dr Smita Patel, Consultant Clinical Immunologist, Oxford University Hospitals NHS Foundation Trust.

Further reading

1. Bousfiha A, Jeddane L, Al-Herz W, et al. The 2015 IUIS Phenotypic Classification for Primary Immunodeficiencies. Journal of Clinical Immunology 2015;35(8):727–38.
2. Lehman H, Hernandez-Trujillo V, Ballow M. Diagnosing primary immunodeficiency: a practical approach for the non-immunologist. Current Medical Research and Opinion 2015;31(4):697–706.

Immunosuppressive drugs

Introduction

There is an ever increasing number of immunosuppressive agents in use for treatment of haematological malignancies, multisystem autoimmune diseases, and for anti-rejection therapy in transplant recipients. Such agents may predispose to certain infections based on their particular immune arm target. This chapter covers the key information on the most common of these agents necessary to aid the assessment of an unwell patient who may be taking one or more of these agents. This is, however, a rapidly evolving field.

• The details (individual components, sequence, and timing) of the immunosuppressive prescription are crucial to the assessment of the patient presenting with suspected infection.

• Potential interactions between immunosuppressive agents and antimicrobials must be carefully considered before starting prophylaxis or treatment of a suspected infection.

• The infective differential can be wide, particularly in patients receiving drugs that have broad effects on the immune system.

• The relative predisposition to different infections must be considered in the wider context of the patient's net state of immunosuppression (e.g. age, comorbidities, organ dysfunction, anatomical defects, mucocutaneous integrity, and other mechanisms of immune compromise).

Corticosteroids

Mechanism of action

Steroids have been a key component of anti-rejection therapy since the earliest days of solid organ transplant (SOT), but are also used across a wide range of inflammatory conditions. Their mechanisms of action are anti-inflammatory and immunosuppressive (Figure 4.1).

Anti-inflammatory

- Complex effects on leucocytes; increase circulating neutrophil levels but reduce accumulation at sites of infection/inflammation. Reduce numbers of circulating lymphocytes and increase ratio of B:T cells, and CD8:CD4.
- Inhibit monocyte/macrophage activation and ability to recognize antigen.
- Inhibit all arachidonic acid metabolites, e.g. prostaglandins, leukotrienes, and other mediators of vasodilatation, reducing vascular permeability.
- Inhibit *in vivo* expression of pro-inflammatory cytokine production (e.g. IL-1, -12, -3, -4, -10, TNFα, and IFNγ). Increase breakdown of mRNA for IL-1, 3, and GM-CSF. Inhibit IL-2R expression and so inhibit T-cell activation.
- Inhibit inducible nitric oxidase, phospholipase A2, and cyclooxygenase (COX-2).

These factors have a major effect on preventing an effective inflammatory response to microbial invasion, leading to blunted symptoms and signs, blunted X-ray findings, and a very high microbial burden.

Cellular immunosuppression

- Inhibit T-cell activation and proliferation (via suppression of cytokines, e.g. IL-2) and block clonal T-cell expansion in response to antigenic stimulation. This renders patients susceptible to infections including herpes viruses, fungal infections, *Nocardia* spp., mycobacteria, and *Strongyloides stercoralis*, and intracellular organisms such as *Listeria* spp. and *Salmonella* spp.
- Blunt the activation of immature B cells, including the response required to a new vaccine. It is therefore very important to complete vaccinations, where possible, prior to starting steroids (established B-cell responses are not affected by steroids).

Indications

Many, including:

- multiple autoimmune or immune mediated conditions (e.g. asthma, inflammatory bowel disease, rheumatological conditions, eczema and other dermatological conditions, autoimmune renal and haematological conditions, etc.)
- anti-rejection therapy for SOT and haematopoietic stem cell transplantation (HSCT) recipients
- graft-versus-host disease (GvHD).

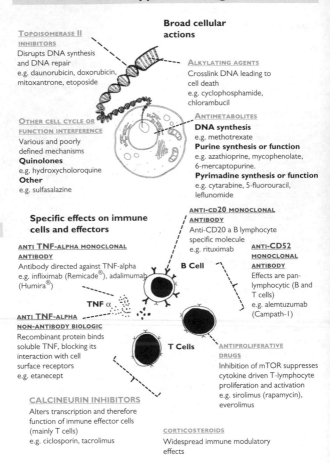

Broad cellular actions

TOPOISOMERASE II INHIBITORS
Disrupts DNA synthesis and DNA repair
e.g. daunorubicin, doxorubicin, mitoxantrone, etoposide

ALKYLATING AGENTS
Crosslink DNA leading to cell death
e.g. cyclophosphamide, chlorambucil

OTHER CELL CYCLE OR FUNCTION INTERFERENCE
Various and poorly defined mechanisms
Quinolones
e.g. hydroxycholoroquine
Other
e.g. sulfasalazine

ANTIMETABOLITES
DNA synthesis
e.g. methotrexate
Purine synthesis or function
e.g. azathioprine, mycophenolate, 6-mercaptopurine.
Pyrimidine synthesis or function
e.g. cytarabine, 5-fluorouracil, leflunomide

Specific effects on immune cells and effectors

ANTI-CD20 MONOCLONAL ANTIBODY
Anti-CD20 a B lymphocyte specific molecule
e.g. rituximab

ANTI TNF-ALPHA MONOCLONAL ANTIBODY
Antibody directed against TNF-alpha
e.g. infliximab (Remicade®), adalimumab (Humira®)

B Cell

ANTI-CD52 MONOCLONAL ANTIBODY
Effects are pan-lymphocytic (B and T cells)
e.g. alemtuzumab (Campath-1)

TNF α

ANTI TNF-ALPHA NON-ANTIBODY BIOLOGIC
Recombinant protein binds soluble TNF, blocking its interaction with cell surface receptors
e.g. etanecept

T Cells

ANTIPROLIFERATIVE DRUGS
Inhibition of mTOR suppresses cytokine driven T-lymphocyte proliferation and activation
e.g. sirolimus (rapamycin), everolimus

CALCINEURIN INHIBITORS
Alters transcription and therefore function of immune effector cells (mainly T cells)
e.g. ciclosporin, tacrolimus

CORTICOSTEROIDS
Widespread immune modulatory effects

Fig 4.1 Summary of some of the more common immunosuppressive agents. Non-biological agents are represented in light grey; biological agents are represented in dark grey.

Side effects

Numerous including:

• neuropsychiatric: anxiety, depression, and psychosis
• cardiovascular: fluid retention and hypertension
• metabolic: fat redistribution

- endocrine: hyperglycaemia, insulin resistance, and diabetes
- steroid-induced osteoporosis
- skin damage, cataract, and retinopathy.

Associated infections

- Bacteria: common organisms including *Staphylococcus aureus*, Gram negatives plus *Nocardia* spp., mycobacteria, and intracellular organisms such as *Listeria* and *Salmonella* spp.
- Fungi: *Candida* spp., *Aspergillus* spp., and *Pneumocystis jirovecii*.
- Viruses: reactivation of hepatitis B/C, herpes viruses.
- Parasites: *S. stercoralis* hyperactivation.

Because of the potentially severe effect of steroids with respect to infection, steroid-sparing agents have become increasingly important. The combination of biological agents and high doses of steroids, in particular, needs to be used carefully and, if possible, avoided in patients with additional risk factors such as older age or comorbid conditions.

Cytotoxic chemotherapeutic agents

Cyclophosphamide

Alkylating agent: nitrogen mustard.

Mechanism of action
- Cross-links DNA leading to cell death, reduces T and B cell lymphocytes, and inhibits immunoglobulin synthesis.
- Other alkylating agents with a similar mechanism of action and side effect profile include chlorambucil and melphalan.

Indications
- Treatment of many haematological malignancies (e.g. lymphoma, as part of R-CHOP regimen: rituximab + cyclophosphamide, doxorubicin, vincristine, and prednisolone; or R-EPOCH regimen: R-CHOP + etoposide).
- Treatment of neuroblastoma, ovarian adenocarcinoma, and retinoblastoma.
- Treatment of minimal change nephrotic syndrome in children (steroid unresponsive).
- Treatment of rheumatological disease (e.g. systemic lupus erythematosus (SLE) or vasculitis).

Side effects
- Alopecia (reversible).
- Amenorrhoea, azoospermia, gonadal suppression, oligospermia (oogenesis impaired), sterility.
- Abdominal pain, anorexia, diarrhoea, mucositis, nausea/vomiting (dose related), stomatitis.
- Haemorrhagic cystitis.
- Anaemia, leucopenia (dose related; recovery 7–10 days after cessation), myelosuppression, thrombocytopenia.
- Cardiotoxicity.
- Secondary malignancies: dose-dependent risk of acute leukaemia due to long-term bone marrow damage.
- Rarely: pulmonary injury and progressive pneumonitis.

Associated infections
- Bacterial infections: broad range of increased susceptibility.
- Fungal infections, e.g. *Pneumocystis jirovecii*.
- Herpes viruses, e.g. varicella zoster virus (VZV) and cytomegalovirus (CMV).

Cytarabine (Ara-C)

Antimetabolite.

Mechanism of action
- Metabolized to its active compound, aracytidine triphosphate, a pyrimidine analogue which is incorporated into DNA (responsible for drug activity and toxicity).
- Inhibits DNA polymerase resulting in decreased DNA synthesis and repair.
- Cytarabine is specific for the S phase of the cell cycle (blocks progression from the G1 to the S phase).

Other cytotoxic antimetabolites with a similar mechanism of action include fludarabine, 5-fluorouracil, and 6-mercaptopurine.

Indications
- acute myeloid leukaemia (AML): remission induction, consolidation, and salvage treatment (in combination with other chemotherapy medications).
- acute lymphoblastic leukaemia (ALL): treatment.
- chronic myeloid leukaemia (CML): treatment.
- Meningeal leukaemia: prophylaxis and treatment.

Side effects
- Fever.
- Rash.
- Gastrointestinal (GI): anal inflammation/ulceration, anorexia, diarrhoea, mucositis, nausea, and vomiting.
- Myelosuppression (major toxicity): neutropenia, anaemia, and bleeding.
- Hepatic dysfunction and increased transaminases (acute).
- Local thrombophlebitis.
- Central nervous system (CNS), ocular, and pulmonary toxicities also occur: more commonly with high-dose regimens and in patients with pre-existing renal or hepatic impairment.

Associated infections
As for cyclophosphamide; broad range of increased susceptibility.

Daunorubicin
Anthracycline.

Mechanism of action
- Inhibits DNA and RNA synthesis by intercalation between DNA base pairs and by steric obstruction.
- Inhibits DNA repair through topoisomerase II inhibition.

Other anthracyclines with a similar mechanism and side effect profile include doxorubicin (Adriamycin®), epirubicin, and idarubicin.

Indications
Treatment of ALL and AML (with combination therapy).

Side effects
- Transient electrocardiogram (ECG) abnormalities (supraventricular tachycardia, S-T wave changes, atrial or ventricular extrasystoles); generally asymptomatic and self-limiting.
- Congestive cardiac failure; dose related, may be delayed for 7–8 years after treatment.
- Alopecia (reversible).
- Radiation recall and, less commonly, skin flare at injection site.
- Mild nausea or vomiting, stomatitis. Less commonly GI ulceration, pain, and diarrhoea.
- Discoloration of urine (red), sometimes saliva, sweat, and tears.
- Myelosuppression: primarily leucopenia, thrombocytopenia, and anaemia.

Associated infections
As for other cytotoxic drugs; broad range of increased susceptibility.

Mitoxantrone
Anti-tumour antibiotic.

Mechanism of action
- Intercalates into DNA resulting in cross-links and strand breaks. Binds to nucleic acids and inhibits DNA and RNA synthesis by template disordering and steric obstruction.
- Decreases replication by binding to DNA topoisomerase II (cell-cycle non-specific).

Indications
- Initial treatment of acute non-lymphocytic leukaemias.
- Treatment of advanced hormone-refractory prostate cancer.
- Secondary progressive or relapsing–remitting multiple sclerosis.

Side effects
Similar to the anthracyclines. Myelosuppression is a major toxicity.

Associated infections
Broad range of increased susceptibility to bacterial, viral, and fungal pathogens.

Etoposide (VP-16)
Topoisomerase II inhibitor.

Mechanism of action
- Topoisomerase II inhibitor, causes DNA strand breaks.
- Delays transit of cells through the S phase and arrests cells in late S or early G2 phase. May inhibit mitochondrial transport at the NADH dehydrogenase level or inhibit uptake of nucleosides.

Indications
- Treatment of lung cancer and testicular cancer.
- Treatment of non-Hodgkin lymphoma (NHL).
- Off-label use for AML induction therapy, HSCT conditioning, and some refractory malignancies.

Side effects
- Commonly: alopecia, myelosuppression, and GI upset.
- Less commonly: hypotension (infusion effect), hypersensitivity reactions, peripheral neuropathy, and hepatotoxicity.

Associated infections
Broad range of increased susceptibility to bacterial, viral, and fungal pathogens.

Autoimmune/connective tissue disease suppressive therapies

Azathioprine

Purine analogue: precursor of 6-mercaptopurine.

Mechanism of action
- Inhibits purine metabolism and DNA/RNA synthesis.
- Greatest inhibitory effect is on actively dividing lymphocytes responding to antigenic stimulation (it has minimal effects on memory/end-stage lymphocyte function).
- Inhibits T-cell responses and NK cell activity.
- Inhibits B-cell proliferation and antibody synthesis.
- Causes neutropenia, therefore increasing the risk of bacterial sepsis and invasive fungal infections.

Indications
- Renal transplantation: adjunctive therapy in prevention of rejection of kidney transplants.
- Crohn's disease and ulcerative colitis.
- Multiple autoimmune conditions including rheumatoid arthritis, immune thrombocytopenia, lupus nephritis, multiple sclerosis, recurrent pericarditis, psoriasis, uveitis, dermatomyositis/polymyositis, and pemphigus vulgaris.
- Adjunct in prevention of rejection of SOT (non-renal) transplants.

Side effects
- Bone marrow toxicity can be severe in individuals deficient in the enzyme thiopurine S-methyltransferase. Testing for activity of this enzyme is now becoming routine prior to commencing any of the thiopurine drugs.
- Severe leucopenia can occur if xanthine oxidase inhibitors (e.g. allopurinol or febuxostat, used to treat hyperuricaemia/gout) are used with azathioprine.
- Thrombocytopenia.
- Neoplasia, e.g. skin cancer.
- Nausea and vomiting, diarrhoea.
- Hepatotoxicity, increased serum alkaline phosphatase, increased serum bilirubin, and increased serum transaminases.
- Fever and myalgia.
- Very rarely (<1%): progressive multifocal leucoencephalopathy (PML), Sweet's syndrome.

Associated infections
- Bacterial infections including *Nocardia* spp., mycobacteria, and intracellular bacteria.
- Fungal infections.
- *Strongyloides stercoralis* hyperactivation syndrome.
- Herpes viruses, e.g. VZV, and papillomaviruses (particular role in human papillomavirus (HPV) infection), and reactivation of hepatitis B.

Sulfasalazine (SSZ)

Metabolized to 5-aminosalicylic acid (5-ASA).

Mechanism of action

- In the colon, SSZ is reduced by the bacterial enzyme azoreductase to sulfapyridine and 5-ASA. The latter is excreted in the faeces, hence its utility in inflammatory bowel disease.
- Impairment of polymorphonuclear and macrophage adhesion and cell migration (through increasing production of adenosine at sites of inflammation).
- Reduces lymphocyte responses by blocking lymphocyte DNA synthesis and cell cycle progression *in vitro* so preventing clonal expansion of potential pathogenic T- and B-cell populations. 5-ASA also prevents the accumulation of the early T-cell activation gene for IL-2, so inhibits both T-cell proliferation and subsequent activation and differentiation.
- Inhibits cytokine synthesis, e.g. TNFα expression via macrophage apoptosis.
- Inhibits prostaglandin and leukotriene synthesis.
- Inhibits angiogenesis.
- Free radical scavenging.

Indications

- Rheumatoid arthritis: used as combination therapy with other disease-modifying antirheumatic drugs.
- Inflammatory bowel disease (Crohn's, ulcerative colitis).

Side effects

Either idiosyncratic (e.g. hypersensitivity related or immune related) or dose related:

- Idiosyncratic side effects:
  - Skin reactions (rash very common).
  - Hepatitis.
  - Pneumonitis.
  - Agranulocytosis.
  - Aplastic anaemia.
  - Haemolytic anaemia: may be more common in glucose-6-phosphate dehydrogenase (G6PD)-deficient individuals. When such reactions occur, the drug should be immediately stopped, and the patient should not be re-challenged.
- Dose-related side effects—may resolve with dose reduction, or may lead to treatment withdrawal:
  - GI upset (nausea very common).
  - CNS symptoms.
  - Leucopenia, haemolytic anaemia, megaloblastic anaemia.
  - oligospermia.

Associated infections

Broad range of bacterial and fungal infections may occur with SSZ-induced agranulocytosis, neutropenia, or myelosuppression.

Methotrexate

Antimetabolite and antifolate drug.

Mechanism of action

- Inhibits metabolism of folic acid via dihydrofolate reductase—blocks further purine/thymidylate synthesis.
- Reduces neutrophil adhesion, inhibits phagocytosis and intracellular killing by granulocytes.
- Reduces monocyte production and macrophage activation.
- Reduces immunoglobulin synthesis.
- Suppresses cell-mediated immunity but has little effect on T-cell function.

Indications

- GvHD prophylaxis.
- Disease-modifying agent for various autoimmune diseases, including rheumatoid arthritis, psoriasis, sarcoidosis, Crohn's disease, eczema, and many forms of vasculitis.
- Chemotherapy for various solid organ cancers, leukaemia, and lymphoma.

Side effects

Common:
- Hepatotoxicity.
- GI upset: nausea and abdominal pain.
- Elevated creatinine.
- Ulcerative stomatitis and cutaneous side effects, e.g. alopecia, psoriasis, and photosensitivity.
- Leucopenia.
- Fatigue, fever, and dizziness.
- Acute pneumonitis.

Rarely:
- Pulmonary fibrosis and renal failure.
- Cutaneous side effects at high doses.
- CNS reactions (when given via intrathecal route), neurological damage, and memory loss.

Associated infections

Broad range of bacterial, viral, and fungal infections, especially *Pneumocystis jirovecii* and reactivation of hepatitis B.

Hydroxychloroquine

Quinoline antimalarial.

Mechanism of action

- Increases lysosomal pH in antigen-presenting cells, inhibiting lysosomal enzymes.
- In inflammatory conditions, blocks Toll-like receptors on plasmacytoid dendritic cells, reducing cell activation.
- Effects of above-listed mechanisms reduce presentation of antigen to T cells.
- Inhibits IL-1 release and polymorphonuclear and lymphocyte responses.

Indications
- Malaria.
- Q-fever.
- Rheumatoid arthritis, SLE, and Sjögren's syndrome.
- Porphyria cutanea tarda.

Side effects
GI upset is common. With chronic use only:
- Eye and skin pigmentation, cutaneous inflammation, and acne.
- Anaemia and blood disorders.
- Vertigo, tinnitus, and alopecia.
- Hepatotoxicity.
- Muscle paralysis and weakness/atrophy.
- Exacerbation of psoriasis.
- Chloroquine retinopathy.

Associated infections: few
On balance, chloroquine and hydroxychloroquine do not result in any meaningful increase in susceptibility to infection. Both have antibacterial, antifungal, and antiviral effects beyond their antiparasitic activity. The first two effects are exerted by pH-dependent iron deprivation and by increasing lysosomal pH, leading to growth inhibition of intracellular organisms. The antiviral effect is mediated by the inhibition of pH-dependent steps of viral replication and by the alteration of post-translational modifications of newly synthesized proteins.
  In vitro activity against the following pathogens has been demonstrated:
- *Staphylococcus aureus, Mycobacterium tuberculosis, Salmonella typhi,* and *Escherichia coli.*
- *Histoplasma* spp., *Cryptococcus* spp., and *Aspergillus* spp.
- Hepatitis A, B, C, HIV, influenza, and some herpes viruses.

Hydroxychloroquine has shown a protective role against major infections in patients with SLE.

Leflunomide

Pyrimidine synthesis inhibitor.

Mechanism of action
Inhibits dihydro-orate dehydrogenase, leading to depletion of intracellular pyrimidine. This results in antiproliferative and anti-inflammatory effects. Leflunomide is a prodrug; the active metabolite is responsible for activity. In CMV, it may interfere with virion assembly.

Indications
- Rheumatoid arthritis and juvenile idiopathic arthritis.
- Resistant CMV disease in SOT patients.

Side effects

Wide range, most commonly:

- Headache.
- Alopecia.
- Rash.
- GI upset.
- Respiratory tract infections.

Associated infections

Broad range including opportunistic pathogens such as *M. tuberculosis, P. jirovecii* and *Aspergillus* spp., and reactivation of herpes (simplex and zoster) viruses.

Specific T-cell immunosuppressive drugs

Ciclosporin (cyclosporin)

Calcineurin inhibitor.

Mechanism of action

- A lipophilic cyclic peptide, derived from a fungus, *Cylindrocarpon lucidum*. In use since 1981.
- Calcineurin inhibitors act by binding to cyclophilins in cells and inhibiting calcineurin (a phosphatase) which inhibits translocation of transcription factors (NF-AT). It reduces transcription of multiple early cytokine genes, especially IL-2 (dose related). This potent suppression of T-cell function serves to prevent allograft rejection, but through inhibition of microbial-specific T-cell cytotoxicity, also amplifies the extent and effects of herpes viruses, especially of CMV and Epstein–Barr virus (EBV).
- Inhibits immunoglobulin production by B cells and proliferation of stimulated B cells.

Ciclosporin is metabolized by cytochrome P450 and so has a number of important interactions. Monitoring of daily levels is required post transplant.

Indications

- Main uses in SOT and GvHD.
- Expanding use in autoimmune conditions, e.g. SLE, psoriasis, and rheumatoid arthritis.

Side effects

- Nephrotoxicity.
- Hypertension.
- Neurotoxicity.
- Hyperkalaemia, hypomagnesaemia, and hyperlipidaemia.
- Hirsutism.
- Increased risk of lymphoproliferative disorders and squamous cell carcinoma.

Associated infections

- Increased viral replication, especially CMV and EBV, and reactivation of hepatitis B.
- Early bacterial infections (B-cell depression).
- Gingival infections.
- Intracellular infections: *Legionella* spp., *Pneumocystis jirovecii*, mycobacteria, *Listeria*, and *Salmonella* spp.

Tacrolimus (FK506)

Macrolide, calcineurin inhibitor.

Mechanism of action

- Originally isolated from a fungus (has antifungal activity). In use since 1989.
- Similar mechanism of action to ciclosporin (inhibition of signalling through the T-cell receptor), though inhibits calcineurin via binding to

FK506 binding proteins rather than cyclophilins. It is also 10–100 times more potent.
- Inhibits immunoglobulin production by and proliferation of stimulated B cells, resulting in blunted vaccine responses.
- Also metabolized by cytochrome P450.

Indications
- Main use in SOT. First line for liver transplant. Now also approved for kidney transplantation. Associated with less acute rejection episodes than ciclosporin.
- Expanding use in autoimmune conditions.

Side effects
As for ciclosporin plus increased risk of new-onset diabetes mellitus after transplant (NODAT) (may result in decreased allograft survival in some patients). Reported differences in non-renal toxicity as compared with ciclosporin include the following:
- More prominent neurological side effects: tremor and headache.
- More frequent diarrhoea, dyspepsia, and vomiting.
- Hypertrophic cardiomyopathy (reported in children).
- More frequent alopecia.
- Increased proclivity to polyoma virus infection.
- Less frequent hirsutism, gingival hyperplasia, and hypertension.
- Severe neutropenia.

Box 4.1 Important interactions between calcineurin inhibitors and antimicrobials

- Rifampicin, nafcillin, and isoniazid can upregulate the hepatic metabolism of calcineurin inhibitors, reducing blood levels for a given dose of drug.
- Levels of tacrolimus and ciclosporin must therefore be closely monitored and doses adjusted accordingly.
- Macrolides (erythromycin > clarithromycin > azithromycin) and azoles (ketoconazole > itraconazole/voriconazole > fluconazole) can downregulate the hepatic metabolism of calcineurin inhibitors, therefore increasing the blood levels for a given dose of drug. This results in an increased risk of over-immunosuppression, infection, and nephrotoxicity.
- High doses of ciprofloxacin or trimethoprim–sulfamethoxazole (TMP-SMX) can lead to renal dysfunction in patients taking calcineurin inhibitors.
- Even low doses of amphotericin and aminoglycosides can result in an accelerated nephrotoxicity. Aminoglycosides and amphotericin are therefore usually avoided (where possible) with preferential use of extended-spectrum beta lactams and azoles in the treatment of bacterial and fungal infections.
- Occasionally, single doses of gentamicin/amphotericin/intravenous (IV) TMP-SMX can lead to oliguric renal failure in those on calcineurin inhibitors.

Associated infections
- Increased viral replication.
- Early bacterial infections (B-cell depression).
- Gingival infections.
- Intracellular infections: *Legionella* spp., *P. jirovecii*, mycobacteria, *Listeria*, and *Salmonella* spp.

Mycophenolate mofetil (MMF)
Purine synthesis inhibitor.

Mechanism of action
In use since the 1990s, derived from penicillin. It is a prodrug, metabolized to the active agent mycophenolic acid. Inhibits a crucial enzyme in the synthesis of guanine (IMPDH), preventing cells from synthesizing GTP or d-GTP and replicating. This is the pathway required by proliferating lymphocytes as they lack a key enzyme of the guanine salvage pathway. This results in a prolonged inhibition of the proliferative response of B and T cells to allospecific stimulation. It also inhibits lymphocyte migration to sites of inflammation.

It has a more potent anti-rejection effect than azathioprine but without a major increase in infections or lymphomas. It has a lower incidence of neutropenia-related infection than azathioprine.

Indications
- SOT (~86% of renal transplant recipients receive it).
- Autoimmune conditions (e.g. SLE, vasculitis, and retroperitoneal fibrosis).

Side effects
- GI toxicity > bone marrow suppression.
- Particular risk of reactivation of BK virus nephropathy (can present with haemorrhagic cystitis/stenosis of ureters).
- Allograft failure.

Associated infections
- Early bacterial infections (B cell depression).
- Potential role in late onset CMV.
- Potential protective effect against certain pathogens. In transplant recipients, a possible protective effect against *P. jirovecii* pneumonia and Coxsackie virus has been observed.

Sirolimus (rapamycin) and everolimus
mTOR inhibitors.

Mechanism of action
- From a bacterium *Streptomyces hygroscopicus* (has antifungal activity against yeasts and filamentous fungi).
- Structurally similar to tacrolimus but has a different cytoplasmic target. Acts on a protein called mammalian target of rapamycin (mTOR). The mTOR inhibits IL-2-mediated signal transduction, resulting in cell-cycle arrest in the G1–S phase, so inhibiting synthesis of ribosomal proteins and progression to DNA synthesis. In this way sirolimus and

everolimus block the response of T- and B-cell activation by cytokines, which prevents proliferation of T cells, B-cell immunoglobulin synthesis, ADCC, and also NK cell activation.
• Inhibits growth factor providing an antiproliferative effect (this helps to prevent and treat allograft injury).

Indications
• Second line in prophylaxis of organ rejection in SOT.
• Often used with ciclosporin to allow reduced ciclosporin dosing and therefore reduced nephrotoxicity.
• Similarly used for steroid-sparing.

Side effects
Less nephro- and neurotoxic than calcineurin inhibitors:
• Bone marrow suppression.
• GI complaints.
• Hyperlipidaemia.
• Hepatic artery thrombosis.
• Rashes.
• Among kidney and kidney–pancreas SOT recipients, an increased mortality risk has been associated with sirolimus- compared with non sirolimus-containing immunosuppressive regimens (from cardiovascular and infection-related deaths).

Associated infections
• Same as for ciclosporin, but less risk of CMV reactivation.
• Idiosyncratic pulmonary syndrome, often with concomitant respiratory pathogens.
• High incidence of *P. jirovecii* pneumonia and aphthous ulcers (but offers some protection against other yeasts and filamentous fungi).

Immunosuppressant antibody therapy

Immunosuppressant antibody therapy has become established as an important and rapidly developing modality in the treatment of a wide range of conditions including cancers, autoimmune and inflammatory conditions, as well as antirejection therapy in transplant recipients. It has the advantage of being able to target specific features of the immune system by targeting particular receptors or signalling molecules. Most therapies now in common usage are targeted at T and B cells directly or their effector molecules. They can be polyclonal, e.g. anti-thymocyte globulin (ATG; Thymoglobulin®), or monoclonal, e.g. alemtuzumab (Campath®-1H) and muromonab-CD3 (Orthoclone OKT®3) (Box 4.2).

Box 4.2 Monoclonal antibody naming conventions

Monoclonal antibodies are named in a specific manner that describes features of the origin and intended target of the drug.

1. *Prefix-* to create a unique name.
2. *Infix representing the target or disease* (e.g. -tu-/-t- = tumour or -li-/-l- = immunomodulator).
3. *Infix indicating source* (e.g. -zu- = humanized, -o- = mouse, -xi- =chimeric).
4. *Stem is used as a suffix,* -mab = monoclonal antibody. Other biologic therapies have different stems (e.g. -kinra = interleukin receptor antagonists, -cept = receptor molecules, etc.).

Polyclonal antibodies

Anti-lymphocyte antibody (e.g. ATG)

Rabbit-derived anti-thymocyte globulin.

Mechanism of action

It is a potent pan T-lymphocyte depleting agent but lacks specificity and can induce neutropenia, thrombocytopenia, and haemolysis, and also allergic reactions to foreign proteins.

Indications

- Treatment of acute renal transplant rejection (that has failed to respond to steroids).
- Renal transplant induction therapy to prevent rejection (avoids use of calcineurin inhibitors for 5–14 days, reducing nephrotoxicity).
- Treatment of acute cardiac transplant rejection.
- Myelodysplastic syndrome.

Side effects

Common (>10%):
- Hypertension, peripheral oedema, and tachycardia.
- Chills, fever (through stimulation of IL-1), headache, malaise, and pain.
- Hyperkalaemia.
- GI upset.
- Leucopenia and thrombocytopenia.
- Dyspnoea and muscle weakness.
- Antibody development (anti-rabbit).

1–10%:
- Dizziness, gastritis, and GI moniliasis.

Uncommon <1%:
- Anaphylaxis.
- Cytokine-release syndrome.
- Neutropenia.
- Post-transplant lymphoproliferative disorder (PTLD).
- Serum sickness (delayed).

Associated infections

- Wide range of bacterial, viral, fungal, and protozoal infections, including reactivation of tuberculosis (TB).
- Reactivation of herpes viruses, especially CMV, EBV, and herpes simplex virus (HSV).

Receptor-targeted antibodies

Alemtuzumab (Campath®-1)

Humanized anti-CD52 pan-lymphocytic (both B and T cells) monoclonal antibody.

Mechanism of action

Targets human CD52 antigen, a GPI-anchored cell surface protein of unknown function. Highly expressed on B and T cells and also on monocytes, macrophages, and eosinophils, and the male reproductive tract. Binds to 95% of normal and malignant blood cells but does not affect early haematopoietic progenitor cell development. Mode of action is via ADCC, complement-mediated cytotoxicity, and caspase-independent apoptosis. Leads to profound long-lasting depletion of mature T and B cells, NK cells, and monocytes, within 2–4 weeks of starting. CD4 count usually <0.05 $\times 10^9$/L at the end of treatment and only starts to rise after 9 months. Increased risk in pre-treated patients, e.g. with fludarabine, or patients who do not respond to alemtuzumab.

Indications

- B-cell chronic lymphocytic leukaemia (first line, and for relapsed/refractory disease).
- Lymphomas: cutaneous and peripheral T cell, prolymphocytic.
- Prevention of GvHD in allogeneic HSCT if patient unable to tolerate highly myeloablative conditioning regimens.
- SOT, and post-SOT rejection—in order to allow lower-dose calcineurin inhibitor use and prevent steroid use.
- Multiple sclerosis (aggressive relapsing forms) and rheumatoid arthritis.

Side effects

- Transfusion reactions.
- GI side effects (diarrhoea, anorexia).
- Rashes.
- Bone marrow suppression—transient neutropenia, anaemia and thrombocytopenia—usually resolves by 2 months.

Associated infections

Typically occur around T cell and neutrophil nadirs, within the first 3 months of therapy, but invasive fungal disease, VZV, and TB have been reported >180 days after treatment.

- Viral: CMV: 60–80% risk of CMV reactivation in those at risk, HSV/VZV reactivation, adenovirus, coxsackievirus, parvovirus, EBV, human herpesvirus (HHV)-6.
- Hepatitis B virus (HBV) reactivation (NB hepatitis B surface antigen (HBsAg) negative, core antibody positive, DNA negative—give prophylaxis for up to 6 months).
- Bacterial: common in first 8 weeks.
- Mycobacterial: TB and non-tuberculous mycobacteria—occur late after treatment (10 months+).
- Treat with isoniazid for 12 months if tuberculin skin test/IGRA positive.

- Fungi: moulds more common than *Candida* (no mucositis or prolonged neutropenia). This should be reflected in broader-spectrum prophylaxis. Majority of mould infections occur within 3 months of treatment but prophylaxis may need extending up to 6 months, or adopt aggressive screening strategy.
- Helminths: *Strongyloides* hyperinfection syndrome can occur—treat with ivermectin prior to starting alemtuzumab if serology positive (always check if from endemic area).

In general, HSV and *Pneumocystis jirovecii* prophylaxis should be continued for at least 2 months after treatment has been discontinued.

Muromonab-CD3 (Orthoclone OKT®3)
Anti-CD3 mouse monoclonal antibody.

Mechanism of action
- More specific alternative to polyclonal Thymoglobulin® that avoids the non-specific adverse effects. However, it can stimulate proinflammatory cytokines, like Thymoglobulin®.
- Directed against the CD3 antigen that is closely associated with the T-cell receptor.
- Immune responses to the murine antibody can produce fever and allergic responses and can interfere with T-cell depletion.

Indications
- Treatment of GvHD.
- Part of preparatory regimen prior to HSCT and prophylaxis of GvHD following HSCT.
- Frequently used in patients with renal dysfunction to avoid the use of nephrotoxic calcineurin inhibitors.

Side effects
- Dose-limiting side effects result from T-cell activation and the high incidence of infection.
- A 'humanized' OKT®3 is becoming available, which does not activate T cells and which retains significant immunosuppressive properties.

Associated infections
- Inhibits microbial-specific T-cell responses, therefore increasing susceptibility to herpes viruses, especially CMV and EBV, fungal infections, and mycobacterial infections.

Rituximab
Chimeric monoclonal antibody against CD20.

Mechanism of action
Anti-CD20 receptor antibody (CD20 is a B lymphocyte-specific molecule found on the B-cell surface). Rituximab causes B-cell depletion through one or more of several antibody-dependent mechanisms including Fc receptor gamma-mediated antibody-dependent cytotoxicity, complement-mediated cell lysis, growth arrest, and B-cell apoptosis.

Indications
Used in treatment of the following:
- GvHD.
- Chronic lymphocytic leukaemia, NHL, Hodgkin's lymphoma (as part of R-CHOP).
- PTLD.
- Antibody-mediated rejection in SOT recipients.
- Autoimmune conditions: rheumatoid arthritis, pemphigus vulgaris.
- Waldenström's macroglobulinaemia.

Side effects
- Impaired responses to inactivated viral or bacterial vaccines (e.g. hepatitis B, influenza, or pneumococcal vaccines). Patients should be immunized at least 4 weeks before rituximab is given. B-cell recovery can take 6–12 months.
- Late-onset neutropenia — typically seen several months after drug administration. Early (within 1 month) neutropenia can also occur, though is less common.
- Rarely: serious mucocutaneous reactions (Stevens–Johnson syndrome, vesiculobullous dermatitis, and toxic epidermal necrolysis)—usually present 1–13 weeks after therapy.
- Serum sickness (delayed type III hypersensitivity) reactions have been reported.

Associated infections
- Increased risk of infection up to 1 year post treatment and if concomitant immunosuppression, e.g. HIV, other immunosuppressants.
- Early bacterial infections (B-cell depression), e.g. *Streptococcus pneumoniae, Staphylococcus aureus*, and *Escherichia coli*. Pneumonia is common.
- HBV reactivation with fulminant hepatitis among patients positive for HBsAg or just anti-HB core positive. Reports are more common among patients with lymphoma or other malignancies and also include some patients with initially only serological evidence of resolved past hepatitis B infection. Patients with evidence of prior hepatitis B infection should be monitored for clinical and laboratory signs of reactivation during therapy and for several months after completion of therapy.
- Other viral infections: rituximab should be discontinued in patients with reactivation of CMV, HSV, or VZV. Parvovirus B19 and West Nile virus can occur. PML remains a risk for over a year (though this is uncommon, PML is much more frequently associated with deficient cellular immunity).
- Some reports of severe *P. jirovecii* and cryptococcal meningitis.

Anti-TNFα antibodies

Infliximab (Remicade®) and adalimumab (Humira®)
Anti-TNFα monoclonal antibodies.

Mechanism of action
Human–murine chimeric monoclonal antibody directed against TNFα (also golimumab, certolizumab pegol). Combines with TNFα and downregulates endothelial cell adhesion molecules.

Indications
- Autoimmune conditions including rheumatoid arthritis, inflammatory bowel disease, psoriatic arthritis, severe plaque psoriasis, and ankylosing spondylitis.
- Off-label use in hidradenitis suppurativa, blistering diseases, pyoderma gangrenosum, and acute GvHD.

Side effects
- Injection site and infusion reactions, cutaneous reactions.
- Demyelinating disease.
- Heart failure.
- Malignancy.
- Induction of autoimmunity.

Associated infections
- Bacterial including *Listeria* spp.
- Mycobacterial (TB and non-tuberculous mycobacteria)—most cases occur in the first 3–6 months of treatment. All patients should be screened/assessed for TB prior to starting, and latent TB infection treated.
- Viral: HBV and hepatitis C virus (HCV) reactivation.
- Fungal: *Pneumocystis jirovecii* (need prophylaxis if also on steroids or other immunosuppressants in conjunction with infliximab); reactivation of endemic mycoses, e.g. *Histoplasma* spp., *Blastomycosis*, and *Coccidioides*.

Other anti-cytokine agents (non-antibodies)

Etanercept
Anti-TNF fusion protein.

Mechanism of action
Recombinant DNA-derived protein composed of tumour necrosis factor receptor (TNFR) linked to the Fc portion of human IgG1. Etanercept binds (neutralizes) soluble TNF, blocking its interaction with cell surface receptors: resulting in anti-inflammatory effects.

Indications
- Autoimmune conditions including rheumatoid arthritis, ankylosing spondylitis, psoriatic arthritis, plaque psoriasis, and polyarticular juvenile idiopathic arthritis.
- Off label use for GvHD.

Side effects
- Headache, rash, and GI upset.
- Local injection site reaction.
- Upper respiratory tract infections.
- Antibody development, positive antinuclear antibody titre.

Associated infections
- Reactivation of latent TB infection.
- Invasive fungal infections.
- Bacterial opportunistic infections including *Legionella* spp. and *Listeria* spp.
- Reactivation of hepatitis B.

Anakinra
IL-1 receptor antagonist.

Mechanism of action
Prevents immunological responses of endogenous IL-1, including degradation of cartilage (loss of proteoglycans) and stimulation of bone resorption.

Indications
- Disease-modifying antirheumatic drug-insensitive rheumatoid arthritis.
- Periodic/recurrent inflammatory conditions, e.g. neonatal-onset multisystem inflammatory disease (NOMID).

Side effects
- Headache.
- Local injection site reactions.
- Arthralgia.
- Fever.
- GI upset.
- Neutropenia.

Associated infections
- Reactivation of latent TB infection.
- Variety of opportunistic infections.

Further reading

1. Koo S, Marty FM, Baden LT. Infectious complications associated with immunomodulating biologic agents. Infectious Disease Clinics of North America 2010;24:285–306.
2. Rubin RH, Ikonen T, Gummert JF, Morris RE. The therapeutic prescription for the organ transplant recipient: the linkage of immunosuppression and antimicrobial strategies. Transplant Infectious Disease 1999;1(1):29–39.
3. Kang I, Park SH. Infectious complications in SLE after immunosuppressive therapies. Current Opinion in Rheumatology 2003;15(5):528–34.

HIV infection

Introduction

The human immunodeficiency viruses (HIV-1 and HIV-2) are enveloped, icosahedral RNA retroviruses. Both cause the acquired immunodeficiency syndrome (AIDS); HIV-1 is responsible for the vast majority of infections worldwide, while HIV-2 is, for the most part, limited to West Africa. HIV-2 causes less severe immunodeficiency and progresses more slowly. HIV-2 is also constitutionally resistant to an entire class of antiretrovirals (non-nucleoside reverse-transcriptase inhibitors (NNRTIs)).

HIV epidemiology

According to the Joint United Nations Programme on HIV and AIDS (UNAIDS), by the end of 2014, there were 36.9 million people globally living with HIV infection, 25.8 million of these were in sub-Saharan Africa. In the year 2014, 1.2 million people died from AIDS related illness globally. It is estimated that 17.1 million people worldwide are infected, but unaware of it (Figure 5.1).

HIV is truly a global pandemic. First recognized in 1981, HIV has exploded across the globe to become one of the greatest modern-day health disasters. In a familiar pattern, HIV disproportionately affects the poor, disenfranchised, and most vulnerable people in society, with the least access to education and healthcare. Despite this, there has been an unprecedented global collaborative response, and the epidemic now appears to be in decline. According to UNAIDS, new HIV infections have fallen by 35% since 2000 (by 58% among children) and AIDS-related deaths have fallen by 42% since the peak in 2004.

HIV biology

The HIV viral particle (virion) is 120 nm in diameter and consists of a viral envelope enclosing a capsid, which in turn encloses two single-stranded positive sense RNA molecules (see Figure 5.2).

The viral envelope is a lipid bilayer derived from the host cell and is punctuated by viral proteins. These are responsible for binding to host cells— Gp 120 (glycoprotein 120) binds to CD4 receptors on host immune cells (helped by co-receptors CCR5 or CXCR4 on some cells), and fusion with the host cell membrane—Gp 41. The capsid is composed of the viral protein p24 (protein 24). This enclosures three enzymes, reverse transcriptase (p51 and p66), integrase (p32), and protease (p11), and two copies of single-stranded RNA associated with nucleocapsid proteins (p7 and p6).

Briefly, the viral replicative cycle is as follows (see Figure 5.3); the viral particle via Gp120 binds to a CD4 receptor on a host immune cell. On helper T cells or macrophages, co-receptors are important in facilitating binding (CCR5 or CXCR4). The viral envelope fuses with the host cell membrane (Gp41) and the viral capsid is released into the cell. The enzyme reverse transcriptase is then responsible for transcribing, from the single-stranded RNA, a double-stranded DNA molecule. This is then integrated into the host cell DNA (with the aid of the enzyme integrase). Once incorporated into the host cell DNA, the process of transcription and translation of the proviral DNA is carried out by host cells proteins to form new viral RNA particles and viral proteins. These are assembled in the cytoplasm and

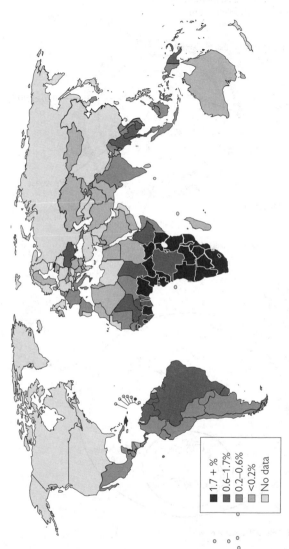

Fig 5.1 Global HIV prevalence 2016. Reproduced with permission from UNAIDS. Number of people living with HIV. Copyright © 2016 UNAIDS. Available at: ℗ http://aidsinfo.unaids.org/.

1.7 + %
0.6–1.7%
0.2–0.6%
<0.2%
No data

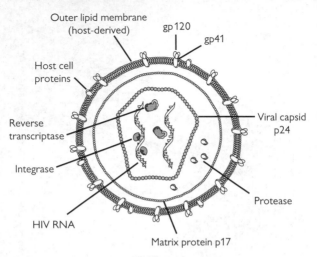

Fig 5.2 The HIV viral particle.

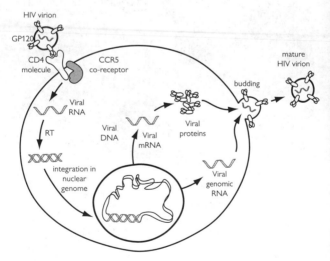

Fig 5.3 The viral replicative cycle.

translocated to the host cell membrane in order to bud off as mature virions (aided by the enzyme protease).

The HIV virus is genetically extremely variable, both within and between infected individuals. The replicative process is particularly error-prone, but highly active with 10^8–10^{10} viral particles produced each day in the untreated individual. HIV-1 is divided into four 'groups': M, N, O, and P. Group M is responsible for the global pandemic (>90%) and is in turn divided into at least nine genetically distinct subtypes (A, B, C, D, F, G, H, J, and K). Subtype B is the most common in the UK.

Transmission

The most important mode of transmission of HIV is through unprotected sexual intercourse with an infected partner. Other modes include injection, transfusion of contaminated blood products or other human tissue, sharing of needles and injecting paraphernalia, and maternofetal (during pregnancy, birth, or breastfeeding). Occupational infections in healthcare workers have occurred, but it appears to carry a low risk particularly if post-exposure prophylaxis is employed (Table 5.1).

Table 5.1 Relative risks of different exposures

Type of exposure		Risk per 10,000 exposures	Type of exposure		Risk per 10,000 exposures
Parenteral	Blood transfusion	9250	Sexual	Receptive anal intercourse	138
	Needle-sharing (during drug use)	63		Insertive anal intercourse	11
	Percutaneous (needle-stick)	23		Receptive penile-vaginal intercourse	8
				Insertive penile-vaginal intercourse	4
				Receptive oral intercourse	Low
				Insertive oral intercourse	Low

Source: data from Patel, P. et al. Estimating per-act HIV transmission risk: a systematic review. *AIDS*. 2014. 28(10), 1509–1519. Copyright © 2014 Wolters Kluwer Health.

Testing for HIV

The diagnosis of HIV infection can be established by the following methods: serology, detection of viral antigens, detection of viral RNA or DNA, and virus culture. Screening is most commonly carried out by serology (detection of antibodies to the virus; third-generation tests) or combined antibody/antigen tests (combination or fourth-generation tests). This is usually carried out on the blood sample, but can be carried out on saliva. Antigen detection tests for the p24 viral capsid protein. Antibody tests are not accurate until 3 months after exposure, due to the 'window period' prior to the development of antibodies.

Confirmatory tests include PCR for viral RNA and DNA. This also allows for specific testing for genotypes and resistance markers.

Basics of antiretroviral treatment

Antiretroviral drugs ('antiretrovirals' (ARVs)) interrupt the viral replicative cycle at various points in order to suppress or eliminate viral replication. Due to the rapid development of resistance, these are always used in combination. There are several preparations now that have combined drugs in a single pill.

ARVs can be broadly divided into five main groups (Figure 5.4):

- *Nucleoside reverse transcriptase inhibitors* (NRTIs) (also known as nucleoside analogues) block reverse transcriptase. Often included in this group are the nucleotide reverse transcriptase inhibitors (NtRTIs), e.g. tenofovir.
- *Non-nucleoside reverse transcriptase inhibitors* (NNRTIs) block reverse transcriptase by binding directly to the enzyme. HIV–2 is constitutionally resistant to most NNRTIs.
- *Protease inhibitors* (PIs) bind to and block the action of viral proteases. As these have poor oral bioavailability, they are often given in combination with a second PI (e.g. ritonavir): or a specific enzyme inhibitor (e.g. cobicistat), which inhibits both gut wall and liver metabolism of other PIs. This is known as boosting.
- *Integrase inhibitors* block the action of integrase.
- *Fusion/entry inhibitors* interfere with the binding, fusion, and entry of the HIV virion to the human cell.

There are several factors that influence the selection of the most appropriate regimen; these include side effects, drug interactions, adherence and 'pill burden', virological resistance, and cost.

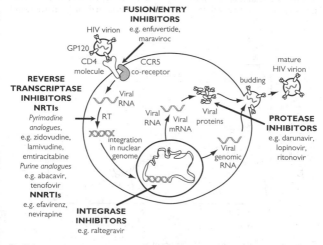

Fig 5.4 Mechanism of action of antiretroviral drugs.

Natural history of infection

HIV infection elicits a broad immune response that is both adaptive and innate. This response is usually capable of significant suppression of viral activity, sometimes for years following initial infection, but is insufficient to prevent ongoing viral replication or to eradicate the infection.

Immune response

CD4-positive T-cell decline is the key immunological feature of HIV illness and leads to susceptibility to opportunistic infection. HIV, however, has a widespread effect on the immune system. Mucosal dendritic cells (Langerhans cells) are likely to be the first immune cells that are encountered and infected. These virus-infected cells then transport the infection to the local lymph nodes where virus amplification occurs in CD4-positive T cells. There is significant immune stimulation including activation of NK cells, up-regulation of CD8-positive T cells and cytotoxic T cells, and activation of B cells resulting in the development of an antibody response.

Immune response and therefore progression of HIV varies among individuals; HLA subtype has an important impact on the host's ability to control viral replication as do polymorphisms in chemokine receptors (e.g. CCR5 receptor).

Following transmission, HIV infection progresses through three stages (Figure 5.5):

Acute seroconversion or early infection

This period relates to symptomatic early infection in the 6 months or so following transmission. Usually occurs 2–6 weeks after exposure. This is characterized by a period of rapid viral replication and infection of CD4 cells. Plasma viral load is usually high. This period may be asymptomatic or present as a flu-like illness with fever, headache, myalgia, arthralgia, malaise, and

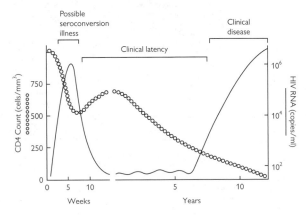

Fig 5.5 A schematic illustrating the history of HIV.

sore throat. Maculopapular rash and lymphadenopathy can also occur and may alert the physician to the possibility of acute seroconversion. Rarely, an acute meningoencephalitis can occur.

Latent infection or chronic infection in the absence of AIDS

Progression from acute seroconversion to chronic latent infection is reached following the establishment of a viral 'set point'; the adaptive immune response gains some measure of control of viral replication and induces a period of dynamic equilibrium between viral replication and immunological control. Plasma viral load drops to low levels, but is still detectable. This period lasts for 8–10 years on average, but is affected by factors such as comorbidity (including co-infection, e.g. TB/hepatitis), nutritional status, viral subtype, host genetics, and increasing host age. Largely asymptomatic, although many will have lymphadenopathy on examination. HIV-associated lymphadenopathy is usually bilateral, symmetrical, and painless. The term persistent generalized lymphadenopathy applies to lymphadenopathy in at least two areas of the body for at least 3 months, and is part of a spectrum of lymphadenopathy that occurs during this stage.

Clinical disease

Progressive immune dysfunction and decline eventually results in the presentation of clinical disease due to opportunistic pathogens. This usually occurs once the CD4 count falls to <200 cells/μL. Although most of the opportunistic pathogens associated with HIV will present as CD4 counts <200 cells/μL, there is still significant immunosuppression at CD4 counts higher than this and infections, including more usual pathogens, occur at a much higher frequency in this population (Figure 5.6a and 5.6b).

Primary HIV Infection
- Asymptomatic
- Acute retroviral syndrome

Clinical Stage 1
- Asymptomatic
- Persistent generalized lymphadenopathy

Clinical Stage 2
- Moderate unexplained weight loss (<10% of presumed or measured body weight)
- Recurrent respiratory infections (sinusitis, tonsillitis, otitis media, and pharyngitis)
- Herpes zoster • Angular cheilitis • Recurrent oral ulceration • Papular pruritic eruptions
- Seborrheic dermatitis • Fungal nail infections

Clinical Stage 3
- Unexplained severe weight loss (>10% of presumed or measured body weight)
- Unexplained chronic diarrhea for >1 month • Unexplained persistent fever for >1 month (>37.6°C, intermittent or constant) • Persistent oral candidiasis (thrush)
- Oral hairy leukoplakia • Pulmonary tuberculosis (current) • Severe presumed bacterial infections (e.g., pneumonia, empyema, pyomyositis, bone or joint infection, meningitis, bacteremia) • Acute necrotizing ulcerative stomatitis, gingivitis, or periodontitis
- Unexplained anemia (hemoglobin <8 gidL) • Neutropenia (neutrophils <500 cells/μL)
- Chronic thrombocytopenia (platelets <50,000 cells/μL)

Clinical Stage 4
- HIV wasting syndrome, • *Pneumocystis* pneumonia • Recurrent severe bacterial pneumonia • Chronic herpes simplex infection (orolabial, genital, or anorectal site for >1 month or visceral herpes at any site)
- Oesophageal candidiasis (or candidiasis of trachea, bronchi, or lungs) • Extrapulmonary tuberculosis • Kaposi sarcoma • Cytomegalovirus infection (retinitis or infection of other organs)
- Central nervous system toxoplasmosis • HIV encephalopathy • Cryptococcosis, extrapulmonary (including meningitis) • Disseminated nontuberculosis mycobacteria infection • Progressive multifocal leukoencephalopathy • Candida of the trachea, bronchi, or lungs • Chronic cryptosporidiosis (with diarrhea) • Chronic isosporiasis • Disseminated mycosis (e.g, histoplasmosis, coccidioidomycosis, penicilliosis) • Recurrent nontyphoidal *Salmonella* bacteremia • Lymphoma (cerebral or B-cell non-Hodgkin) • Invasive cervical carcinoma • Atypical disseminated leishmaniasis • Symptomatic HIV-associated nephropathy • Symptomatic HIV-associated cardiomyopathy • Reactivation of American trypanosomiasis (meningoencephalitis or myocarditis)

Fig 5.6a Summary of WHO Clinical Staging of HIV disease.

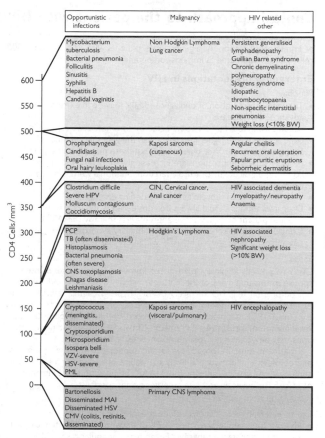

	Opportunistic infections	Malignancy	HIV related other
600 / 550 / 500	Mycobacterium tuberculosis Bacterial pneumonia Folliculitis Sinusitis Syphilis Hepatitis B Candidal vaginitis	Non Hodgkin Lymphoma Lung cancer	Persistent generalised lymphadenopathy Guillian Barre syndrome Chronic demyelinating polyneuropathy Sjogrens syndrome Idiopathic thrombocytopaenia Non-specific interstitial pneumonias Weight loss (<10% BW)
450 / 400	Orophpharyngeal Candidiasis Fungal nail infections Oral hairy leukoplakia	Kaposi sarcoma (cutaneous)	Angular cheilitis Recurrent oral ulceration Papular pruritic eruptions Seborrheic dermatitis
350	Clostridium difficile Severe HPV Molluscum contagiosum Coccidiomycosis	CIN, Cervical cancer, Anal cancer	HIV associated dementia /myelopathy/neuropathy Anaemia
300 / 250 / 200	PCP TB (often disseminated) Histoplasmosis Bacterial pneumonia (often severe) CNS toxoplasmosis Chagas disease Leishmaniasis	Hodgkin's Lymphoma	HIV associated nephropathy Significant weight loss (>10% BW)
150 / 100 / 50	Cryptococcus (meningitis, disseminated) Cryptosporidium Microsporidium Isospera belli VZV-severe HSV-severe PML	Kaposi sarcoma (visceral/pulmonary)	HIV encephalopathy
0	Bartonellosis Disseminated MAI Disseminated HSV CMV (colitis, retinitis, disseminated)	Primary CNS lymphoma	

CD4 Cells/mm³

Fig 5.6b CD4 count at which important complications first start to occur.

Clinical approach to the patient with HIV

The key consideration in the approach to the patient with HIV is the degree of immunosuppression. As a general rule, patients with a CD4 count >500 cells/μL can be treated as immunocompetent.

Emergency presentations in HIV

Principles

- The initial presentation of undiagnosed HIV may be in extremis with advanced HIV disease.
- Patients living with HIV are still affected by common diseases; indeed, they contract them with higher frequency than the general population (e.g. *Streptococcus pneumoniae* pneumonia), but these may present atypically.
- Non-infective complications are increasingly important and more common e.g. acute myocardial infarction, pulmonary embolism, and acute pancreatitis.
- Drug toxicities can present as life-threatening emergencies.
- Drug interactions should always be considered when treating the HIV-infected patient on highly active antiretroviral therapy (HAART).
- Consider immune reconstitution inflammatory syndrome (IRIS) in patients who have started HAART within the last year.

Sepsis

Likely to present atypically in advanced immune compromise; blunted response means that many of the features normally associated with SIRS may not be present (e.g. lack of fever, ↑WBC, hyperglycaemia, etc.). Sources of infection may be poorly localized. Atypical organisms may be present, e.g. fungi (PCP, *Cryptococcus*, disseminated candidiasis), parasites (e.g. *Toxoplasma*), or viruses (e.g. HSV, VZV, CMV). Several simultaneous infections may be occurring; 'Occam's razor' does not apply.

Treatment must be broad; sepsis and septic shock in the absence of microbiological information is likely to require broad-spectrum antibiotic, antifungal, and possibly antiviral (not HAART) medication. The introduction of HAART is never an absolute emergency: get specialist help.

Drug toxicity

Life-threatening complications include the following:

- *Abacavir hypersensitivity reaction*: 3.7% of patients, usually within the first 2 months after starting abacavir. Fever, maculopapular rash, malaise, arthralgia progressing to multi-visceral involvement (pneumonitis, hepatitis, mucositis, myocarditis, interstitial nephritis). Less common now where patients are tested for HLA B*5701 prior to treatment.
- *Stevens–Johnson syndrome and toxic epidermal necrolysis*: particularly with nevirapine started at high CD4 counts. Associated with TMP–SMX.
- *Mitochondrial toxicity*: due to inhibition of mitochondrial DNA polymerase. Associated with NRTIs (particularly stavudine, didanosine). Can lead to lactic acidosis, hepatic steatosis, and acute pancreatitis.
- *Hepatic toxicity*: a potential with most ARVs and is often a result of interactions.
- Nephrotoxicity and acute kidney injury, particularly associated with tenofovir and indinavir.

Intensive care and HIV

With correct management, HIV disease is eminently treatable. Patients should be offered intensive care support if necessary. Specialist and multi-disciplinary input is vital early. Acute respiratory failure is the most common reason for intensive care unit (ICU) admission. There are several potential drug interactions between HAART/opportunistic infection therapy and many of the drugs commonly used in intensive care.

Fever with no focal signs

Differential is wide and becomes wider with ↓CD4 count. Every effort should be made to identify a source of infection; although with severe immune compromise, more than one infection may be present. In the absence of a CD4 count, a clinical assessment can provide useful information about the degree of immunosuppression; examining the mouth and skin may be helpful in identifying HIV-related manifestations associated with ↓CD4 count (e.g. candidiasis, Kaposi's sarcoma). The most common causes for fever in HIV depend on CD4 count, treatment and prophylaxis, and local epidemiology (Box 5.1).

Common causes
- *Bacterial infection*: particularly *S. pneumoniae, Staphylococcus aureus*.
- *Mycobacteria*: TB—both pulmonary and extrapulmonary; non-tuberculous mycobacteria (NTM).
- *Fungal*: PCP pneumonia, cryptococcal meningitis, and cryptococcosis.
- *Viral*: acute HIV seroconversion, CMV.
- *Malignancy*: NHL, visceral Kaposi's sarcoma.
- *Tropical infections*: malaria, leishmaniasis.

Investigations to consider
- *Blood*: full blood count, urea and electrolytes, liver function tests (LFTs), bone profile, amylase, C-reactive protein, CD4 count, viral load, resistance markers. Malaria microscopy ± rapid diagnostic test; blood cultures; serology: hepatitis A, B, C, E, CMV, EBV, VZV, cryptococcal antigen, *Toxoplasma* serology.
- *Sputum* (± BAL): microscopy for acid-fast bacilli, PCP DNA.
- *Urine*: culture and microscopy, including for acid-fast bacilli, nucleic acid amplification tests (NAAT).
- *Stool*: culture and microscopy (ova, cysts, and parasites).
- *Lumbar puncture*: microscopy (Gram stain, India ink, Ziehl–Nielsen), PCR (CMV, JC virus, HSV, VZV), protein, glucose, *Cryptococcus* antigen, cytology.

Box 5.1 Consider tropical and travel-associated infections

(This subject is covered in more detail in ➔ Chapter 10.)
- Malaria: any exposure in a region of known malaria transmission.
- Legionnaire's disease (*Legionella pneumophila*): exposure to air conditioning/cooling towers etc.
- Leishmaniasis: travel in Mediterranean and tropics.
- Enteric fever (*S. typhi/S. paratyphi*), histoplasmosis, coccidiomycosis, Chagas disease (*Trypanosoma cruzi*), penicilliosis, and *Strongyloides* hyperinfection.

- *Other aspirates*: ascites, pleural effusion, pericardial effusion, joint (synovial fluid), lymph node aspirate, bone marrow, splenic aspirate. For microscopy and culture, cytology.
- *Skin and histological biopsy*: histological examination.
- *Endoscopy*: oesophagogastroduodenoscopy (OGD)/colonoscopy.
- *Imaging*: chest X-ray, skeletal plain films, echocardiography, ultrasound thorax, abdomen, CT head, chest and abdomen, and pelvis. MRI brain, soft tissue, positron emission tomography scanning.

Neurological presentations

Neurological complications are common in HIV, in up to 30% of presentations. Key organisms to consider in addition to HIV are *Toxoplasma gondii*, *Cryptococcus neoformans*, CMV, VZV, and JC virus (PML). Primary CNS lymphoma is an important differential. Imaging of the CNS (CT/MRI) is almost always indicated. CD4 count helps predict the likely causative organism (See Figure 5.6b).

Causes (See Table 5.2)

- Cryptococcal meningitis, *Toxoplasma* encephalitis, acute HIV seroconversion, HIV-associated dementia, *M. tuberculosis*, VZV, PML (JC virus), CMV, syphilis, *M. avium* complex, neurocysticercosis. Staphylococcal, streptococcal, or *Salmonella* infection. Less common pathogens (*Nocardia, Aspergillus, Rhodococcus*).
- Primary CNS lymphoma is common (when CD4 is low), metastatic extra-CNS lymphoma (NHL), neuro-IRIS.
- Side effects of ARV medication (esp. stavudine, didanosine, efavirenz). Consider more usual causes of neurological disease as well as comorbid psychiatric disorders.

Clinical features

Altered mental state

Acute encephalopathy with rapid progression, particularly if associated with very low CD4 count, suggests toxoplasmosis/cryptococcosis/CMV/VZV. Patients on co-trimoxazole prophylaxis have a greatly reduced risk of

Table 5.2 Differential for CNS lesions

Space-occupying lesion	Diffuse brain disease	
	Meningitis	Encephalitis
Toxoplasma	Cryptococcal meningitis	Acute HIV
Primary CNS lymphoma	Tuberculous meningitis	HIV dementia
Tuberculoma	Bacterial meningitis	*Toxoplasma* encephalitis
PML		CMV
Abscess		VZV
Metastatic NHL		HSV
Cryptococcoma		Neurosyphilis
Syphilitic gumma		

toxoplasmosis. HIV-associated dementia (otherwise known as AIDS dementia complex, HIV-associated neurocognitive disorders (HAND)) generally have a more subacute presentation with progressive impairment of concentration, attention, psychomotor speed, and memory. Language relatively unaffected.

Seizures
A careful examination for focal neurology is important. Most likely causes: toxoplasmosis, primary CNS lymphoma, or PML.

Headache
Common and important presentation. Acute seroconversion may present as 'aseptic' meningitis. Cryptococcal meningitis and tuberculous meningitis are key considerations. Cryptococcosis presents sub-acutely with worsening headache, meningism, and fever over ~2 weeks. CD4 count usually <100 cells/μL. May develop altered mental state, cranial nerve lesions, features suggesting raised intracranial pressure. TB meningitis presents in a similar manner, can be acute or chronic, and may occur at any CD4 count.

Focal signs
Usually associated with a space-occupying lesion on imaging. *Toxoplasma* and primary CNS lymphoma main differentials. Progressive hemiparesis/cerebellar signs/hemianopia/dysphasia associated with cognitive decline is suggestive of PML. Consider intracerebral abscess.

Peripheral neurology
TB/cryptococcal meningitis can present with cranial nerve palsies. At low CD4 counts, CMV can cause a lumbosacral plexopathy. HIV-associated neuropathy may present as a Bilateral symmetrical polyneuropathy or as a mono neuritis multiplex. HIV vacuolar myelopathy and myelitis are common with advanced HIV disease (CD4 <50 cells/μL) and present with gait abnormalities, abnormal proprioception, ataxia, and paraparesis. Acute seroconversion illness can present as Guillain–Barré syndrome.

Investigation
Neurological imaging (See Figure 5.7)
Early cross-sectional imaging is important (CT ± contrast and/or MRI). Most space-occupying lesions can be detected with contrast CT but MRI is much more sensitive and specific, particularly with pathology of the base of the skull and leptomeninges. MRI is essential for the diagnosis of spinal cord and plexus disease.

CSF examination (See Table 5.3)
Unless contraindicated, lumbar puncture is almost always useful. Measurement of opening pressure is particularly important (normal opening pressure 6–25 cmH$_2$O). Cryptococcal meningitis classically generates high opening pressures (> 25 cmH$_2$O)

Consider the following tests:
- *Biochemistry*: protein, glucose (with paired plasma glucose).
- *Microbiology*: white cell count, Gram stain, India ink stain, Ziehl–Neelsen or auramine stain. CSF cryptococcal antigen, PCR: VZV, CMV, EBV, JC virus, TB, syphilis, HIV CSF viral titre.
- *Cytology*: send at least 10–15 mL CSF, positive in 25–35% cases of primary CNS lymphoma.

Toxoplasma: typically multiple hypodense, ring enhancing lesions that favour the basal ganglia, thalamus and corticomedullary junction. May be associated with mass effect.
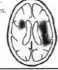

TB: basilar meningeal enhancement, hydrocephalus, ring enhancing lesions (tuberculoma). May show no abnormality.
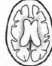

PML: periventricular and sub-cortical low attenuation lesions, focal and asymmetrical.
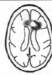

HIV dementia: cerebral atrophy, favours basal ganglia (particularly the caudate)
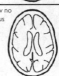

Primary CNS lymphoma: may be solitary or multiple, usually periventricular, hyperdense or isodense and well defined.

Cryptococcus: May show no abnormality. Hydrocephalus sometimes. Cryptococcal masses (cryptococcomas) favour the midbrain and basal ganglia.

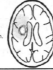
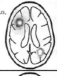

Fig 5.7 Some classical illustrative CT appearances of CNS infections in HIV.

Table 5.3 CSF interpretation

	Protein	Glucose	Cell count	Microscopy	Further tests
Toxoplasma	↑↑	↔	↑lymphs	Rarely tachyzoites detected on cytology	PCR has poor sensitivity
Cryptococcus	↔ or ↑	↓	↔ or ↑ lymphs	India ink stain	CrAg PCR
PML	↑	↔	↔ or ↑lymphs	Nil	JC virus PCR
TB	↑	↔ or ↓	↑lymphs	Ziehl–Neelsen or auramine stain	MTB PCR
CMV	↑	↔	↔ or ↑ lymphs	Nil	CMV DNA PCR
CNS lymphoma	↑	↔ or ↓	↑lymphs	Cytology, flow cytometry, immuno-histochemistry	EBV DNA PCR (of dubious utility)
VZV	↑	↔	↔ or ↑ lymphs	Nil	VZV PCR
Bacterial (e.g. pneumococcal)	↑↑	↓↓	↑↑PMNs	Gram stain	PCR available

CrAg cryptococcal antigen; lymphs lymphocytes; MTB *Mycobacterium tuberculosis*; PMNs polymorphonuclear neutrophils.

Blood tests
Routine blood tests including blood cultures. Serology: syphillis, toxo-plasma. Toxoplasma encephalitis is mainly caused by re-activation of prior infection; almost all will be plasma *Toxoplasma* IgG positive (a negative result does not rule it out, but should prompt a reconsideration of the diagnosis).

Therapeutic trial
In the absence of mass effect, a therapeutic trial of anti-*Toxoplasma* treatment may be diagnostic and avoids a brain biopsy. Deterioration after 3 days of treatment is strongly suggestive of an alternative diagnosis. Rescanning after 2 weeks of treatment should show marked improvement.

Brain biopsy
Stereotactic brain biopsy may provide the definitive diagnosis and is the gold standard.

Management

Toxoplasmosis
Pyrimethamine and sulphadiazine are first line (NB Ideally patient should be screened for G6PD deficiency). Alternative agents include clindamycin, tri-methoprim, atovaquone, and dapsone. Steroids are not recommended routinely but may be considered if raised intracranial pressure. Antiepileptics are similarly not recommended routinely in the absence of seizures (See Table 5.3) (➔ Also See '*Toxoplasma gondii*', p.289).

Cryptococcus
Induction with liposomal amphotericin B, usually combined with flucytosine followed by maintenance with fluconazole. An alternative regimen is flu-conazole ± flucytosine as induction followed by fluconazole maintenance. Raised intracranial pressure may require daily lumber punctures, aiming to maintain intracranial pressure <20 cmH$_2$O. (➔ See '*Cryptococcus spp*', p.323).

CMV
Ganciclovir ± foscarnet induction followed by valganciclovir maintenance. (➔ See 'Cytomegalovirus (CMV/ HHV- 5)', p.244).

PML
HAART; no specific treatment has improved clinical outcomes. (➔ See 'progressive multifocal leucoencephalopathy (PML)', p.285).

CNS TB
See Table 5.2 and Figure 5.7.
➔ Also see '*Mycobacterium tuberculosis* complex (MTBC)' p.337.

Respiratory presentations

Common and account for a significant burden of disease in HIV (>60% will have some respiratory complication as part of their disease). Key organisms are *Pneumocystis jirovecii* (PCP), bacterial pneumonia (e.g. *Streptococcus pneumoniae*), and *Mycobacterium tuberculosis*. The use of HAART and co-trimoxazole prophylaxis is significantly reducing the prevalence of PCP disease in populations with access to treatment. Millions of people worldwide with HIV are co-infected with TB, which has shadowed the HIV pandemic. Achieving a microbiological diagnosis can still be challenging and often treatment must be instituted presumptively (Figure 5.8).

Pneumocystis (PCP): classic 'bat-wing' is a fine reticular interstitial pattern in a perihilar distribution. Particularly with profound immune suppression, CXR can be variable with appearances similar to bacterial pneumonia or the CXR maybe completely normal.

Mycobacterium tuberculosis: the classic finding of primary TB is the Ghon focus, which consists an upper lobe caseating granuloma with or without cavitation accompanied by enlargement of the adjacent hilar lymph nodes. The formation of the granuloma requires a functioning immune response, so this finding does not appear in profound in main suppression. Patchy infiltrates, consolidation or widespread miliary spread is more typical of immune suppression. Can also present with a (usually) unilateral pleural diffusion.

Viral: Can be highly variable, ranging from patchy confluent alveolar infiltrates (HSV, CMV), diffuse alveolar haemorrhage, lobar consolidation to extensive nodular opacities that can eventually calcify (VZV).

Bacterial: Typical appearances include lobar consolidation with air broncograms and para pneumonic effusions. Immunosuppression can delay the appearance of CXR findings, and tend to present with bilateral and multilobar infiltrates.

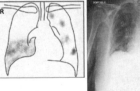

Fig 5.8 Typical chest X-ray (CXR) findings of respiratory infections associated with HIV. Illustrative representations of classical findings in addition to an example x-ray. Reproduced with permission from Desai, S. et al. CXR Pictures Chapter: Air space diseases. In Desai, S. et al. (eds.) *Oxford Specialist Handbook in Thoracic Imaging.* Oxford, UK: OUP. Copyright © 2012, OUP; and Maroune, L. et al. Pulmonary Infections. In Abujudeh, H. et al. (eds). *Emergency Radiology.* Oxford, UK: OUP. Copyright © 2016, OUP.

Causes

- CD4 count helps to predict potential causative organisms. (see Figure 5.6 p.70)
- Most important: *S. pneumoniae*, PCP, TB.
- Bacteria: *S. pneumonia, Haemophilus influenzae, Klebsiella pneumoniae, Pseudomonas aeruginosa, Staphylococcus aureus, Rhodococcus equi.*
- Mycobacteria: *M. tuberculosis, M. avium complex, M. kansasii.*
- Fungi: PCP, *C. neoformans, Aspergillus* spp., *Candida* spp., *Histoplasma capsulatum, Penicillium marneffei.*
- Viruses: CMV, VZV, HSV.
- Parasites: *Strongyloides stercoralis, T. gondii.*
- Malignancy: Kaposi's sarcoma, NHL, broncogenic carcinoma,
- Other: pulmonary embolic disease, lymphocytic interstitial pneumonitis, non-specific interstitial pneumonitis, cryptogenic organizing pneumonia, primary pulmonary hypertension.

Clinical features

- *Acute breathlessness*: spontaneous pneumothorax (450× increased risk in AIDS); may be primary or associated with infection (PCP), pulmonary embolus (significantly increased risk in HIV). Bacterial pneumonia may present acutely with acute respiratory failure and/or sepsis. HIV and ARV treatment are strong risk factors for coronary artery disease; consider cardiac causes.
- *Subacute and chronic breathlessness*: PCP tends to present sub-acutely with increasing breathlessness on exercise, weight loss, dry cough, and night sweats at CD4 counts <200 cells/μL. Oxygen saturation will fall precipitously on exercise. TB and bacterial pneumonia can present at any CD4 count, but occur more frequently and more floridly with progressive immuno-compromise. Other causes to consider include anaemia and lactic acidosis.
- *Cough*: classically PCP causes a dry cough, while bacterial pneumonia causes a more productive cough.
- *Haemoptysis*: mycobacterial disease, but can present in other pulmonary infections and in non-infectious causes (e.g. pulmonary embolism).

Investigations

- Near-patient testing: pulse oximetry and ABG; desaturation on exercise is sensitive for PCP, as is a widened A–a gradient. Spirometry and pulmonary function tests are useful in determining severity and response to treatment.
- Sputum analysis: microscopy/PCR/immunohistochemistry for mycobacteria and PCP, PCR for CMV.
- Imaging: chest X-ray—important test; may be normal, but often informs the diagnosis (see Figure 5.8). CT—more sensitive and specific than chest X-ray.
- Bronchoscopy: allows for BAL; increases sensitivity of microscopy for TB and PCP. Examination and biopsy of bronchial lesions (e.g. Kaposi's sarcoma)
- Invasive sampling: transbronchial biopsy, open lung biopsy.

Management

- *P. jirovecii* (PCP): mild to moderate disease—oral TMP–SMX; moderate to severe PCP—high-dose IV TMP–SMX (NB Ideally patients should be screened for G6PD deficiency). Alternative agents include clindamycin,

primaquine, dapsone, and pentamidine. Steroids are indicated if PaO_2 <9.3 kPa (<70 mmHg) or SpO_2< 92%.
- *Bacterial pneumonia*: as per national guidelines for community-acquired pneumonia in HIV-negative individuals (e.g. amoxicillin and/or clarithromycin).
- *Pulmonary TB*: ➔ see section on TB in HIV, p.90.
- *Pulmonary Mycobacterium avium-intracellulare infection (MAI)*: macrolide (clarithromycin/azithromycin) + ethambutol + rifampicin or rifabutin. (➔ See section on MAI, p.339)
- *CMV pneumonitis*: ganciclovir. Alternatives include valganciclovir, foscarnet, cidofovir. (➔ See section on CMV, p.244)

Gastrointestinal presentations

The entire GI tract, from mouth to anus, is vulnerable to opportunistic infections and HIV-related malignancy. With progressive immunodeficiency, multiple infectious causes become more common. Key organisms are *Cryptosporidium, Candida*, CMV, and *M. tuberculosis*. Co-infections with hepatitis viruses are common and important to recognize as this worsens prognosis and affects treatment strategy (Figure 5.9 and Figure 5.10).

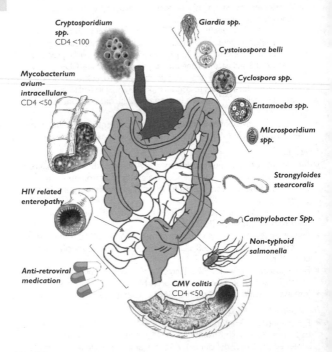

Fig 5.9 Causes of diarrhoea in HIV.

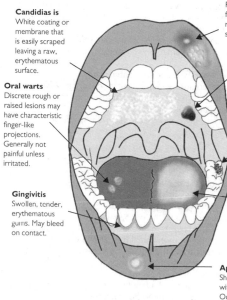

Herpes simplex
Painful orolabial fluid filled vesicles that rupture leaving superficial ulcers.

Candidias is
White coating or membrane that is easily scraped leaving a raw, erythematous surface.

Kaposi sarcoma
Dark purple to red-brown lesions. Can be flat or raised. Often found on hard palate but also occur on gums. May bleed on contact.

Oral warts
Discrete rough or raised lesions may have characteristic finger-like projections. Generally not painful unless irritated.

Dental caries and abscesses

Oral hairy Leukoplakia
White 'hairy' or fuzzy patches, usually on side or on top of tongue. Does not scrape off with light scraping.

Gingivitis
Swollen, tender, erythematous gums. May bleed on contact.

Apthous ulceration
Shallow painful ulcers with erythematous 'halo'. Occur on mucosal surfaces without immediate underlying bony attachment.

Fig 5.10 Oral complications in HIV.

Causes
- *Mouth*: candidiasis, HSV ulceration, aphthous ulcers, angular cheilitis, HPV disease (warts), oral hairy leucoplakia (EBV). Periodontal disease, gingivitis, necrotizing stomatitis. Kaposi's sarcoma, NHL, TB (See Figure 5.10)
- *Oesophageal*: candidiasis, CMV oesophagitis, HSV, Kaposi's sarcoma, histoplasmosis.
- *Weight loss*: may be due to anorexia, nausea/vomiting, diarrhoea or all of these. Anorexia and nausea are common in advanced HIV disease; possibly related to cytokine production, drug therapy, opportunistic infections, oral or oesophageal pain, malabsorption.
- *Hepatopancreatobiliary*: co-infection with HBV and/or HCV, CMV, EBV hepatitis, HIV-associated cholangiopathy; drugs—ARVs, anti-mycobacterial medication, etc.; Kaposi's sarcoma, NHL, alcohol/illicit drugs. Acalculous cholecystitis. Acute pancreatitis (CMV, cryptococcosis, toxoplasmosis).

- *Diarrhoea*:
  - Parasitic: *Cryptosporidium parvum, Giardia lamblia, Microsporidium, Cystoisospora belli* (previously known as *Isospora belli*), *Entamoeba, Leishmania donovani*.
  - Bacteria: non-typhoidal *Salmonella, Salmonella typhi, Campylobacter, E. coli, Clostridium difficile*, small-bowel overgrowth, *Vibrio parahaemolyticus*, MAI.
  - Viruses: CMV colitis, HIV-associated enteropathy.
  - Other: chronic pancreatitis with malabsorption, drugs (ARVs), malignancy (NHL, colonic carcinoma). Lactose intolerance. HIV-associated enteropathy (See Figure 5.9).
- *Anorectal*: HPV (warts), HSV, gonorrhoea, chlamydia, syphilis, anal carcinoma.

Clinical features
- *Mouth*:
  - Candidiasis: white plaques; can be scraped off to reveal underlying erythematous mucosa, painful.
  - HSV ulcers: painful vesicular lesions, usually on the lips but can spread to the gums and hard palate.
  - Oral hairy leucoplakia—white plaques, adherent and usually non-painful. Does not spread into the oesophagus.
  - Oral Kaposi's sarcoma: bluish-mauve lesion, nodular or flat.
- *Swallowing*: dysphagia is common and almost always caused by candidiasis. Therapeutic trial of antifungals is a reasonable first step. If this is ineffective, then further investigation may be necessary, particularly to exclude malignancy.
- *Weight loss*: usually multifactorial; identify oropharyngeal problems and/or dysphagia, lack of taste leading to poor nutritional intake. Nausea and vomiting are important symptoms; these are common drug side effects. Malabsorptive symptoms include diarrhoea, flatulence, pale or foul smelling stool.
- *Hepatopancreatobiliary*: jaundice, pruritus, right upper quadrant (RUQ) pain, signs of chronic liver disease. Malabsorption. HIV-associated cholangiopathy occurs at low CD4 counts (<100 cells/μL) presents with RUQ pain, fever ± jaundice.
- *Diarrhoea*:
  - Acute: more likely to be bacterial and can be severe with profound dehydration. Can lead to toxic megacolon; severe abdominal pain and distension needs urgent assessment and management.
  - Chronic: often more than one pathogen at CD4 counts <200 cells/μL, consider malabsorption, drug side effects.
- *Anorectal*: common in men who have sex with men; anal warts are generally non-tender growths, perianal pain or discomfort is usually caused by HSV, proctitis presents with pain, tenesmus, mucus and blood, may be due to gonorrhoea or chlamydia. Anal carcinoma is important to exclude, presents with bleeding, tenesmus, palpable mass. Usually originates at the dentate line (epithelial transitional zone) between upper two-thirds and lower-third of the anal canal). Associated with HPV-16 and -18 in a manner similar to cervical cancer.

Investigation

- *Mouth*: examination, biopsy.
- *Upper GI*: OGD, contrast swallow, biopsy.
- *Hepatopancreatobiliary*: blood tests (including LFT and amylase), tissue transglutaminase antibodies, viral serology (Hep A IgM, HBsAg, HBcAb, Hep C antibody, CMV IgM, Epstein–Barr nuclear antigen), faecal fat and elastase. Ultrasound liver.
- *Weight loss*: accurate measurement and documentation of weight is important. Detailed history of nutritional input. Symptoms direct investigation; e.g. swallowing difficulties, diarrhoea. Often cross-sectional imaging necessary if obvious causes are not found.
- *Diarrhoea*: stool and blood culture, stool microscopy for ova, cysts and parasites. *C. difficile* toxin. Faecal fat and elastase.
- *Anorectal*: examination and proctoscopy, microbiological swabs for gonococcus, biopsy.

Management

- *Candidiasis*: fluconazole, itraconazole is an alternative. (➔ See 'Candida spp.', p.321).
- *CMV colitis*: ganciclovir, alternative is foscarnet. (➔ See section on CMV, p.244).
- *Cryptosporidium*: optimize HAART, nitazoxanide (evidence for efficacy in severely immunocompromised individuals is poor). (➔ See 'Cryptosporidum', p.292).
- *Giardiasis*: metronidazole or tinidazole.
- *Amoebiasis*: metronidazole + diloxanide or paromomycin (to eradicate luminal infection). (➔ See 'Entamoeba histolytica', p.296).
- *Cyclosporiasis*: TMP–SMX. (➔ See 'Cyclospora cayetanensis' p.294).
- *C. belli*: TMP–SMX. (➔ See 'Cystoisospora belli', p.295).
- *Strongyloides stercoralis*: ivermectin or albendazole. (➔ See 'Strongyloides stercoralis' p.307)

Genitourinary presentations

As HIV is mainly transmitted sexually, co-infection with other sexually transmitted infections (STIs) is common. The presence of other symptomatic STIs that breach the genital mucosa greatly increases the infectivity of infected individuals as well as the risk of transmission to uninfected individuals. Detection and treatment of concomitant STIs is therefore important in reducing transmissibility. STIs can be asymptomatic therefore all HIV-infected individuals should be screened regardless. Local sensitivities are important in determining treatment.

Urethral discharge and urethritis

- Discharge, burning on urination, irritation of distal urethra.
- Causes: *Chlamydia trachomatis, Neisseria gonorrhoeae*, HSV, *Trichomonas vaginalis, Mycoplasma genitalium, Ureaplasma urealyticum.*
- Diagnosis: microscopy, culture, NAAT.
- Example empiric treatment: ceftriaxone + azithromycin.

Vaginal discharge

- Discharge, odour, pruritus, dysuria.
- Causes: bacterial vaginosis, candidiasis, *Trichomonas vaginalis.*
- Diagnosis: vaginal pH, microscopy.
- Example empiric treatment: metronidazole + fluconazole.

Cervicitis
- Cervical discharge, erythema, contact bleeding, intermenstrual and post-coital bleeding.
- Causes: *C. trachomatis, N. gonorrhoeae. HSV.*
- Diagnosis: microscopy, culture, NAAT, PCR.
- Example empiric treatment: ceftriaxone + azithromycin.

Genital ulcers
- Ulcers may be painful or painless, dysuria, inguinal lymphadenopathy.
- Causes: HSV, chancroid (*Haemophilus ducreyi*) (usually painful), syphilis, LGV (*C. trachomatis* L1–L3), Granuloma inguinale/Donavanosis (*Klebsiella granulomatis*) (usually painless).
- Diagnosis: microscopy, culture, HSV PCR, treponemal specific enzyme immunoassay (EIA), NAAT.
- Example empiric treatment: aciclovir, benzylpenicillin, azithromycin.

Scrotal pain/swelling
- Usually unilateral, may be overlying erythema, discharge, fever.
- Causes: *C. trachomatis, N. gonorrhoeae*, coliforms, mumps orchitis, TB.
- Diagnosis: microscopy, culture, NAAT.
- Example empiric treatment: ceftriaxone + doxycycline.

Pelvic inflammatory disease
- Lower abdominal pain, fever, deep dyspareunia, abnormal menstrual bleeding, cervical motion tenderness.
- Causes: exclude ectopic pregnancy, appendicitis, etc. *N. gonorrhoeae, C. trachomatis*, anaerobic bacteria (e.g. *Bacteroides* spp.).
- Diagnosis: β-human chorionic gonadotropin, microscopy, culture, NAAT.
- Example empiric treatment: ceftriaxone + doxycycline + metronidazole.

Dermatological presentations

Over 90% of patients infected with HIV will have a dermatological presentation at some point during their illness. Dermatological complications of HIV often play an important role in the clinical diagnosis of HIV disease where laboratory testing is difficult to access. With advanced disease, dermatological presentations are often florid and atypical (e.g. multi-dermatomal shingles) (Figure 5.11).

Causes
- *Infection:*
  - Bacterial: *S. aureus* (cellulitis, abscesses, folliculitis, bullous impetigo, ecthyma, hidradenitis, pyomyositis), *Pseudomonas aeroginosa*, bacillary angiomatosis (*B. henselae and B. quintana*), cutaneous mycobacterial disease, syphilis.
  - Fungal: candidiasis, dermatophytosis (tinea), cryptococcosis, histoplasmosis, sporotrichosis, aspergillosis.
  - Viral: molluscum contagiosum, HSV, VZV, oral hairy leucoplakia (EBV), HPV (warts), cytomegalovirus infection. HIV seroconversion.
  - Infestation/parasitic: scabies, acanthamoebiasis, leishmaniasis, strongyloidiasis.

Candida: white plaques, will scrape off leaving raw/bleeding red mucosa. Oral, angular chelitis, vaginal, balanitis, intertrigo. CD4 <300.
Treatment: Nystatin/Fluconazole

Oral hairy leukoplakia: white plaques, adherent to mucosa, will not scape off. EBV related, benign, occurs CD4 <400.
Treatment: Topical podophyllin, aciclovir.

Kaposi's sarcoma: discrete red-mauve-blue-purple patches, bilaterally symmetric lesions. Lower extremity, oral mucosa.
Treatment: Local radiotherapy/intralesional chemotherapy.

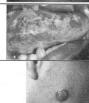

Bacillary angiomatosis (B. henselae and B. quintana): Single or multiple red-purple or colourless papules. Vary in size from 1 mm to >10 mm. Important differential of Kaposi's sarcoma. Treatment: Erythromycin or doxycycline for >3 months.

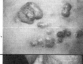

Varicella zoster virus: usually reactivation of latent infection, vesicular/maculopapular eruption, may be mutli-dermatomal, occurs CD4 <250. Treatment: acyclovir, famciclovir

Herpes simplex virus: Vesicular and ulcerative lesions leading to crusting erosions. Usually painful. Common sites are the lips, gums, tongue and genitals. Treatment: Aciclovir

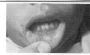

Primary HIV (seroconversion): usually 2–4 weeks post initial infection, widespread, non pruritic morbilliform rash, usually fades within 1–2 weeks.

Molluscum contagiosum: single or multiple pearly-white dome-shaped papules. Often involves the face (eyelids) or groin with >CD4, becomes extensive and sometimes overwhelming once CD4 <50.
Treatment: lance lesions, cryotherapy.

Syphilis: Primary disease; open sore or ulcer (chancre), painless. Common sites are genitals, mouth, rectum.
Secondary disease; maculopapular rash, usually on the palms of the hands and soles of the feet.
Treatment: Benzylpenicillin

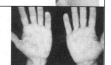

Fig 5.11 Important dermatological conditions in HIV. Reproduced courtesy of Susanne Theresia Dürr, MD, University of Regensburg, Germany; Deborah Greenspan, DSC, BDS, University of California San Francisco; Toby A. Maurer, MD, University of California, San Francisco; Paul A. Volberding, MD, University of California San Francisco; and Arthur Ammann, MD, Global Strategies for HIV Prevention. Available at: ℘ https://www.hiv.va.gov/provider/image-library/.

- *Malignancy*: Kaposi's sarcoma, NHL, basal cell carcinoma, melanoma.
- *Autoimmunity/inflammatory*: psoriasis, reactive arthritis (Reiter's syndrome), pityriasis rosea, seborrhoeic dermatitis, bullous pemphigoid, xerosis, ichthyosis, vasculitis, pyoderma gangrenosum.
- *Medication related*: abacavir-related hypersensitivity; Stevens–Johnson syndrome, toxic epidermal necrolysis.
- *Other*: manifestations of nutritional deficiency.

Patterns of disease
- *Maculopapular rash*: acute HIV seroconversion illness, drug reactions (particularly NNRTIs), VZV, EBV, secondary syphilis, pityriasis rosea, viral exanthem.
- *Erythroderma* (involving >90% skin): drug reaction, psoriasis, scabies
- *Ulcer*: HSV, VZV, EBV, CMV, mycobacteria, leishmaniasis, aphthous ulcer, BCC, melanoma, primary syphilis, chancroid (*H. ducreyi*), LGV, Donovanosis (*K. granulomatis*), deep fungal infection.
- *Pruritus*: folliculitis, dermatophytosis, scabies, xerosis, ichthyosis, prurigo nodularis, atopic dermatitis, seborrheic dermatitis, eczema, psoriasis, eosinophilic folliculitis, drug reactions, liver failure, renal failure, systemic lymphoma, idiopathic HIV-pruritus.
- *Vesicles/blistering*: HSV, VZV, molluscum contagiosum, bullous impetigo, Stevens–Johnson syndrome, toxic epidermal necrolysis.

Ophthalmological presentations

Up to 70% of patients living with HIV will have some form of ocular involvement during the course of their illness. All aspects of the eye can be affected. Accessibility of the eye to examination allows for clinical diagnosis of HIV and gives information about the degree of immunosuppression in the absence of timely laboratory testing. Patients with a CD4 count <200 cells/μL need detailed retinal examination (Figure 5.12).

Adnexa and anterior segment
Corneal infection (HSV, VZV, bacterial, fungal and protozoal infection. Kaposi sarcoma involves the eyelids and conjunctiva in 20% of HIV-associated cases. Anterior uveitis can occur.

Posterior segment including retina
The major opportunistic pathogens that involve the retina are CMV and toxoplasma. VZV and HSV also cause retinitis. Immune reconstitution is an important cause of sight-threatening retinitis.

HIV retinopathy is a non-infectious microvascular complication with retinal findings not dissimilar to chronic systemic hypertension. Increasingly common with progressive immunosuppression (~70% with advanced HIV disease). (➔ See 'Cytomegalovirus (CMV/ HHV- 5)', p.244).

CMV retinitis occurs at a CD4 count <50 cells/μL, patients with CD4 count <100 cells/μL are very unlikely to have CMV retinitis. Progressive invasion of retinal cells results in retinal haemorrhage and necrosis that characteristically follows the vascular arcades. Retinal detachment can occur (flashes). Presentation depends on site of retinal involvement; can present as blurred vision, blind spots, floaters as well as with sudden decrease in vision. Usually presents in one eye first with both eyes found to be affected

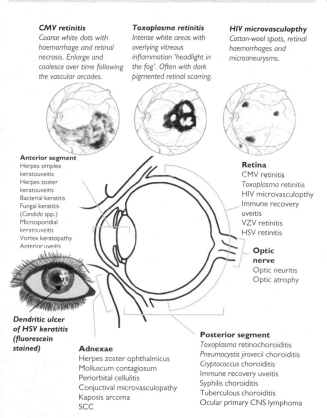

CMV retinitis
Coarse white dots with haemorrhage and retinal necrosis. Enlarge and coalesce over time following the vascular arcades.

Toxoplasma retinitis
Intense white areas with overlying vitreous inflammation 'headlight in the fog'. Often with dark pigmented retinal scarring.

HIV microvasculopthy
Cotton-wool spots, retinal haemorrhages and microaneurysms.

Anterior segment
Herpes simplex keratouveitis
Herpes zoster keratouveitis
Bacterial keratitis
Fungal keratitis (Candida spp.)
Microsporidial keratouveitis
Vortex keratopathy
Anterior uveitis

Retina
CMV retinitis
Toxoplasma retinitis
HIV microvasculopthy
Immune recovery uveitis
VZV retinitis
HSV retinitis

Optic nerve
Optic neuritis
Optic atrophy

Dendritic ulcer of HSV keratitis (fluorescein stained)

Adnexae
Herpes zoster ophthalmicus
Molluscum contagiosum
Periorbital cellulitis
Conjuctival microvasculopathy
Kaposis arcoma
SCC

Posterior segment
Toxoplasma retinochoroiditis
Pneumocystis jirovecii choroiditis
Cryptococcus choroiditis
Immune recovery uveitis
Syphilis choroiditis
Tuberculous choroiditis
Ocular primary CNS lymphoma

Fig 5.12 Ophthalmic manifestations of HIV.

in up to 50% of patients. Treatment is with systemic anti-CMV treatment (e.g. valganciclovir), which provides prophylaxis to the asymptomatic eye. Disease threatening the macula may require intravitreal treatment. Retinal screening is recommended 3-monthly while CD4 count <50 cells/µL. (➲ See 'Cytomegalovirus (CMV/ HHV-5)', p.244).

Toxoplasma retinochoroiditis
Causes a necrotizing retinitis with overlying vitreous inflammation ('headlight in the fog'). Occurs when CD4 count <200 cells/µL. Presents typically with unilateral impaired or blurred vision, floaters. Treated in the same way as CNS disease with systemic anti-toxoplasma therapy (TMP–SMX). (➲ Also See 'Toxoplasma gondii', p.289).

HSV/VZV retinitis
Usually reactivation of latent infection. Causes rapidly progressive retinal necrosis. In the immunocompetent, a vigorous immune response causes acute retinal necrosis (ARN) whereas with significant immune suppression (CD4 count <100 cells/μL) there is less inflammation and therefore a more silent presentation termed progressive outer retinal necrosis (PORN). Treatment is with systemic antivirals (aciclovir or valaciclovir). (➔ See section on HSV/VZV in p.256,258)

Haematological presentations

All cell lines can be potentially affected in HIV disease. The prevalence of haematological abnormality increases with increasing immunosuppression. Progressive impairment of immune surveillance makes haematological malignancy increasingly prevalent with advanced disease.

Red cell disorders
Anaemia is common (~70% with CDC-defined AIDS are anaemic) largely caused by decreased haemopoiesis; due to HIV infection alone or opportunistic infections (e.g. parvovirus B19, MTB, MAI, PCP), ARV or antimicrobial medication (e.g. zidovudine, TMP–SMX, ganciclovir, dapsone), malignancy (NHL). Assess iron stores (serum iron, total iron-binding capacity, and ferritin), vitamin B12, folate, TSH and reticulocyte count. Consider haemoglobinopathies in appropriate ethnic backgrounds (sickle cell, thalassemia traits, G6PD deficiency, hereditary spherocytosis). Further tests may include investigation for haemolysis (lactate dehydrogenase, haptoglobins, serum bilirubin, antiglobulin (Coombs) test, blood film), review of patient medications (NB methaemoglobinaemia), bone marrow examination.

White cell disorders
Lymphopenia due to CD4+ cell destruction is a common finding. Granulocytopenia and granulocyte dysfunction is also common and appears to mirror CD4 decline. Opportunistic infection (e.g. parvovirus B19, MTB, MAI) may contribute to marrow dysfunction. Drug-induced neutropenia (particularly zidovudine) is an important cause to consider. Bone marrow examination may be necessary if cause is unclear. Granulocyte colony stimulating factors may be of benefit in certain circumstances. Lymphoma (NHL and Hodgkin lymphoma) need always be considered in HIV. (➔ See 'HIV-associated malignancy' p.93.)

Platelet disorders
Thrombocytopenia is present in ~40% of untreated patients; the risk increases with degree of immunosuppression. The mechanism is thought to be immune-mediated platelet destruction due to immune dysregulation. In addition, bone marrow suppression may contribute to ineffective platelet production. Introduction of effective ARV treatment may be sufficient to restore normal platelet function. Otherwise treatment is similar to the treatment of ITP in non-HIV-infected individuals; corticosteroids and/or IV immunoglobulin may be necessary.

Coagulation disorders
HIV infection confers a significant independent risk factor for thrombosis. There is also an increased frequency of anti-phospholipid antibodies and proteins S and C dysfunction/deficiency.

Cardiovascular presentations

As prognosis of HIV infection and management of opportunistic infections improves, cardiovascular complications are becoming more important (particularly in the economically developed world). The inflammatory state associated with HIV infection, even if controlled by ARV medication, is a potent risk factor for accelerated atherosclerosis (incidence of myocardial infarction 1.5× age- and sex-matched controls).

Causes
- Coronary artery disease: accelerated atherosclerosis.
- Valvular disease: endocarditis; *S. aureus* most common organism, usually related to risk activities such as IV drug using.
- Myocardial disease: myocarditis (HIV, Coxsackie B viruses, CMV), HIV-associated cardiomyopathy. Medication-related cardiotoxicity (e.g. zidovudine).
- Rhythm disorders: prolonged QT due to medication (PIs, e.g. saquinavir, atazanavir).
- Pericardial: most important cause of cardiac disease in resource-limited settings, vast majority are due to *M. tuberculosis* (>90%) and present with a pericardial effusion. Other causes include NTM, *S. aureus*, *S. pneumoniae*, *Nocardia*, *Cryptococcus*, *Aspergillus*, NHL, and Kaposi's sarcoma.
- Primary pulmonary hypertension and venous thromboembolic disease both occur at higher frequency in the HIV-positive population.

Clinical features
Heart disease in HIV largely presents in the same way as heart disease in the non-HIV population. Pericardial disease usually presents as an effusion that may progress to tamponade; breathlessness, pleuritic chest pain, pericardial friction rub, fever. Beck's triad (tamponade) hypotension, engorged neck veins, and distant heart sounds.

Investigation
In general, carried out in a manner similar to cardiac disease in the non-HIV population (ECG, blood tests including troponins, echocardiography). Ischaemic heart disease should be investigated in the normal manner with dynamic testing (exercise test, stress echo, myocardial perfusion scanning) ± coronary angiography. Right heart catheterization may be necessary for measuring pulmonary artery pressures.

Management
Similar to the non-HIV population. Once pericardial disease has become symptomatic, it is likely to require drainage of the pericardium (pericardiocentesis).

Renal presentations

HIV-associated renal disease is becoming more apparent with improved prognosis. HIV is also an important risk factor for acute kidney injury as concomitant illness can result in pre-renal states.

The majority of renal disease in HIV is caused by pre-renal acute kidney injury precipitated by hypovolaemia and poor renal perfusion. This may be exacerbated by the concomitant use of nephrotoxic drugs.

- *Drug-induced nephrotoxicity*: ARVs—tenofovir (NtRTI), indinavir and atazanavir (PIs).
- *Drugs used to treat opportunistic infection*: aciclovir, foscarnet, trimethoprim (TMP–SMX), co-trimoxazole, pentamidine, amphotericin, itraconazole.
- *HIV-associated nephropathy (HIVAN)*: a glomerular condition causing focal segmental glomerulosclerosis (FSGS) causing rapidly progressive renal failure. Presents with nephrotic-range proteinuria, uraemia, normal blood pressure, normal/large-sized kidneys. The majority of patients have a CD4 count <200 cells/μL.
- *HIV-associated immune complex kidney disease (HIVICK)*: basement membrane reaction possibly due to of circulating immune complexes.
- *Co-infection*: hepatitis C can cause a membranoproliferative glomerulonephritis (MPGN) both on its own and in combination with HIV.

Management
- *Acute*: key priorities are maintaining adequate renal perfusion and treatment of hypovolaemia, excluding renal or bladder outflow obstruction, withholding nephrotoxic drugs, and dose adjustment of renally cleared drugs
- *Chronic*: optimizing ARV and concomitant opportunistic infection treatment, angiotensin-converting enzyme inhibition, renal replacement therapy.

Endocrine and metabolic presentations

As the prognosis of HIV disease due to ARV therapy approves, metabolic complications have become an increasingly important problem. At the same time, advanced immunosuppression and opportunistic infection causes significant endocrine and metabolic dysfunction. HIV infection and treatment leads to a significantly higher risk of diabetes and dyslipidaemia, contributing to a greatly elevated cardiovascular risk. HIV-associated lipodystrophy occurs as a result of ARV medications (particularly PIs and thymidine analogue NRTIs). Bone metabolism is strongly affected by dysfunctional immune regulation leading to defective skeletal renewal and bone loss. The result is osteopenia and eventually osteoporosis and fragility fractures.

Additional important aspects of HIV management

Monitoring the well-controlled patient

Non-infective disease and problems related to drug treatment form the main emphasis in this group. Chronic HIV infection is an inflammatory state and a significant risk factor for coronary artery disease. Long-term treatment with ARV drugs can result in dyslipidaemia, hepatic dysfunction, and the development of type 2 diabetes mellitus. Pharmacists and support workers form an important part of the therapeutic team.

Routine care involves the following considerations
- *Psychosocial issues*: depression is common; relationship and sexual issues are a common cause of psychological distress.
- *Education*: understanding of disease, transmission, treatment, etc.
- *Medication*: check drug adherence and tolerability/side effects.
- *Non-infectious comorbidities*: e.g. diabetes, cardiovascular disease.
- *Co-infection*: screen on initial presentation for hepatitis B, hepatitis C, and syphilis. Determine immunological status of toxoplasma, CMV, EBV, and VZV. STD screening.
- *Vaccination and prophylaxis*: see 'immunization and prophylaxis' (next section).
- *Screening*: cervical cytology, diabetes, cardiovascular and bone fragility risk assessment.
- *HIV specific*: HLA-B*57:01, viral tropism.
- *Routine blood tests* (full blood count, urea and electrolytes, LFTs, lipids, fasting glucose) should be monitored. Other blood tests may need monitoring depending on drug regimen (creatine kinase and plasma lactate).
- Urinalysis including urine protein: creatinine ratio.
- *Viral monitoring*: viral load (usually 6–12 monthly in stable patients), CD4 count (usually 12 monthly in stable patients).

Immunization and prophylaxis

Vaccination is important in HIV and should include routinely offered vaccines. Response to vaccination may be inadequate or suboptimal; altered schedules may be necessary. In addition to the routine vaccinations, hepatitis B virus, pneumococcal and influenza vaccination should be carried out. Live (replicating) vaccines may pose a risk and are contraindicated at CD4 counts <200 cells/μL (e.g. varicella, measles, mumps, and rubella (MMR)). These may be used following restoration of immune function. BCG and live attenuated typhoid vaccine are contraindicated in HIV.

Chemotherapeutic prophylaxis is recommended for:
- *Toxoplasma* (if positive serology) and PCP at CD4 count <200 cells/μL with TMP–SMX (prophylaxis dose). This may be offered at a higher CD4 count if there are other markers of immunosuppression (e.g. oral candidiasis).
- MAI at CD4 count <50 cells/μL: azithromycin once weekly.
- CMV and cryptococcal prophylaxis are not routinely recommended.

HIV in pregnancy and children

Pregnancy

Individuals diagnosed with HIV infection in pregnancy should be started on ARV therapy as soon as practicable (regardless of CD4 count). Patients who conceive while on ARVs should continue their treatment regimen. Opportunistic infections should be diagnosed and treated in a manner similar to the non-pregnant population (although some drug regimens may be avoided/altered). These patients should be managed by an obstetric unit with experience of HIV.

Mother-to-child transmission

Vertical transmission can occur during pregnancy (*in utero*), during labour and delivery, and from breastfeeding. The use of ARVs can significantly reduce (but not eliminate) the risk. Ideally, all women diagnosed in pregnancy should be established on full ARV treatment to be continued for life. In parts of the world where this is not possible, ARV therapy may be used briefly in order to reduce the risk of mother-to-child transmission. The choice of mode of delivery depends on the degree of maternal viral suppression. If the viral load is undetectable (at 36 weeks) then vaginal birth is recommended. If there is detectable viral load or if the delivery occurs in an emergency, then a caesarean section is recommended. Where possible (available clean water etc.), baby formula feed is recommended in preference to breastfeeding to reduce the risk of transmission by this route. In parts of the world where this is not possible, exclusive breastfeeding is encouraged along with prophylactic ARV therapy for the baby while breastfeeding.

HIV in children

Largely because of vertical transmission, there are 2.6 million children living with HIV (in 2015), mostly in sub-Saharan Africa. Significant reductions in vertical transmission have been achieved, however, by measures to avoid mother-to-child transmission. Presentation is usually with failure to thrive, growth failure, and developmental delay along with recurrent and/or unusual infections. The World Health Organization now recommends that ARV treatment should be started as soon as possible following diagnosis and should be offered lifelong, regardless of CD4 count.

Tuberculosis in the HIV-infected patient

Anywhere between 50% and 80% of patients with active TB in sub-Saharan Africa are also infected with HIV. TB is the most common cause of death in HIV-infected individuals globally. The central role of T-cell-mediated immunity in host defence against TB makes HIV infected individuals particularly vulnerable to a relapse of previous infection or active disease following a new infection. HIV-infected individuals are at significantly increased risk of developing active TB, and the disease process is greatly accelerated. The risk increases with declining CD4 count, but active TB can occur at any CD4 count. Patients with a normal CD4 count remain at increased risk of TB, compared to the non-HIV-infected population. Previous BCG vaccination is not protective. (➲ See Mycobacterium tuberculosis complex (MTBC), p.337).

Clinical features

Presentation is significantly affected by the degree of immunosuppression; patients with ↑/↔ CD4 counts present like the non-HIV infected population while presentation at ↓CD4 counts is often atypical.

- *Pulmonary*: fever, cough, lymphadenopathy, and weight loss. Cavitation is a result of immune response to TB; therefore, becomes less common with declining CD4 count. With ↓CD4 count, may present with much less localized pulmonary disease and widespread pulmonary infiltrates. May mimic bacterial pneumonia. Haemoptysis less likely due to lack cavitation.
- *Extrapulmonary*: more common in HIV disease (up to 50% co-infections), the risk increases with ↓CD4 count. Can progress to overwhelming disseminated infection. Common sites include lymph nodes (lymphadenitis, cervical lymphadenitis = 'the King's scrofula'), CNS (meningitis, space-occupying lesion), GI tract (ascites, chronic diarrhoea 'tuberculous enteritis'), urinary tract ('sterile' pyuria), cardiovascular system (pericarditis), pleural space (pleural effusion), adrenal glands (Addisonian syndrome), and skeletal system (joints; tuberculous arthritis, spinal TB; 'Pott's disease of the spine', tuberculous osteomyelitis).
- *TB-IRIS*: TB is particularly associated with IRIS following the initiation of HAART. (→ See 'Immune reconstitution inflammatory syndrome (IRIS)' p.93.)

Diagnosis

Sputum or histological sample for direct microscopy and culture is always preferable. Sputum microscopy is less sensitive in HIV. BAL may be necessary to obtain diagnostic samples. Urine/synovial fluid/pleural fluid/peritoneal fluid as appropriate.

Tuberculin skin testing is not reliable due to defective cell-mediated response. Nucleic acid amplification techniques (Xpert® MTB/RIF). IGRAs are sensitive but not specific. Chest X-ray is almost always helpful, but rarely definitive. CT is far more sensitive.

Treatment

HIV/TB co-infection presents particular management challenge. In the absence of multidrug-resistant (MDR)/extensively drug-resistant (XDR) TB, regimens are the same as for HIV-negative individuals. Sensitive TB is treated with quadruple therapy (rifampicin, isoniazid, pyrazinamide, and ethambutol) + pyridoxine. The initial 2 months is with four drugs (induction phase), followed by two drugs, isoniazid and rifampicin (continuation phase). Treatment duration for pulmonary and extrapulmonary disease (with the exception of CNS disease) is for 6 months. Treatment of CNS disease is for a total of 12 months (with a 10-month continuation phase). → See 'Mycobacterium tuberculosis complex (MTBC)' p.337.

Anti-TB drugs can interact with ARVs, rifampicin in particular is a powerful enzyme inducer (cytochrome P450), and can significantly alter the metabolism of other drugs. In general, NRTIs/NtRTIs do not have major interactions, NNRTIs (e.g. efavirenz) and PIs (e.g. lopinavir, saquinavir) may result in toxicity, and require dose adjustments and/or drug monitoring.

MDR/XDR TB

MDR TB: resistance to at least two anti-tubercular drugs (usually isoniazid and rifampicin), estimated 5% of TB cases worldwide.

XDR TB is MDR TB + resistance to fluoroquinolones and one of capreomycin, kanamycin or amikacin. Represents ~10% of MDR TB cases. Risk factors for MDR/XDR TB include previous TB treatment, poor compliance, contact with MDR/XDR TB, coming from a high prevalence region (Eastern Europe/former Soviet Union, India, South Africa, and China).

Viral hepatitis in the HIV-infected patient

Viral hepatitis, principally HBV and HCV, are common co-pathogens in HIV due to shared routes of transmission. In addition, the prevalence of HBV and HCV is highest in regions of the world with the highest prevalence of HIV (sub-Saharan Africa and Asia) where co-infection rates can approach 20–30%. Chronic liver disease and liver failure in these populations is a significant cause of death in co-infected patients. There is also an increased risk of hepatotoxicity of HAART. Consider acute viral hepatitis (hepatitis A, hepatitis E) in acute worsening of LFTs. All patients should be encouraged to moderate or abstain from alcohol.

Hepatitis B

HBV complicates ~10% of HIV infections worldwide. Risk higher in sub-Saharan Africa, men who have sex with men, and IV drug users.

Almost all aspects of HBV disease are exacerbated by HIV infection. HBV DNA levels are higher than in HBV infection alone and there is a significantly increased risk of liver cirrhosis and liver failure. HIV-infected adults who are challenged with HBV infection are less likely to spontaneously clear the virus. Risk of hepatocellular carcinoma likely to be higher. There is an increased risk of drug-induced liver injury; close monitoring is required while using ARV and anti-tuberculous drugs. Test for hepatitis D infection (defective virus that requires HBV to replicate) as prognosis is worse with HDV.

Patients infected with HIV and HBV should be treated for both viruses, regardless of CD4 count. ARV regimens should contain agents active against HBV. Usually the anti-HBV component will be tenofovir (either alone or in combination with lamivudine or emtricitabine). Vaccinate against hepatitis A.

Hepatitis C

Particularly common in IV drug users due to shared transmission route, therefore proportion of patients with HIV co-infected with HCV is higher in North America and Europe. Progression to fibrosis and liver failure is accelerated, and are likely at higher risk of development of hepatocellular carcinoma. HIV-positive patients who are infected with HCV are less likely to clear the infection spontaneously. It is not clear how HCV infection affects the progression of HIV disease.

Patients co-infected with HIV/HCV should be treated with HAART, regardless of CD4 count. Treatment for HCV may be delayed until established on HAART. Treatment regimen for HCV is the same as for HCV mono-infection, i.e. direct-acting antiviral combination depending on genotype.

Immune reconstitution inflammatory syndrome (IRIS)

With the restitution of immune function brought about by HAART, a paradoxical clinical deterioration can occur. This is thought to be due to an antigen-specific T-cell-mediated inflammatory reaction to pre-existing antigens that have hitherto escaped the attentions of a depleted immune system. Can occur days to months after starting HAART, but usually in the first 1–2 months. Occurs in anything from 10% to 30% of patients starting HAART. Most common opportunistic infections involved: TB, *Cryptococcus*, MAI, HSV, VZV, and CMV. TB is the most important. There is no firm definition of IRIS; loosely:

- Follows the initiation, reintroduction or alteration of HAART + usually accompanied by an increase in CD4 cell count and/or a rapid decrease in viral load and/or clinical improvement (e.g. ↑ weight).
- *Plus* symptomatic worsening of known conditions (e.g. pulmonary TB) and/or development of new presentations (e.g. cryptococcal meningitis) hitherto clinically undetected. Characterized by an exaggerated inflammatory response. This may also involve worsening of HIV-associated malignancy (e.g. Kaposi's sarcoma) and/or presentation of autoimmune conditions (e.g. Graves' disease).
- *HIV/TB co-infection*: decision as to when to start HAART/anti-TB treatment is complicated by lack of definitive evidence. Current British HIV Association (BHIVA) recommendations:
  - CD4 count <100 cells/μL start HAART as soon as practicable.
  - CD4 count of 100–350 cells/μL start as soon as practicable, but can wait until after completing 2 months of TB treatment, especially when there are difficulties with drug interactions, adherence and toxicities.
  - CD4 count >350 cells/μL at physician's discretion.

Presentations
- Neurological: altered mental state, meningitic symptoms.
- Respiratory: breathlessness, wheeze, cough.
- Systemic: fever, lymphadenopathy, sepsis/systemic inflammatory response.
- Other: hepatitis, folliculitis, visual deterioration, autoimmunity.

Treatment
- Do not stop HAART unless absolutely necessary.
- Symptomatic (e.g. non-steroidal anti-inflammatory drugs), corticosteroids.
- Specific treatment of opportunistic infections.

HIV-associated malignancy

As well as providing protection from pathogens, an important function of the immune system is to recognize and destroy neoplastic cells: immune surveillance. Progressive immunodeficiency depletes the ability of the immune system to fulfil this role. In addition, several viruses (oncoviruses) have been shown to promote the development of cancer by interfering with host cell replicative machinery. The combination of these two factors makes malignancy a common occurrence in HIV disease. With HAART, the proportion of all HIV-related deaths attributable to cancer has risen to 25–30%. HIV infection is particularly associated with four malignancies (AIDS defining): Kaposi's sarcoma, intermediate or high-grade B-cell NHL, primary CNS lymphoma, and invasive cervical cancer. In addition, HIV infection substantially increases the risk of Hodgkin lymphoma, and anal, liver, and lung cancer.

Kaposi's sarcoma

Most common HIV-related malignancy; sarcoma of vascular origin, associated with HHV-8. Variable clinical course; often indolent but can be very aggressive. Most commonly a cutaneous presentation with reddish–mauve–black lesions usually affecting face, mouth, ears, genitals, or lower legs (including soles of feet). Appear as 'bruise-like" macules early in disease. May progress to papules or nodules and ulcerate. Biopsy all suspicious lesions. Visceral disease classically affects the lungs and/or GI tract.

Treatment: HAART + local radiotherapy or intralesional vinblastine for early stage, advanced stage treated with HAART plus chemotherapy (first line: liposomal anthracyclines; second line: paclitaxel).

Non-Hodgkin lymphoma

Second most common HIV-related malignancy; strongly associated with EBV infection. Two most frequent subtypes are diffuse large B cell lymphoma (DLBCL) and Burkitt's lymphoma. Present with widespread disease (may involve GI tract, CNS, bone marrow, liver, lungs) and usually at CD4 counts <100 cells/μL. 'B' symptoms (weight loss, night sweats, fatigue etc.) common. Should be diagnosed histologically. High risk of CNS disease (especially Burkitt's lymphoma).

Treatment: HAART + usually require systemic combination chemotherapy e.g. R-CHOP (rituximab + cyclophosphamide, doxorubicin, vincristine, prednisolone). CNS involvement requires intrathecal chemotherapy (methotrexate + cytarabine). Prophylactic intrathecal chemotherapy should be offered to patients with high risk of CNS involvement or with Burkitt's lymphoma.

Primary CNS lymphoma

Almost all associated with EBV infection. Usually present at CD4 counts <50 cells/μL. Assess for ocular involvement. Carries a poor prognosis; median survival 2–4 months from diagnosis.

Treatment: HAART + whole brain radiotherapy + corticosteroids.

Cervical cancer

Closely associated with HPV, particularly HPV-16 and HPV-18. Risk of cervical at least five times higher in HIV infection. HIV-positive women should be screened 6–12-monthly. Treated with excision/surgery ± chemotherapy/radiotherapy.

Hodgkin lymphoma

Tenfold increase in risk in HIV infection. Strongly associated with EBV infection. Appears to be more common in patients where transmission of HIV has been by IV drug use. Treated with HAART + combination chemotherapy (e.g. R-CHOP).

Anal cancer

Patients infected with HIV are 25 times more likely to develop anal cancer; particularly men who have sex with men. Associated with HPV in a manner similar to cervical cancer. Treated with HAART ± resection ± chemoradiotherapy.

Hepatic cancer

HIV infection alone confers a five times higher risk, co-infection with hepatitis B or C greatly increases this risk as these viruses are powerful risk factors for hepatic cancers. Treated with surgery and percutaneous ablative therapies.

Lung cancer

Three times higher risk in HIV infection, particularly if combined with smoking cigarettes. Treatment as per non-HIV population.

Acknowledgement

This chapter was kindly reviewed by Dr Nicola Jones, Consultant in Infectious Diseases, Oxford University Hospitals NHS Foundation Trust.

Further reading

1. Current guidelines on all aspects of HIV are available online. British HIV Association (BHIVA) and British Infection Association (BIA): ℘ http://www.bhiva.org/Guidelines.aspx and Infectious Diseases Society of America (IDSA): ℘ http://www.idsociety.org/PracticeGuidelines/

Neutropenic sepsis in patients with leukaemia, lymphoma, and solid organ tumours

Introduction

Leukaemias, lymphomas, and solid organ tumours represent a widely diverse range of cancers. Until recently, the general approach to treating them was to administer cytotoxic anticancer drugs that damage proliferating cells by interfering with mitosis and cellular replication. A major disadvantage of this approach is the lack of specificity of cytotoxic drugs—they destroy actively dividing normal cells as well as malignant cells. As a result, achieving maximum tumour killing using high doses of these agents is often offset or prevented by collateral damage to normal tissues. Two common adverse effects are profound neutropenia, due to disruption of haematopoiesis in the bone marrow, and mucositis, resulting from injury to the GI mucosal barrier. Mucositis potentiates the translocation of normal and colonizing GI flora into the bloodstream. In the setting of neutropenia, where there is a paucity of effector cells to contain serious infections, bacteraemia may cause severe morbidity and mortality. *Chemotherapy-related neutropenia is defined as an absolute neutrophil count of <0.5 × 10⁹ cells/L.* It is considered the single most significant risk factor for the development of invasive bacterial and fungal infections in the patient undergoing treatment for cancer. The degree of infection risk depends on:

1. *The depth of neutropenia*: risk of infection is inversely related to absolute neutrophil count: if $<0.1 \times 10^9$ cells/L, infection is very common; if $>1 \times 10^9$ cells/L, there is little added risk of infection.
2. *The duration of neutropenia*: neutropenic periods lasting several weeks may be seen with induction therapy for AML, and they are associated with increased risk for bacterial bloodstream infections and pneumonias as well as invasive mould infections (e.g. aspergillosis and mucormycosis). Mould infections typically occur when neutropenia lasts for 14 days or more. Treatment of solid tumour or lymphomas is generally associated with a briefer neutropenic period, lasting from a few days to a week, depending on the type and dose of cytotoxic chemotherapy, and severe infections are less common than during treatment of AML.

Neutropenia occurs most frequently because of cytotoxic chemotherapy but it is also seen in patients with haematological malignancy, HIV infection, or bone marrow infiltration by malignant disease. Several forms of congenital neutropenia also occur which may or may not result in serious infections.

Neutropenic sepsis definition (NICE guidelines)

Neutropenic sepsis = neutropenia ($<0.5 \times 10^9$/L (500/cm^3) *plus* fever $>38°$C *or* other signs or symptoms consistent with clinically significant sepsis.

Studies link these parameters to the risk of serious infection, mortality, and intensive therapy unit admission, but the evidence is low quality. There is a single study showing a high negative predictive value for bacteraemia when the neutrophil count is >0.5 10^9/L. Raising the temperature threshold above $38°$C reduces the negative predictive value. Caveats are that sepsis can present with hypothermia or normothermia and it is therefore important to diagnose neutropenic sepsis in patients receiving anti-cancer treatment whose neutrophil count is $\leq0.5 \times 10^9$/L and who have symptoms or signs suggestive of significant infection regardless of temperature.

Spectrum of infections

Before the 1960s, infections were predominantly due to Gram-negative organisms. The 1970–1990s saw a higher prevalence of Gram-positive infections, including coagulase-negative staphylococci, followed by the emergence of fungi. The year 2000 onwards has seen an increasing number of resistant Gram-negative organisms, including extended-spectrum beta-lactamase (ESBL)-producing coliforms and, more recently, carbapenemase-producing Enterobacteriaceae (CPE).

Attributable mortality ranges from zero to >40%. It is particularly high in infections due to *Candida* species, *Pseudomonas*, and multi-resistant Enterobacteriaceae. Immunocompromised patients are more likely to have received antibiotics and are more likely to acquire resistant organisms. Only 25–30% of fevers have microbial documentation. Infection may progress rapidly; there is often no time to wait for culture results and robust treatment protocols are necessary (Table 6.1).

Table 6.1 Infectious aetiologies by site of involvement in neutropenic sepsis

	Common	Less common
Skin/soft tissue/ line	*Staphylococcus aureus*, coagulase-negative staphylococci, HSV, *Candida* spp.	*Pseudomonas aeruginosa*, *Acinetobacter* spp., *Serratia* spp., *Corynebacterium* spp., *Bacillus* spp., *Capnocytophaga* spp., atypical mycobacteria, mucormycosis, *Fusarium* spp., *Trichosporon* spp.
Central nervous system	Streptococci, *Listeria*, herpes viruses including CMV, *Mycobacterium tuberculosis*, *Aspergillus* spp.	Gram negatives, atypical mycobacteria, *Nocardia asteroides*, VZV, mucormycosis
Respiratory tract	Streptococci, *S. aureus*, *Legionella* spp., *Mycoplasma* spp., CMV, influenza, parainfluenza, rhinovirus	*Candida* spp., *Aspergillus* spp., *P. aeruginosa*
Cardiac (endocarditis)	Staphylococci, streptococci, enterococci	Gram negatives including *Pseudomonas* spp., HACEK, fungi, mycobacteria
Gastrointestinal tract	Enterococci, *Escherichia coli*, *Klebsiella* spp., *Clostridium difficile*	*Clostridium septicum*, *Bacteroides* spp.
Genitourinary tract	*E. coli*, *Klebsiella* spp., *P. aeruginosa*	*Candida* spp., *Aspergillus* spp.

Clinical and investigative approach

If possible, the approach to treatment should be targeted rather than empiric; however, this is rarely possible. The aim should be to 'start smart and then focus'. Blood cultures plus cultures from any potentially involved clinical site should be taken before starting antibiotics.

Common sites for focal infection include IV lines, the oral cavity, the lungs, skin, sinuses, perianal region, GI tract, and urinary tract. When faced with a neutropenic patient with apparent undifferentiated fever, a thorough clinical assessment of all these sites should be performed.

Empirical management

Guidelines from the National Institute for Health and Care Excellence (NICE) recommend monotherapy with piperacillin–tazobactam (Tazocin®) as the initial empiric antibiotic therapy in patients with suspected neutropenic sepsis, unless there are patient-specific or local microbiological contraindications (e.g. significant penicillin allergy or local resistance patterns), or a clear source of infection allowing more targeted therapy. Refer to local guidelines in case of penicillin allergy.

Based on a large meta-analysis, NICE and the European Conference on Infections in Leukemia do not recommend offering an aminoglycoside, either as monotherapy or dual therapy. Despite this, the use of single-dose aminoglycoside (gentamicin) alongside piperacillin–tazobactam (Tazocin®) as empiric therapy remains widespread practice in the United Kingdom. Meta-analysis also shows no benefit for empirical vancomycin or teicoplanin usage unless a resistant Gram-positive organism has been identified. However, many of the included studies predated the emergence of methicillin-resistant *Staphylococcus aureus* (MRSA), and it is important to incorporate screening and surveillance to inform empirical microbial policy. Guidelines recommend not to offer empiric glycopeptide antibiotics to patients with vascular devices *in situ* unless there are patient-specific or local microbiological indications, e.g. MRSA colonization, MRSA outbreaks, or if there is clinical evidence of a line infection.

Guidelines also do *not* recommend removal of central venous devices as part of the initial empiric management of suspected neutropenic sepsis, as the evidence for line removal is weak. A pragmatic approach is required; line removal should be considered in septic patients who do not respond to fluid resuscitation or if signs of tunnel/pocket infection are present. Removal should also be considered if cultured organisms are suggestive that the line is the source of infection, if specific organisms identified are difficult to treat without line removal (e.g. *Candida* spp., *Pseudomonas* spp.) or if treatment options are less effective (e.g. vancomycin-resistant enterococci (VRE), CPE).

Fever and respiratory symptoms

Classical signs of infection such as purulent sputum and focal chest findings may be absent. The pattern of chest X-ray abnormalities may be helpful in formulating a differential diagnosis and deciding on treatment (➜ see Table 8.2, Chapter 8), but often X-ray changes are also absent. It is important to remember that these patients can be very compromised by common viral respiratory infections, in a way that immunocompetent patients are usually not. Consideration of influenza is especially important as this has a specific treatment (although there is no randomized controlled trial evidence) and has infection control implications. In general, the choice of empirical therapy should depend upon the risk for specific infections, whether the presentation is community or hospital acquired, and the local susceptibility patterns. For example, an appropriate empirical regimen for a community-acquired presentation with focal consolidation on X-ray would be piperacillin–tazobactam with clarithromycin (an antipseudomonal penicillin plus a macrolide to cover atypicals).

History
A full history covering preceding upper respiratory tract symptoms or exposure to those with symptoms (e.g. family members) is crucial. Remember to ask about occupational exposures, animals, and travel. Consider the possibility of reactivated infection such as TB or endemic mycoses (e.g. histoplasmosis). ➐ See Chapter 7 for a detailed approach to history-taking.

Examination
This may reveal little but must be thorough and include all systems including the skin and oral mucosa, to maximize the chances of making an accurate diagnosis. For example, skin nodules of cryptococcosis can be a helpful finding when respiratory signs are non-specific and cultures negative.

Investigations
Take a viral throat swab (for multiplex PCR), in addition to urine for *Legionella* antigen. If the patient is non-productive but very unwell with bilateral infiltrates on chest X-ray, have a low threshold for a CT scan and bronchoscopy, especially if antibiotics do not make any improvement within 24–48 hours. Viral (especially CMV) and fungal infections become more likely and more important to exclude. A full viral respiratory panel (including CMV PCR) can be run on BAL fluid as can cultures for fungi and mycobacteria. Consider CMV PCR on a blood EDTA (ethylenediamine tetraacetic acid) and serum cryptococcal antigen (CrAg). Sputum should always be sent for acid-fast bacilli and TB culture if there is any suspicion of TB (indolent history, previous exposure, endemic area, upper lobe X-ray changes, especially if cavitation).

Fever and gastrointestinal symptoms

History and examination
It is important to consider *Clostridium difficile* infection in addition to commoner causes of gastroenteritis (viral/bacterial), as neutropenic patients have often been heavily exposed to antibiotics. Diarrhoea is common in these patients and may also be related to drugs or chemotherapy (details and temporal relation of these must be explored in the history). For this reason, due consideration must be given to the possibility that the fever may be a sign of a separate infective process (dual pathologies in these patients are not uncommon). Details of recent antibiotic therapy and hospitalizations, travel history, and symptomatic contacts must be elicited.

Investigations

Stool for microscopy, culture, and sensitivity; *C. difficile* toxin, ova, cysts and parasites ± viral PCR.

Neutropenic enterocolitis (typhlitis) is a serious complication of neutropenia in which the bowel (usually caecum) becomes ulcerated, oedematous, and necrotic. It is associated with *Clostridium septicum* and *Pseudomonas aeruginosa* bacteraemia and presents with fever, shock, and abdominal pain, usually in the right ilia fossa requiring surgical resection.

Fever and neurological symptoms

History and examination

The history should include any prior neurological symptoms or signs, immunosuppressive agents, other drugs (e.g. analgesics, psychiatric agents, or antimicrobials), and epidemiological exposures. Review of blood tests is crucial to exclude any contributing metabolic disturbance.

A thorough clinical examination, in addition to neurological assessment, should aim to elicit any signs of a possible metastatic infection, e.g. pneumonia, cardiac murmur, sinusitis, or skin lesions. ⮕ See Chapter 7 for a detailed approach.

Investigations

All immunocompromised patients should have blood cultures if presenting with neutropenic fever and CNS signs (e.g. encephalitis/altered Glasgow Coma Scale score/focal neurological signs). Early brain imaging (CT within 24 hours) should be performed if symptoms/signs are not fully explained by non-CNS clinical findings. This should be followed by a lumbar puncture ± MRI where indicated (see proposed algorithm in Figure 6.1). If the patient has signs of sepsis (source unclear) empirical IV antibiotics with CNS cover should be started as soon as blood cultures have been taken (e.g. vancomycin 1 g BD + meropenem 2 g TDS). Any unexplained skin lesions should be biopsied for culture and histopathology.

If there is no explanation for the patient's symptoms/signs on CT, cerebrospinal fluid (CSF), blood cultures, urine cultures, or on multi-systems examination, then a MRI brain scan should be obtained within 24 hours (Figure 6.1).

Fever and evidence of tunnelled line infection (e.g. red exit site, positive line cultures)

Take blood cultures peripherally and from any lines. Treat empirically with a glycopeptide, e.g. vancomycin or teicoplanin—to cover MRSA, methicillin-sensitive *Staphylococcus aureus* (MSSA), and coagulase-negative staphylococci. The best chance of cure lies with line removal but sometimes precious lines can be salvaged in the context of less virulent pathogens (e.g. coagulase-negative staphylococci) where a minimum of 2 weeks of antibiotics are recommended, followed by surveillance blood cultures. Less commonly, line infections can be due to Gram-negative organisms or fungi, where line removal is usually necessary, hence the importance of blood cultures at the outset.

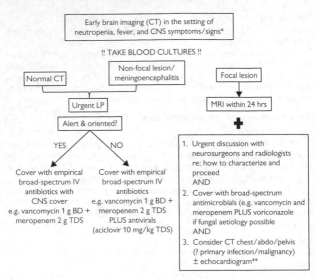

Fig 6.1 Suggested algorithm for investigation of neutropenic fever with CNS symptoms/signs. BD, twice daily; CNS, central nervous system; CT, computed tomography; LP, lumbar puncture; MRI, magnetic resonance imaging; TDS, three times daily.

Fever and cellulitis

If the patient is unwell or febrile, ensure blood cultures are taken prior to starting antibiotics, even if the cellulitis does not appear severe. Refer to local antibiotic guidelines for treatment choice, an example empirical regimen is flucloxacillin (or ceftriaxone if non-severe penicillin allergy, vancomycin/teicoplanin if severe penicillin allergy). Oral options (if the cellulitis is mild with no systemic complications) include flucloxacillin or clindamycin. Watch closely for response to treatment and if limited response or progression on empirical treatment, consider early imaging to exclude complications, such as abscess formation. Less commonly, skin and soft tissue infections can be due to Gram-negative organisms, especially in neutropenic patients who are heavily hospital-exposed. The results of blood cultures may be very useful in such cases.

Fever and positive blood culture

Any source of infection can be accompanied by bacteraemia or this can result primarily by direct translocation of bacteria (commonly aerobic Gram-negative rods) across the barriers between the GI tract and the bloodstream. Treatment should be targeted to the blood culture isolate.

Empirical antifungal treatment

Empirical antifungal treatment has been considered standard of care for years but is not covered in the NICE guidelines and is not supported by any evidence base. More recently its use has been restricted to a targeted or pre-emptive strategy. The incidence of invasive fungal disease remains low in haematological malignancy (<2% incidence of invasive candidiasis, slightly higher incidence of invasive aspergillus of ~0.5–12%). However, symptoms and signs are often very non-specific, diagnostic tools are limited, and infection is associated with considerable morbidity and mortality, a poorer outcome being associated with treatment delays. Table 6.2 aids in the assessment of a patient with regard to their risk of developing an invasive fungal infection. Always consult an infectious diseases specialist or haematologist before starting a patient on empirical antifungal therapy (Table 6.2).

Resolution of fever

This is frequently delayed; 6–8 days in documented Gram-negative infection and 7–12 days in documented Gram-positive infection. 30% of patients will have unresponsive fever at 5 days, and even when 'responding' (e.g. improving parameters including temperature trend, haemodynamic status,

Table 6.2 Risk of invasive fungal infection in neutropenic patients

Low risk	Period of neutropenia <10 days
	Autologous bone marrow or peripheral stem cell transplant treated with growth factors
Medium risk	Corticosteroid therapy
	Period of neutropenia 10–21 days
	Treatment with purine analogues (e.g. fludarabine)
	Severe mucositis
	Chronic pulmonary disease
High risk	Allogeneic bone marrow transplant, especially with prolonged neutropenia, mismatched, or graft-versus-host disease
	Period of neutropenia >21 days
	Bacteraemic during period of neutropenia
	Colonized with Candida tropicalis
	Colonized with Aspergillus spp.
	Fungal infection during previous neutropenic episode

Source: data from Wilks D et al The Infectious Diseases Manual Second Edition Black-well Publishing Oxford UK Copyright © 2003 by Blackwell Science Ltd.

and inflammatory markers), >50% remain pyrexial at 3 days. Patients with persistent fever require daily evaluation and diagnostic workup, bearing in mind 'occult' sites of infection (e.g. the sinuses, teeth, perianal region, and the prostate). However, changes to treatment should depend on clinical status and results; empirical antibiotics should not be switched in patients with purely unresponsive fever, unless there has been a clinical deterioration or a microbiological indication (e.g. positive blood culture not covered by current antimicrobials). Fever remains unexplained in >50% with no clinical or microbiological cause found. When this occurs, possible explanations include occult bacterial infection, viral infection, fungal infection, or febrile mucositis (disruption to the mucosa is very common after cytotoxic therapy, leading to cytokine release and fever).

Prevention and prophylaxis

NICE guidelines recommend that adult patients with acute leukaemia, stem cell transplant, or solid tumours in whom neutropenia is anticipated for >14 days, should all be offered prophylaxis with a quinolone. Meta-analyses and economic analysis show that this strategy reduces short-term mortality and neutropenic sepsis, and that this effect outweighs the potential for antibiotic resistance over such a timeframe. It is the most cost-effective intervention in solid tumour patients (number needed to treat (NNT) to prevent one episode of neutropenic sepsis = 11; NNT to prevent one infection death = 59; NNT to induce additional resistant infection = 77). There are no recommendations for antifungal prophylaxis in neutropenic sepsis, but antifungal prophylaxis is used in certain patient groups (➔ see Chapters 7 and 8 for further information).

Acknowledgement

This chapter was kindly reviewed by Dr Jaimal Kothari, Consultant in Haematology, at Oxford University Hospitals NHS Trust, and by Dr Bhuvan Kishore, Consultant in Haematology, at University Hospitals Birmingham NHS Foundation Trust.

Further reading

1. Apostolopoulou E, Raftopoulos V, Terzis K, Elefsiniotis I. Infection Probability Score, APACHE II and KARNOFSKY scoring systems as predictors of bloodstream infection onset in hematology-oncology patients. BMC Infectious Diseases 2010;10:135.

2. Furno P, Bucaneve G, Del Favero A. Monotherapy or aminoglycoside-containing combinations for empirical antibiotic treatment of febrile neutropenic patients: a meta-analysis. Lancet Infectious Diseases 2002;2(4):231–42.

3. National Institute for Health and Care Excellence (2012). Neutropenic Sepsis: Prevention and Management of Neutropenic Sepsis in Cancer Patients. London: NICE.

Infections in solid organ transplant recipients

Introduction

Despite advances in prevention and treatment, infection is the most frequent cause of death in the first year post solid organ transplant (SOT). In liver transplant recipients, it is the leading cause of death over the first 1–3 years, with the majority occurring in the first 3–6 months. Infection is also the main cause of death in kidney transplantation in the immediate post-transplant period.

Infection established prior to transplant is difficult to treat in the post-transplant recipient and significant antimicrobial toxicities are common, often due to compromised renal or hepatic function and drug interactions. It is therefore crucial to detect and eliminate any potential pathogens whenever possible prior to transplantation or to design effective prophylactic strategies to prevent the re-emergence of latent infections after transplantation.

Post transplant, there are three main categories of infection in SOT recipients:
1. Surgical complications/perioperative.
2. Epidemiological exposures.
3. Infections present in the recipient or donor that clinically manifest post SOT.

The risk of infection in SOT recipients is determined by the interaction between the above-listed factors and the net state of immune suppression. There is a broadly typical expected timeline by which infections tend to present post transplant. However, it does not always apply and excessive epidemiological exposure or a change in the immunosuppressive regimen may alter this. Similarly, if an unexpected infection is identified, ensure a full epidemiological investigation is pursued. Clinical features of infection are frequently subtle so a prompt and aggressive approach to 'minor' skin lesions, illnesses, and any radiographic abnormalities is warranted.

Consideration must be given to the immunosuppressive regimen when tailoring an individual antimicrobial prophylaxis strategy. It is also important to consider and recognize any indirect effects of an infectious process (e.g. allograft injury/rejection, modulation of other infections, and oncogenesis). Antimicrobial prophylaxis has significantly altered the incidence and severity of post-transplant infections. Restarting prophylaxis should be considered during periods of repeat neutropenia or intensified immune suppression.

Risk of infection in transplantation

Transplant-specific surgical features

The following are all risk factors for bacterial infection in the early post-transplant period and are common to all SOT patients:
- Central venous lines.
- Urinary catheters.
- Abdominal drains.
- Mechanical ventilation.
- Use of broad-spectrum antibiotics.

There are also certain features related to the specific surgical technique that alter the risk of bacterial infection after SOT.

Renal grafts

Urinary tract infection is the most common infectious complication after renal transplantation. Grafts are usually implanted in the iliac fossa without removing the native kidneys and the ureter is directly connected to the native bladder. After surgery, ureteric stenosis or vesicoureteric reflux may result in urine flow alterations. In addition, some renal transplant patients have underlying urological abnormalities (e.g. chronic vesicoureteral reflux) that increase the risk of infection after transplant. Recipients from cardiac-death (non-heart-beating) donors are more likely to have delayed graft function compared to grafts from living or deceased (heart-beating) donors, which in turn increases the need for dialysis and the incidence of infection.

Liver grafts

Biliary infections and peritonitis can occur following the bile duct reconstruction that occurs during transplant. Bile duct reconstruction can be performed in three ways: duct-to-duct reconstruction (by far the most frequent), choledochojejunostomy and hepaticojejunostomy. Bile duct reconstructions other than duct-to-duct carry a higher risk of biliary infection and peritonitis.

Liver grafts may come from deceased (heart-beating), cardiac-death (non-heart-beating), or living donors. Living donor livers are used in adult-to-adult right lobe liver transplantation, which is more frequently associated with biliary complications such as leaks, as well as anastomotic and non-anastomotic strictures. Liver transplantation from cardiac-death donors has an increased risk of ischaemic cholangiopathy.

Pancreas grafts

Simultaneous kidney–pancreas transplantation from a deceased donor is the most frequent transplant strategy used for young diabetic patients with end-stage renal failure. Exocrine drainage of the donor pancreas is made through a duodenal stump from the donor that can be attached to the jejunum (intestinal drainage) or to the bladder (bladder drainage). The latter is associated with a higher risk of infection. As pancreas transplantation involves intestinal manipulation, there is a high risk of peritonitis and abdominal collections.

Small bowel grafts
Typically, patients offered this have intestinal failure and complications of parenteral nutrition, and many such patients will have had multiple abdominal operations and previous bowel resections, leading to heavy scarring of the abdominal wall. This may cause technical difficulties during transplantation and later complications. Often, small bowel and liver transplantation are combined when irreversible liver damage develops due to long-term parenteral nutrition. Patients undergoing small-bowel transplantation have a higher incidence of infectious complications than other SOT recipients because of a high microbial load in the intestinal graft and because they require a greater degree of immunosuppression (the small bowel is rich in lymphoid tissue, which increases the risk of allograft rejection). Bacterial translocation or peritoneal contamination during surgery can cause intra-abdominal abscesses.

Cardiac grafts
The transplanted cardiac graft does not have any direct contact with the environment (unlike renal or hepatic transplants, for example). However, postoperative mediastinitis can complicate the sternotomy performed at transplant surgery.

Lung grafts
These take three main forms: double-lung, single-lung, or double heart–lung transplantation. The most frequent site of infection is the lung, as the graft is exposed to the environment through the airway. Bacteria are the most frequent pathogens causing respiratory infections after lung transplantation, but environment-acquired tracheobronchial aspergillosis and aspergillosis of the bronchial anastomosis are other complications related to the anatomy of lung transplantation.

Epidemiological exposures
Apart from infections related to organ-specific anatomical abnormalities due to the transplant surgery or perioperative infection, the major determinant of risk of infection after transplantation depends on two fundamental factors: epidemiological exposures and the 'net state of immunosuppression'. Epidemiological exposures of a transplant recipient include community exposures, hospital environment exposures, donor-derived infection, and host-derived reactivation of infection. These must always be sought in the clinical assessment of any febrile SOT recipient.

Community exposures
- Respiratory viruses, e.g. influenza, parainfluenza, adenovirus, Respiratory syncytial virus (RSV), and rhinovirus.
- GI pathogens causing more persistent infection, e.g. norovirus, *Cryptosporidium* spp., *Salmonella* spp., *Listeria monocytogenes*, and hepatitis E.
- Common bacteria, e.g. *Streptococcus pneumoniae*, *Mycoplasma pneumoniae*, and *Legionella pneumophila*.
- Common environmental pathogens causing opportunistic infection, e.g. *Cryptococcus neoformans*, *Aspergillus* spp., *Stenotrophomonas maltophilia*, and *Nocardia* spp.

- Endemic fungi in certain geographic regions, e.g. *Histoplasma capsulatum* and *Coccidioides* spp.

Hospital environment exposures

Acquired from the environment via vascular access catheters, endotracheal tubes, or open surgical wounds, etc. Carbapenem-resistant *Klebsiella pneumoniae* is an increasingly common cause of infection in SOT recipients. These infections are most common in those colonized prior to transplant, notably in lung, liver, and intestinal transplant recipients. Some may manifest well after transplantation and may follow complications of transplantation such as bleeding, or GI procedures or *Clostridium difficile* colitis.

- Gram negatives, e.g. *Legionella* spp., *Pseudomonas aeruginosa*, carbapenem-resistant *K. pneumoniae, S. maltophilia*, and *Burkholderia cepacia*.
- Resistant Gram positives, e.g. VRE and MRSA.
- Fungi, e.g. *Aspergillus* spp. and non-albicans or azole-resistant *Candida* spp.
- *C. difficile.*

Donor-derived infection

- Viruses: herpesvirus (HSV, VZV, EBV, CMV, HHV-6), hepatitis B and C, HIV, human T-cell lymphotropic virus (HTLV), HPV, and rabies.
- Bacteria: TB and non-tuberculous mycobacteria (NTM), meningococcus, syphilis, and bacteraemia at the time of donation.
- Fungi: *Candida* spp., *Aspergillus* spp., *C. neoformans*, and endemic fungi.
- Parasites: *Toxoplasma gondii, Plasmodium falciparum, Strongyloides stercoralis*, and *Leishmania* spp.

Host-derived reactivation of infection

It is important to consider recent and remote exposures:

- Common viral infections: HSV, CMV, VZV, hepatitis B, C, papillomavirus, and BK virus.
- Endemic systemic mycoses (e.g. histoplasmosis, coccidioidomycosis, and blastomycosis).
- TB and NTM.
- Parasitic infections: *S. stercoralis, Leishmania* spp., and *Trypanosoma cruzi*.

Net state of immunosuppression

The 'net state of immunosuppression' is a concept encompassing all patient factors that contribute to the risk of infection. In SOT recipients these include the following:

- Pre-existing immune deficits.
- Critical illness malnutrition.
- Organ dysfunction (uraemia, cirrhosis, chronic obstructive pulmonary disease (COPD)/cystic fibrosis, heart failure).
- Diabetes.
- Colonization with antimicrobial-resistant pathogens, hospitalization.
- Immunosuppressive therapies (current and pre-transplant): consider timing, dose, and sequence in predicting risk of infection.
- Acquired immune deficiencies (e.g. splenectomy, hypogammaglobulinaemia).

- Prior therapies (chemotherapy, antimicrobials).
- Mucocutaneous barrier integrity (catheters, IV lines, drains).
- Fluid collections (blood, lymph, urine, bile, pus).
- Anatomical deficits (e.g. chronic sinusitis; portal for CNS infection).
- Neutropenia, lymphopenia.
- Viral co-infection (e.g. CMV, EBV, HCV, HBV, HIV).

The timing of post-transplant infections reflects the relationship between the recipient's epidemiological exposures and immunosuppressive strategy employed.

Immunosuppressive therapy

There are two key components to the post-transplant therapy for SOT patients:
1. An immunosuppressive regimen to prevent and treat rejection.
2. An antimicrobial strategy to prevent and treat infection and make the immunosuppressive regimen safer.

Both are dependent on and modulate the response to the other.

Most centres have traditionally used a variation of standard 'triple immunosuppression' (prednisolone, calcineurin inhibitor (e.g. ciclosporin or tacrolimus), and an antimetabolite (e.g. MMF), but have more recently moved towards a variety of 'induction' regimens (T-cell depletion and co-stimulatory blockade) with calcineurin inhibition and/or mTOR inhibition (e.g. sirolimus), often with an antimetabolite. These changes in immunosuppressive regimens, together with changes in routine antimicrobial prophylaxis and graft survival, have changed the timeline of infection.
- The use of induction therapy with lymphocyte depletion produces prolonged B- and T-cell deficits and alters T-regulatory cell subsets, antibody function, and NK cell function. This results in a prolonged risk for (late) viral (especially CMV) and fungal infections and increased risk for PTLD and other malignancies.
- Steroid-sparing regimens and anti-*Pneumocystis* prophylaxis have made *Pneumocystis jirovecii* infection less common.
- Antiviral prophylaxis has led to fewer herpesvirus infections.
- Incorporation of antibody depletion (plasmapheresis), bortezomib, or splenectomy in desensitization protocols, has increased the risk of infection due to encapsulated bacteria and yeasts (due to decreased opsonization).
- Use of sirolimus-based regimens has been associated with a non-infectious pneumonitis, easily confused with viral pneumonia or *P. jirovecii*, and also poor wound healing.

Drug interactions

Where antimicrobials are required, the possibility of drug interactions with the two mainstays of modern immunosuppression, ciclosporin and tacrolimus, is very real and significantly affects the choice of agent. There are three categories of such interaction (➋ see Chapter 4):
- The antimicrobial agent (e.g. rifampicin, isoniazid) up-regulates the metabolism of the immunosuppressants, resulting in decreased blood levels and an increased possibility of allograft rejection.

- The macrolides erythromycin, clarithromycin, and, to a lesser extent, azithromycin or the azoles (ketoconazole, itraconazole, and, to a lesser extent, fluconazole) down-regulate the metabolism of the immunosuppressants, which results in increased blood levels and an increased possibility of nephrotoxicity and over-immunosuppression.
- There may be synergistic nephrotoxicity when therapeutic levels of the immunosuppressants are combined with therapeutic levels of aminoglycosides, amphotericin, vancomycin, high therapeutic doses of trimethoprim–sulfamethoxazole (TMP–SMX), and/or fluoroquinolones.

The net effect of these various considerations is to emphasize the prevention of infection, with prophylactic or pre-emptive strategies, in conjunction with technically high-quality surgery, environmental protection, and appropriate immunosuppressive therapy.

Pre-transplant considerations

The pre-transplant evaluation is central to the prevention of postoperative infection.

- Each combination of donor and recipient should be assessed individually.
- Active infections in donors do not necessarily preclude organ donation. Donors with certain infections may be suitable for donation with close monitoring and pre-emptive or prophylactic measures.
- Nucleic acid testing (NAT) should be used to test for HIV and HCV infection in high-risk donors.
- Origin and travel history of both donor and recipient is important in order to screen for geographically restricted infections.

The following factors are associated with a lower infection risk in the recipient:

- Immunological tolerance.
- Good HLA match.
- Technically successful surgery.
- Good graft function.
- Appropriate surgical prophylaxis.
- Effective antiviral prophylaxis and *Pneumocystis jirovecii* pneumonia prophylaxis.
- Appropriate vaccination.

Risk assessment of the recipient

The clinical evaluation of a patient prior to SOT should focus on the following:

- Exposure history (including travel to endemic areas, place of birth, military service, animal exposures, hobbies, etc.)
- Past medical history, prior hospitalization, prosthetic material, infections (and antimicrobial susceptibility where known), and surgical history (e.g. valve replacement, splenectomy).
- Drug history including recent or current use of immunosuppressants and antimicrobials that would normally be started prophylactically (e.g. TMP–SMX). Use of immunosuppressants in the pre-transplant period can increase the risk of *Pneumocystis jirovecii* or toxoplasmosis in the early post-transplant period, and can therefore affect the choice of both prophylactic and immunosuppressive strategies post transplant.
- Vaccination history.
- Screening cultures for colonization, serology for more distant exposures (Table 7.1).

Pre-transplant screening

The tests listed in Table 7.1 are recommended as part of the pre-transplant screening for potential donors and recipients.

Hepatitis B

All organ donors should be screened for HBV infection. The initial screening test is an immunoassay to surface antigen (HBsAg) and total core antibody

Table 7.1 Recommended microbiological and serological testing for potential recipients and donors

Test or study	Notes and implications for donation
Non-specific tests	
Chest radiograph	Test recommended for both donor and recipient
Bronchoscopy with bronchoalveolar lavage	Test recommended for lung donor and recipient. Positive culture in donor is not an immediate contraindication. Individual evaluation in the case of multidrug resistance, fungal and mycobacterial colonization. Treat the recipient if culture positive
Blood cultures	Test recommended for donor at the time of donation. Positive culture in donor is not an immediate contraindication to donation. Individual decision in the case of MDR bacteria.
Geographically-restricted infections	The epidemiology of infections should be considered in decisions relating to disease transmission (e.g. *Trypanosoma cruzi* etc.)
Specific tests	
Rapid plasma reagin (RPR) or other serological test for syphilis	Test recommended for both donor and recipient; positive evidence of syphilis infection not a contraindication to donation. Treat the recipient with penicillin if donor or recipient is serologically active
Tuberculin skin test/ IGRA	Test recommended in recipient (with no previous history of TB) and consider in donor to screen for latent infection. Active TB is a contraindication to donation; lungs with residual tuberculous lesions should not be used for transplantation
HIV 1/2 antibody	Test recommended for both donor and recipient; HIV is a contraindication for donation but considered for HIV-positive recipient. (The high-risk donor should be screened for HIV infection by NAT.)
Cytomegalovirus IgG antibody	Test recommended for both donor and recipient; positive test is not a contraindication to donation but it is essential to define prophylactic strategy after procedure depending on recipient serology
EBV IgG antibody	Test recommended for both donor and recipient; positive test is not a contraindication to donation but it is essential to monitor EBV-negative recipients
HBsAg	Test recommended for donor and recipient. Donation if positive generally contraindicated but considered for HBsAg+ recipients or HBV protective immunity in recipient.
HBcAb/'HBc alone'	Test recommended for donor and recipient. Donation if positive not contraindicated but consider antiviral prophylaxis for liver and HBV non-immune recipients.

(Continued)

Table 7.1 *Contd.*

Test or study	Notes and implications for donation
HCV antibody	Test recommended for both donor and recipient. Donation if positive generally contraindicated but considered for HCV+ recipients. High-risk donors should be screened for HCV infection by NAT
Hepatitis A virus (HAV) antibody	Test recommended for both donor and recipient. Check recipient IgG positive/ensure vaccinated prior to liver transplantation
Toxoplasma IgG antibody	Test recommended for donor and recipient; if positive donation is not contraindicated but consider prophylaxis for heart transplant

(HBcAb). HBsAg+ organs would only be considered for recipients who are HBsAg+, those with protective immunity (as a result of immunization or natural infection), or in a life-threatening emergency. All recipients of HBsAg+ organs are treated with hepatitis B immune globulin plus an antiviral agent and are monitored for active HBV infection following transplant. Prophylaxis does not prevent transmission of infection in all cases. Organs from donors with serological profiles that suggest previous resolved infection (HBsAg–, HBcAb+, HBsAb+/–) may still be used as the risk of transmission from these donors to a susceptible recipient is low, particularly in non-liver donation. However, HBV non-immune recipients and liver recipients should undergo serial laboratory testing for HBV infection or alternatively receive antiviral prophylaxis.

Organ recipients should be screened in a similar manner to donors. If the candidate is HBsAg negative and has not been previously immunized, they should be vaccinated. Immunity is demonstrated by quantitative determination of anti-HBs antibodies (a value >10 IU/mL suggests immunity).

All cases with potential for HBV transmission should be discussed with the local infectious disease/hepatology specialist.

Hepatitis C

All organ donors and recipients should be screened for HCV with a third-generation EIA. These tests have improved sensitivity (>95%) and reduce the 'window period'. In high-risk donors and in recipients on haemodialysis (in whom antibody tests are less reliable), NAT is recommended. The risk of transmission from an infected donor to a susceptible recipient is high and HCV+ status in the donor is generally a contraindication to donation unless the recipient is HCV+ or in a life-threatening emergency. Living donors should be screened again 7–10 days prior to donation to detect new infections and reduce the 'window period'.

Tuberculosis

(➲ See 'Tuberculosis in SOT' p.134 and ➲ Chapter 14.)

Active TB is a contraindication to organ donation and lungs with residual TB lesions should not be used. Latent TB is not an absolute contraindication, but preventive therapy for recipients may be necessary. Tuberculin testing or an interferon-gamma release assay (IGRA) may be appropriate in living donors to screen for this. TB in post-transplant recipients is mostly due to reactivation and is associated with a significant mortality (~30%). A history of previous TB should be elicited and tuberculin testing or an interferon-gamma release assay (IGRA) should be carried out on recipients to determine the need for preventive therapy. Transplantation should be deferred in recipients with active TB until adequately treated.

Active recipient infections

Active bacterial/fungal/parasitic infections are contraindications to SOT until they are eliminated due to the risk of overwhelming infection and/ or failure of the graft (e.g. infections threaten the vascular anastomoses required at the time of transplantation). It is recommended that a minimum of 2 weeks be allowed to elapse following the resolution of an acute infection prior to transplantation. This can be shortened in the case of life-threatening situations. In some cases (e.g. cholangitis in liver SOT), infection will only be resolved with the procedure and the transplant should therefore not be delayed.

Active donor infections

Use of organs from an infected donor must be considered in the clinical context of the intended recipient, balanced against the virulence of the organism, antimicrobial susceptibility, time course of infection, and response to treatment. Informed consent of the recipient is crucial. Bacterial and fungal colonization or infection is frequently identified in potential organ donors as a result of intensive care and invasive resuscitative efforts. This can result in potentially fatal early post-transplant complications in the recipient, such as bacteraemia, myocarditis, or mycotic aneurysm. Organisms including *Staphylococcus aureus, Pseudomonas aeruginosa*, and *Candida* spp. are particular causes of these serious complications.

Infections without systemic spread are not a contraindication for transplant, with the exception of the infected organ. Bacteraemia and focal infections, including meningitis and endocarditis, are not absolute contraindications to organ donation if the cause is identified and appropriate antimicrobials are administered to donors for 48 hours or more and infection is clinically controlled. Generally, recipients who receive organs from bacteraemic/fungaemic donors should receive targeted antimicrobials for a period of 7–14 days. However, there are several infections which constitute exclusion criteria for donation (Table 7.2). To detect subclinical infection, organ perfusate and transport media should be cultured and blood cultures taken from the donor pre-terminally/at time of organ procurement, especially if the donor has been hospitalized for >48 hours.

Table 7.2 Exclusion criteria in organ donor screening

Bacterial

Active TB

Untreated focal infection, e.g. pneumonia

Untreated bacterial sepsis

Untreated syphilis

Viral

Acute viraemia (HSV, adenovirus, lymphocytic choriomeningitis virus (LCMV), HAV, West Nile virus), influenza[a]

Active shingles or herpesvirus pneumonitis/encephalitis

Acute EBV

HIV (serology or PCR positive)

Active hepatitis B or C (relative contraindications)

HTLV

Severe acute respiratory syndrome (SARS)

JC virus

Rabies

Parasitic

Active *Trypanosoma cruzi*

Active toxoplasmosis

Leishmaniasis

Strongyloidiasis

Fungal

Untreated fungal sepsis/disseminated fungal infection

Cryptococcal infection of any site

Other

Encephalitis/meningitis of unknown aetiology

Multiorgan failure due to overwhelming sepsis or gangrenous bowel

Creutzfeldt–Jakob disease

[a] Confirmed or suspected influenza infection is a contraindication to lung and intestinal transplantation. Recipients of other organs from infected donors (treated or not) should receive prophylactic treatment with neuraminidase inhibitors.

Source: data from Kontoyiannis, D.P. Antifungal prophylaxis in hematopoietic stem cell transplant recipients: the unfinished tale of imperfect success. *Bone Marrow Transplantation*. 46(2), 165–73. Copyright © 2011 Nature Publishing Group.

Pre-transplant vaccination

Both living donors and adult SOT recipient candidates should be up to date with vaccines based on age, immune status, and exposure history. MMR, varicella (VAR), and zoster (ZOS) vaccine administration should be avoided within 4 weeks of organ donation. Vaccination of donors for the recipient's benefit is not recommended (Table 7.3).

Table 7.3 Recommended vaccines for SOT recipients

Vaccine	Scheme/recipient group	Before Tx	After Tx	Booster
Varicella	2 doses ≥3 months apart	Last dose 1 month pre-Tx	Contraindicated if active immunosuppression[a]	—
Zoster	SOT candidates aged ≥60 years and varicella-positive candidates aged 50–59 years not severely immunocompromised	Last dose 1 month pre-Tx	Contraindicated if active immunosuppression	
MMR	2 doses (0, 1 month)	Last dose 1 month pre-Tx	Contraindicated if active immunosuppression	—
Streptococcus pneumoniae	All should receive PCV13 (1 dose). Recipients aged ≥2 years should receive 1 dose of PPSV23 if they have not received a dose within 5 years and have not received 2 lifetime doses. When both PCV13 and PPSV23 are indicated, PCV13 should be completed 8 weeks prior to PPSV23	Last dose 2 weeks pre-Tx	2–6 months after Tx	Once after 5 years
Influenza	1 dose	Last dose 2 weeks pre-Tx	After 6 months of Tx	Every year
HBV	Fast (0, 1, 2, 6–12 months)	Last dose 2 weeks pre-Tx	After 6 months of Tx	If anti-HBs
	Accelerated (0, 7, 21 days, 12 months)			<10 IU/L (double dose revaccination)

(Continued)

Table 7.3 Contd.

Vaccine	Scheme/recipient group	Before Tx	After Tx	Booster
	Double dose if high immunosuppression or on haemodialysis (and aged ≥20 years)			
HAV[b]	For HepA-unvaccinated, -undervaccinated, or -seronegative SOT candidates (particularly liver transplant candidates) aged >12 months: 2 doses (0, 6 months)			Once in non-responders (anti-HAV <10 IU/L)
dT	According to previous immunization status			Every 10 years (dT or dTpa)
HPV	Administer to recipients aged 11–26 years			

dT diphtheria and tetanus; dTpa diphtheria tetanus and pertussis; Tx transplantation.

[a] Except for varicella in children without evidence of immunity who are renal or liver transplant recipients are receiving minimal or no immunosuppression and have no recent graft rejection. [b] Combined HepA–HepB vaccine can be used for SOT candidates aged ≥12 years of age in whom both vaccines are indicated

Source: data from Len et al. on behalf of the ESCMID Study Group of Infection in Compromised Hosts (ESGICH). *Clinical Microbiology and Infection.* 2014. 20(7) 10–18. Copyright ©️ 2018 Elsevier Inc. All rights reserved.

Clinical and investigative approach

Two important factors that inform the clinical and investigative approach to infection in SOT recipients are the timeline following transplant and the predominant organ system, if any, involved.

Timeline of infection

The timeline is used to establish a differential diagnosis for infectious syndromes at various stages following SOT. Infections occurring outside the usual period or of unusual severity suggest excessive immunosuppression or epidemiological hazard. It is important to remember that the timeline is not rigid. In addition, when treatment of graft rejection is started or immunosuppression intensified (e.g. bolus corticosteroids or T cell depletion), the timeline is reset to the period of greatest risk for opportunistic infection (Figure 7.1).

Phase I: 1–4 weeks post SOT

Infections during this period are generally donor or recipient derived (colonization, viraemia, candidaemia, catheter, or wound associated) or associated with technical complications of surgery (infected haematoma, peritonitis, infection related to vascular insufficiency of the graft, or complications of critical care). Because of the technical complexity associated with liver, lung, and heart–lung transplantation, this first month is the critical time period in terms of life-threatening infections for these types of transplant.

Opportunistic infections are relatively rare during this initial period as prolonged immunosuppression has yet to become established. If one occurs, it strongly suggests a particular epidemiological exposure. Unexplained early infectious syndromes (hepatitis, pneumonitis, encephalitis, rashes, leucopenia) usually reflect donor-derived infections. *Clostridium difficile* colitis is common. Early graft injuries (e.g. ischaemia to bile ducts or pulmonary reperfusion injury) may manifest as foci for liver or lung abscesses.

Immunomodulating viral infections are unusual during this period; CMV rarely causes disease within the first 20 days, especially in those on antiviral prophylaxis. After the first 4 weeks, the general pattern of infections becomes very similar for all forms of SOT.

Phase II: 1–6 months post SOT

Viral pathogens and graft rejection are responsible for the majority of febrile episodes in this period. Herpesviruses are uncommon in the face of antiviral prophylaxis but may emerge subsequently. Other viral infections commonly seen include BK virus (causing a nephropathy or ureteric stenosis), adenovirus (frequently multiorgan involvement), and recurrent HCV. In addition to immediate or 'direct' tissue invasive disease, some viruses may have 'indirect' pleotropic effects. Indirect effects may include systemic or local immune suppression predisposing to or enhancing other opportunistic infections (e.g. *Pneumocystis jirovecii* or aspergillosis), PTLD, or acute and chronic graft injury and rejection due to antigenic provocation.

The use of TMP–SMX during this period should prevent most urinary tract infections and opportunistic infections such as *Listeria monocytogenes, P. jirovecii, Toxoplasma gondii,* and most *Nocardia* spp. Some infections (pneumonia, *C. difficile*, cholangitis) may persist from the perioperative period.

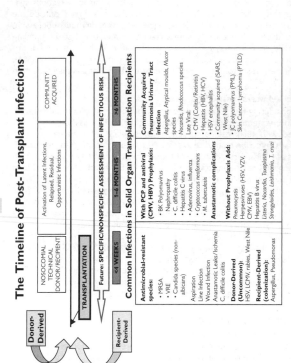

Fig 7.1 The timeline of post-transplant infections. Reproduced with permission from Fishman, J.A. et al., and the AST Infectious Diseases Community of Practice. Introduction: Infection in Solid Organ Transplant Recipients. *American Journal of Transplantation*, 9, 3–6. Copyright © 2009 John Wiley & Sons, Inc. All Rights Reserved.

The main recipient-derived infections that reactivate during this period are *Aspergillus* spp., endemic fungi (e.g. *Histoplasma capsulatum*), *T. gondii*, *Cryptococcus neoformans*, *Trypanosoma cruzi*, and *Strongyloides* spp.

Phase III: >6 months post SOT

In general, the risk of infectious disease decreases as immunosuppression reduces in those with good graft function. However, these patients continue to suffer more severe manifestations of the usual community-acquired infections. Chronic viral infections are seen in some patients and can lead to graft injury (e.g. cirrhosis from HCV-infected livers and accelerated vasculopathy in heart transplants from CMV) or malignancy (PTLD, skin or anogenital cancers). Patients with less adequate graft function continue to receive intense immunosuppression and suffer recurrent infections as a result (sometimes known as the 'chronic never-do-wellers'). These patients are at particularly increased risk for *Listeria* spp., *Nocardia* spp., invasive fungal pathogens, and more unusual organisms such as *Rhodococcus* spp. They may also exhibit more subtle signs of infection and can deteriorate very quickly, so a high degree of clinical suspicion in these patients is paramount. These patients may benefit from lifetime TMP–SMX and antifungal prophylaxis.

Clinical assessment

Identification of the predominant organ system involved (if any) informs the approach to investigation and treatment. Management of SOT recipients with infectious complications requires close collaboration between the transplant team, infectious disease specialists, intensivists, specialty physicians, and physiotherapists.

Undifferentiated fever

SOT recipients generally have fewer clinical manifestations of infection and few or even absent findings on conventional radiography. Classic features of infections (e.g. leucocytosis, erythema, cough, etc.) may be replaced by non-specific and poorly localizing manifestations (e.g. altered mental status, elevation of blood liver function tests, unexplained hypotension, etc.).

In the first few weeks post SOT, the following should be excluded in any episode of unexplained fever:

- A technical problem involving the graft vascular tree.
- A technical problem involving anastomoses, e.g. biliary in liver transplant.
- A deep wound infection; e.g. deep perinephric space infections can present subtly post renal transplant. Early imaging ± aspiration, drainage, and antibiotics are key. Sometimes graft nephrectomy may be required to facilitate drainage of collections and prevent catastrophic anastomotic leaks.

There are also multiple non-infectious causes of fever post transplant (➔ see also Chapter 8). In the first 4 weeks post SOT, the key ones are as follows:

- Allograft rejection (in renal transplant, fever can precede a rise in serum creatinine, especially in children).

- Anti-lymphocyte antibody therapy (e.g. OKT®3 or ATG). This causes fever secondary to cytokine release, especially TNF, and occasionally can lead to hypotension, febrile pulmonary oedema, or aseptic meningitis/encephalopathy.
- Pulmonary embolism.
- Drug reactions; although drug fevers and rashes are less common in SOT patients compared to the normal population due to the anti-inflammatory effects of immunosuppressants.

Following the initial phases post transplant, malignant processes creep into the differential of unexplained fever. More sensitive imaging techniques such as CT and MRI including positron emission tomography are essential for assessing the presence and nature of both infectious and malignant processes.

Respiratory presentations
Postoperative respiratory problems are common after liver, heart, and lung transplantation. Early on, non-infectious complications such as effusion, atelectasis, pulmonary oedema, diaphragmatic dysfunction, and acute respiratory distress syndrome (ARDS) are all fairly common causes of respiratory failure and may mimic, coexist with, or mask infection. During the first month, the risk of infection is usually related to surgery, intensive care, invasive procedures, and hospitalization. Nosocomial bacterial infections, including Gram-negative pathogens and MDR microorganisms are frequent, and fungal infections are infrequent but associated with high mortality.

The lung is the leading infectious site in lung and heart transplant recipients, second most common site (after intra-abdominal infection) in liver transplant recipients, and lowest in frequency in kidney transplant recipients. Post-transplant lung infections occur according to a broadly predictable time (Table 7.4).

In renal transplant recipients, infectious problems are not frequently observed early after surgery. Early respiratory failure is mainly non-infectious in origin (cardiogenic pulmonary oedema), but late respiratory failure may occur due to pneumonia within the subsequent months to years.

In lung transplant recipients, acute pulmonary allograft rejection is an important problem in the first few months after transplantation. Patients are often asymptomatic, and when present, symptoms may be non-specific, including fever, shortness of breath, and cough. The diagnosis of rejection is based on the characteristic histopathological changes on transbronchial lung biopsy specimens. The usual treatment is with steroids so it is crucial that infectious differentials are excluded.

Infectious infiltrates account for approximately two-thirds of lung infiltrates observed after transplantation, and lung infiltrates due to MDR bacterial infections are increasing.

During the 1–6 months after SOT (a period of maximum sustained immunosuppression), opportunistic infections and immunomodulating viruses are common. Invasive aspergillosis is a major cause of respiratory infection in this period, with an incidence of 1–15% and a 22% mortality rate. Symptoms are non-specific and radiographic appearances are highly variable.

After 6 months, opportunistic pathogens are less frequent and community-acquired infections become more common as the level of

Table 7.4 Timeline of pulmonary infections post SOT

	0–1 month	1–6 months	>6 months
Bacterial	*Usually nosocomial Gram negatives*, e.g. *Pseudomonas* spp. MDR Enterobacteriaceae and *Acinetobacter* spp. MRSA *Legionella* spp.	*Usually community acquired* *Nocardia* spp. *Listeria* spp. *Mycobacterium tuberculosis*	*Usually community acquired* *Streptococcus pneumoniae* *Haemophilus influenzae* *Legionella* spp. NTM *M. tuberculosis* (renal transplant)
Fungal	*Candida* spp. *Aspergillus* spp. (if recipient colonized)	*Aspergillus* spp. *P. jirovecii* *C. neoformans*	*Aspergillus* spp. Atypical moulds Mucorales
Viral	HSV	CMV, EBV, VZV Influenza, RSV, human metapneumovirus, rhinovirus, adenovirus	Late viral, e.g. CMV

Source: data from Zeyneloglu, P. Respiratory complications after solid organ transplantation. *Experimental and Clinical Transplantation* 2015: 13(2);115–125. Copyright © 2015 Baskent University. All Rights Reserved.

immunosuppression can be reduced with recovery of allograft function. The exception is the subgroup of patients who have immunosuppression increased for rejection.

Lung transplant recipients have the highest risk for respiratory viral infections. The incidence of CMV pneumonitis is 15–55% in lung transplant recipients, as the lung is a major site of CMV latency. CMV pneumonitis occurs in 0–9.2% of liver transplant recipients, 0.8–6.6% of heart transplant recipients and <1% in renal transplant recipients.

NTM pulmonary infections are more common in heart and lung transplant recipients than other SOT recipients, and onset of the infection usually is ≥1 year after transplant.

Pulmonary infiltrates in a SOT recipient

These need to be detected and investigated early, and treated aggressively to prevent multisystem organ failure and increase survival. This involves:
- A thorough examination to cover all possible extrapulmonary clues such as skin lesions for biopsy, evidence of CNS involvement, etc. due to organisms such as *Nocardia* spp., *Aspergillus* spp., or *Cryptococcus* spp.
- In addition to blood cultures, sputum cultures, and chest radiography, a CT of the chest should be performed. Radiological appearance can aid in the differential diagnosis and guide empirical therapy (see Chapter 8, Table 8.2 p.156).

- Due to the potentially wide differential and the poor prognosis associated with incorrect initial therapy, bronchoscopy should be considered early to provide deep respiratory samples for culture/histology.
- Broad-spectrum antimicrobials should be started while awaiting results based on local microbiological data and narrowed as soon as results allow.

Neurological presentations

Neurological complications are common in SOT recipients (~10–85%), variable in presentation, and often difficult to diagnose. Abnormalities range from diffuse neurological disorders to focal deficits. Immunosuppressive therapy blunts classical symptoms, signs, and radiological appearances. The presence of multiple pathologies is common and may involve infective problems, drug toxicities, and complications due to graft rejection and failure.

Comprehensive evaluation is urgent to identify potentially life-threatening processes. The history should explore prior neurological symptoms, immunosuppression, other drugs (e.g. psychiatric agents, antimicrobials) and epidemiological exposures. The majority of patients should have early neuroimaging.

The combination of epidemiology, timeline post transplant, and the 'net state of immunosuppression' helps to identify risk for CNS infections. Important information includes colonization data and baseline viral serology, alongside current prophylaxis and previous antimicrobial use. Identifying community exposures requires detailed history taking, e.g. contact with *M. tuberculosis* (contact with active cases), *Cryptococcus neoformans* (pets), EBV (social contacts), *Listeria monocytogenes* (contaminated food and water), and moulds including *Zygomycetes* and *Scedosporium* species (gardening). A careful travel history is important, e.g. exposure to *Coccidioides* spp. in Southwestern United States (Table 7.5).

There are also a number of potential donor-derived infections, that can be difficult to exclude, but should always be considered in the differential (Table 7.6). If suspected, the organ procurement organization should be contacted regarding other recipients of organs from the same donor. Donor-derived infections, notably with neurotropic viruses, present with clinical disease mainly in the first 1–3 weeks post transplant.

Non-infectious conditions that may mimic infectious complications include glioblastoma multiforme, lymphoma, metastases (e.g. lung cancer, renal cancer) and neurosarcoidosis.

Empiric antimicrobial therapies in SOT recipients with CNS symptoms should account for prior antimicrobial exposures and colonization. In addition, some viruses (e.g. CMV, EBV, and HCV), are associated with increased risk for other opportunistic infections through modulation of the host immune response. Therefore, detection of these must not preclude evaluation for other coexisting pathologies, whether or not antiviral treatment is started in patients with CNS symptoms.

Table 7.5 Incidence and onset of common central nervous system conditions in the solid organ transplant recipient

First 4 weeks	1–6 months	>6 months
Infectious (approx. incidence where known)		
Post-surgical complications → metastatic infection/ metabolic effects:e.g. surgical site infections, anastomotic leaks, *C. difficile* colitis, pneumonia	Opportunistic infections: e.g. cryptococcosis (0.1%), *M. tuberculosis*If no TMP–SMX prophylaxis: *Listeria/ Toxoplasma/Nocardia* If no antifungal (azole) prophylaxis: invasive fungal infections, mainly aspergillosis (0.2%)	Infections post cessation of prophylaxis, determined by:Immunosuppression Epidemiology (new exposures) Recurrent viral infections with atypical process, e.g. JC virus → PML (0.03%)
Donor-derived neurotropic viruses, e.g. CMV, HSV	Viral CNS infection if no CMV prophylaxis: CMV, HSV, EBV, VZV	Fungal infections: cryptococcosis (0.1%), endemic fungi (0.2%), *Scedosporium*, Mucorales (0.04%)
Opportunistic infections *only* if intense epidemiological exposure or anatomical predisposition (e.g. hospital construction/ sinus disease → CNS aspergillosis)		
Non-infectious (approx. incidence where known)		
Cerebrovascular haemorrhage/infarcts (0–8%, more common in lung/heart recipients)	Posterior reversible encephalopathy syndrome (0.49%; usually early onset in liver, lung; later onset in heart, kidney)	Graft dysfunction → metabolic abnormalities
Seizures (1.5–17%)		Tumour
Encephalopathy (0.8–43%)e.g. to drug toxicity (e.g. high calcineurin inhibitor levels, antimicrobials)		CNS PTLD EBV+: median onset 11.5 months EBV−: median onset 69 months (0.1–0.75% (kidney, liver) vs up to 3.75% (lung, intestinal, multivisceral))
Central pontine myelinolysis (liver only, 0.88–1.2%)		

Source: data from Wright A. et al Central Nervous System Syndromes in Solid Organ Transplant Recipients. *Clinical Infectious Disease*. 2014:59(7) 1001–11. Copyright © 2014 Infectious Diseases Society of America.

Table 7.6 Donor-derived transmissions relevant to central nervous system processes in SOT patients

Bacterial	Viral	Fungal	Parasitic
M. tuberculosis	CMV	Aspergillus spp.	T. gondii
MRSA	EBV	H. capsulatum	Babesia microti
L. monocytogenes	Hep B & C	Coccidioides immitus	Balamuthia mandrillaris
	HSV	C. neoformans	Malaria
	HIV	Zygomyces spp.	Naegleria fowleri
	HTLV		T. cruzi
	LCMV		
	Rabies		
	West Nile virus		

Source: data from Wright A. et al Central Nervous System Syndromes in Solid Organ Transplant Recipients. *Clinical Infectious Disease.* 2014;59(7) 1001–11. Copyright © 2014 Infectious Diseases Society of America.

Hepatitis and liver enzyme derangement

Main differentials of liver enzyme derangement in SOT include:

- *Drugs*: azathioprine, ciclosporin, TB drugs, TMP–SMX, azoles (other than fluconazole).
- *Viral infections*: acute hepatitis: HSV, VZV (disseminated disease), CMV, EBV, adenovirus (unusual cause of fulminant hepatitis), hepatitis A, HHV6; chronic hepatitis: hepatitis B, C, and E.
- *Bacterial sepsis*.

Hepatitis E

In the SOT recipient, chronic infection with hepatitis E virus (HEV) is marked by persistent viremia and abnormal liver function with possible eventual progression to cirrhosis. In a multicentre review of 85 cases of acute HEV infection, 65.9% of the SOT recipients developed chronic hepatitis of whom 14.3% developed cirrhosis. The use of tacrolimus compared with ciclosporin was an independent predictor of chronic infection. The majority of HEV infections following SOT result from *de novo* infections and are unlikely to represent virus reactivation. Rare instances of transmission through blood transfusion or the donated graft have been reported.

Treatment of prolonged HEV viremia often involves reducing immunosuppression. Pegylated interferon administration has been shown to induce a sustained virological response in a limited group of patients. However, both approaches to viral control may increase the risk of graft rejection. Ribavirin monotherapy has induced sustained virological responses without the risk of rejection and may represent the first-line agent for treatment.

➜ See Chapter 8 for approach to oesophagitis and other gastrointestinal symptoms, rash/skin lesions, positive blood cultures, and bone marrow suppression.

Specific infections

Invasive fungal infections

(⊃ See also Chapter 13.)

Opportunistic fungi are universally distributed and invasive infections are caused mainly by *Candida* spp., *Aspergillus* spp., and to a lesser extent, by *Cryptococcus* spp., fungi belonging to the Mucorales order, and other filamentous fungi. Invasive diseases due to endemic fungi are usually a result of reactivation, but may occasionally occur as primary infections in patients who live in or visit highly endemic areas.

Approach to investigation

- Take blood cultures (diagnostic if positive for yeasts or filamentous fungi, e.g. *Scedosporium* spp. and *Fusarium* spp.)
- Obtain sterile tissue for histology and culture or sterile fluid (not obtained through drains) for culture/PCR.
- Never exclude pulmonary invasive fungal infection on the basis of a 'normal' chest radiograph.
- A high-resolution CT of the chest and bronchoscopy for tissue ± detection of galactomannan antigen should be performed for the diagnosis of invasive pulmonary aspergillosis (especially if lung transplant patient with a positive sputum culture for *Aspergillus* spp.).
- Brain MRI is the modality of choice for suspected intracranial fungal infection (especially cryptococcomas) and for skin and soft tissue.
- CT and MRI for sinonasal disease.
- Ultrasound, CT, and MRI all have a role in the diagnosis of fungal abscess in liver, kidney, and spleen (CT better for micro-abscesses).
- Treatment response should be monitored by clinical follow-up, and periodic re-imaging should be considered every 7–10 days during the first weeks of therapy in adults.

Candida species

(⊃ See also Chapter 13.)

Candida spp. are the most frequent invasive fungal agents in the SOT recipient, accounting for half of all cases in the transplant population. The rate varies according to the organ transplanted; it is especially high in abdominal SOT such as intestinal, pancreas, and liver transplantation and extremely uncommon after heart transplantation.

The spectrum of infection secondary to *Candida* spp. includes urinary tract infections (uncomplicated or complicated by urinary fungal balls), hepatosplenic candidiasis, candidaemia (usually secondary to gut translocation or IV catheter associated), candida endocarditis, or ocular candidiasis. Presentation is usually non-specific, often just with fever, and the diagnosis is often made on culture of clinical samples taken as part of a fever work-up.

Urinary candidiasis

Symptomatic candiduria does not require treatment unless the patient is having a urological procedure or is neutropenic. Consider imaging to rule out an abscess, fungal ball or urological abnormality. If a urinary fungal ball is diagnosed, surgical removal is strongly recommended. Treatment of

symptomatic patients with candiduria (cystitis) or pyelonephritis is required, with 7–14 days of antifungals and removal or replacement of any urinary catheter.
(➔ See Chapter 13.)

Aspergillus species
(➔ See also Chapter 13.)

European studies have shown an incidence of invasive aspergillosis between 0.2% and 3.5%, depending on the type of transplant. Incidence is highest among lung transplant recipients. Risk factors for the condition (Table 7.7) depend on the type of transplant.

The most common clinical form is invasive pulmonary disease (mortality 67–82%), the clinical presentation of which is usually acute and invasive.

Table 7.7 Risk factors for invasive aspergillosis

	Early invasive aspergillosis	Late invasive aspergillosis (>3 months post transplant)
Liver transplant	Re-transplantation Kidney failure, especially post transplant Haemodialysis Fulminant hepatic failure Complicated surgery or reoperation	More than 6 g of accumulative prednisone in the third month after transplantationPost-transplant renal failure Post-transplant haemodialysis Leucopenia (<500/µL) Chronic graft dysfunction
Lung transplant	Bronchial anastomotic ischaemia or bronchial stent placement Acute rejection Single-lung transplant *Aspergillus* spp. colonization before or during first year post transplant	Chronic graft dysfunction
Heart transplant	*Aspergillus* spp. colonization of the respiratory tract Re-operation Post-transplant haemodialysis Hypogammaglobulinaemia (<400 mg/dL)	ICU readmission Kidney transplantation >2 acute rejection episodes
Kidney transplant	Graft lost and haemodialysis Post-transplant haemodialysis Prolonged high corticosteroid doses CMV infection Over-immunosuppression	

Invasive tracheobronchitis can also occur in single, ulcerative, or nodular forms in lung transplant patients and may affect the bronchial anastomosis, the worst cases resulting in dehiscence of the suture.

Antifungal therapy should be initiated early in SOT patients with suspected invasive aspergillosis. Diagnostic evaluation is essential to confirm the diagnosis. Treatment should be individualized according to type of transplant, sites of involvement, and immunosuppression.

Reduce immunosuppression as an adjunct to antifungal treatment, but without jeopardizing graft viability. Reducing the corticosteroid dose may be key.

Cryptococcus species
(● See also Chapter 13)

Cryptococcosis is the third most common infection after candidiasis and invasive aspergillosis. The lower incidence in SOT recipients may be explained by the antifungal activity of calcineurin inhibitors. The incidence of cryptococcosis is higher in kidney and heart transplantation, and disseminated disease is more likely in patients who have received high doses of corticosteroids or monoclonal antibodies (e.g. alemtuzumab and infliximab). The mortality of cryptococcosis in SOT recipients ranges from 14% to 27%. It occurs late, usually 16–21 months post transplantation. Presentation is often non-specific (fever, malaise) but most SOT recipients with pulmonary infection will have radiographic abnormalities. Appearances may include mass lesions, diffuse infiltrates, cavitation, multiple opacities, and pleural effusions. More than half will have disseminated disease or CNS involvement (insidious progressive meningoencephalitis, or cryptococcomas) and as many as 33% have fungaemia. ~5% of patients may have soft tissue involvement with ulcerative/nodular skin lesions.

Cytomegalovirus
(● See also 'Cytomegalovirus (CMV/HHV-5)' Chapter 11.)

There are three major epidemiological patterns of CMV disease in SOT recipients:
• Primary infection (CMV naïve recipient infected by donor allograft/ CMV-infected blood or community acquisition).
• Reactivation of latent CMV infection in the recipient.
• Superinfection: both donor and recipient infected, disease caused by reactivation of donor strain in recipient. This may have a greater impact than reactivation of the recipient strain in the recipient, as natural infection cannot protect against symptomatic superinfection.

The most important risk factor for the development of CMV disease in SOT recipients is mismatching CMV serology (positive donor and negative recipient), which confers a >50% risk of developing CMV disease in the absence of antiviral prophylaxis or pre-emptive treatment.

The pathogenesis of reactivation is mediated by inflammation, stress, concurrent infections, and immunosuppressive drugs (anti-lymphocyte antibody therapy (OKT®3/ATG) > cyclophosphamide and azathioprine > ciclosporin/rapamycin/tacrolimus). However, once viral replication is present, the latter agents (and steroids) are more effective in promoting dissemination than anti-lymphocyte antibody therapy. The sequence of administered immunosuppression can therefore determine the course of CMV infection. Viral coinfection (e.g. HHV-6) has been shown to increase the risk of CMV disease in the early post-transplant period of liver and kidney transplant recipients.

Most clinical effects of CMV are seen 1–4 months post transplant (median peak 5 weeks) and rarely within the first 21 days. However, it can be delayed to >6 months in patients receiving prophylaxis. Chorioretinitis occurs even later. The effects of CMV in the different SOT populations are very similar with the major exception that CMV disease has far greater effects on the organ transplanted than on native organs. In general, there is a decreasing risk of CMV disease in small-bowel > lung > pancreas > heart > liver/kidney transplant recipients.

Clinical manifestations

CMV syndrome: fever, leucopenia and thrombocytopenia with no splenomegaly, lymphadenopathy, or end-organ disease. Sometimes even fever may be absent and the sole presentation is unexplained hepatocellular dysfunction.

Pneumonitis: this can be subtle in non-lung transplant patients, usually subacute over a few days. The major differential is *Pneumocystis jirovecii*. If an acute deterioration occurs in <12 hours, bacterial or fungal superinfection needs to be considered. Relapsing CMV pneumonia can also occur.

GI tract disease: this is the major manifestation in non-lung transplant patients. CMV of the upper GI tract should always be considered if there is unexplained abdominal pain, particularly mid-epigastric (gastric involvement common). Colitis may be complicated by haemorrhage, ulceration, or even perforation. Tissue biopsies are essential for diagnosis as colitis with undetectable blood CMV PCR is not uncommon. Immunohistochemistry of appropriate clinical biopsies has a high specificity and sensitivity. MMF (at doses of >2 g/day) has been particularly linked to the development of CMV GI disease in kidney transplant recipients. CMV hepatitis can be catastrophic in liver SOT patients. Pancreatitis ± abscesses can occur in pancreatic allografts.

Renal disease: in renal transplant patients, CMV can cause a tubulointerstitial nephritis, ureteral inflammation/necrosis, haemolytic uraemic syndrome, thrombotic microangiopathy, necrotizing/crescentic glomerulonephritis, or renal artery thrombosis.

Chorioretinitis: occurs >6 months post transplant. Most patients present with unilateral eye involvement first, but both eyes are usually affected. Presentation includes blurred vision, scotoma, and reduced visual acuity. The retina has the appearance of a gradually expanding whitish necrotic retinitis. Rarely, acute retinal necrosis can ensue.

Less common manifestations of CMV include endometriosis, epididymitis, encephalitis, transverse myelitis, and skin ulcerations.

Indirect clinical effects of CMV infection

- Superinfection: *Pneumocystis jirovecii*/*Aspergillus*/Gram-negative bacilli in the lung (especially if leucopenic). Septicaemia secondary to, e.g. Gram-negative bacilli, *Candida* spp., and *Listeria* spp.
- Allograft injury and rejection.
- Malignancy: EBV-associated PTLD is increased seven- to tenfold in patients with symptomatic CMV disease (ganciclovir prophylaxis can therefore also reduce incidence of PTLD).

EBV-related post-transplant lymphoproliferative disorder

PTLD encompasses a wide range of B-cell lymphoproliferative conditions associated with EBV infection and post-transplant immunosuppression. The disease can manifest in the recipient or can affect the transplanted tissue. Following SOT, recipient-derived PTLD is most common and is typically a multisystem disease, involving nodal and extranodal sites. In contrast, the disease in HSCT recipients is usually donor derived and more commonly limited to the allograft tissue.

EBV serostatus should be determined for all SOT donors and recipients because an EBV-seronegative recipient with an EBV-seropositive donor is at high risk for development of PTLD. For EBV-negative recipients, the use of T-cell depleting agents should be avoided if possible (anti-CD25 or no induction is preferred).

The incidence of PTLD is higher after intestinal, lung, and heart–lung transplantation, ranging from 2% to 10%, whereas lower rates are reported after liver and kidney transplantation, ranging from 0.2% to 2.5%.

There are several risk factors for PTLD, occurring early (in the first year of SOT) and late (>5 years):

Early PTLD

- Discordant EBV serostatus (positive donor with negative recipient).
- Use of anti-lymphocyte antibodies.
- Maintenance immunosuppression with tacrolimus.

Late PTLD

- Older age (> 60 years).
- Long-term immunosuppression.

Diagnosis

An accurate diagnosis of PTLD requires a high index of suspicion, since it may present subtly and/or extranodally. It should be suspected in a patient presenting with adenopathy, B symptoms (fever, weight loss, night sweats), unexplained haematological or biochemical abnormalities, and signs or symptoms attributable to the infiltration of extralymphatic tissues. It may also cause symptoms similar to those seen with organ rejection or similar to side effects from immunosuppressive medications. Other features may include:

- radiologic evidence of a mass
- elevated serum markers (such as increased LDH levels)
- positive positron emission tomography scanning indicating metabolically active areas
- a rising EBV viral load in the peripheral blood.

Primary CNS PTLD is uncommon, but should be suspected in transplant recipients with mental status changes or new neurological findings. The diagnosis is strongly suggested if:
- gadolinium-enhanced MRI head shows enhancing lesions
- CSF analysis is positive for EBV by PCR
- rising EBV viral load is detected in the peripheral blood.

The diagnosis should be confirmed either by the presence of malignant lymphocytes in the CSF (can be confounded by use of steroids) or by direct lesion biopsy. Biopsy (excision is best) is essential for an accurate diagnosis of non-CNS PTLD (➔ see Chapter 11.)

Monitoring
- Monitoring of EBV DNA titre is useful for EBV discordant (D+/R−) SOT recipients and should be considered in EBV-seropositive recipients of lung and intestinal transplants.
- For asymptomatic EBV-seropositive SOT recipients undergoing acute rejection therapy, EBV load monitoring should be initiated.
- As a general rule, SOT recipients with significantly rising EBV viral loads (usually more than tenfold or >1 $\log_{10}$ cp/mL), regardless of EBV serostatus, should undergo a careful clinical and radiological examination. This may include CT and/or positron emission tomography-CT to search for lymphadenopathy, mass lesions, and other signs of PTLD.

Treatment principles
(➔ See Chapter 11.)
- For asymptomatic EBV-seropositive SOT recipients without clinical or radiological evidence of PTLD, but significantly increasing EBV loads, consider reducing immunosuppression. A change in immunosuppressive therapy towards a regimen based on a mTOR inhibitor may be beneficial, although data supporting the rationale for this approach in the pre-emptive setting are insufficient.
- The efficacy of anti-CD20 antibody (rituximab) as a pre-emptive agent in SOT recipients with persistent and/or increasing EBV DNA titres is not proven (unlike in HSCT patients where its efficacy has been demonstrated). However, many experts would consider this as pre-emptive treatment in the context of rapidly increasing viraemia.

Prevention
The European Society of Clinical Microbiology and Infectious Diseases (ESCMID) study group recommends prophylaxis using IV immunoglobulins and valganciclovir (in EBV-seronegative recipients of EBV-seropositive donor organs).

Tuberculosis in SOT
(➔ See 'Mycobacterium tuberculosis complex (MTBC)' Chapter 14.)
   While TB may be donor transmitted or community acquired, it usually develops as a result of reactivation of latent infection in the SOT recipient. Active TB in the SOT recipient results in a higher rate of morbidity, mortality, and graft loss post SOT.

Most patients develop TB infection in the first year post transplantation but there is a bi-modal distribution, with the incidence of TB peaking at 2 years after SOT. The rate of post-transplant TB is dependent upon the organ transplanted (highest for lung transplant). Other risk factors for post-SOT TB include use of lymphocyte-depleting antibodies, enhanced immunosuppression, chronic renal insufficiency/haemodialysis, diabetes mellitus, HCV infection in kidney transplant recipients, chronic liver disease, increased recipient age, and a positive tuberculin skin test (TST)/IGRA pre-transplant.

Although pulmonary disease is most common, extrapulmonary or disseminated TB incidence is higher than in the general population. Immune reconstitution and haemophagocytic syndrome associated with TB have also been reported.

A high index of suspicion is essential for performing an appropriate diagnostic workup. Invasive procedures may be necessary to obtain specimens from body sites most likely to yield mycobacteria.

Diagnosis of latent TB infection (LTBI)

Because active TB is associated with a high mortality rate in SOT recipients, all transplant candidates should undergo evaluation for LTBI. TST is currently the standard method for identifying subjects at risk. Patients with either positive or negative TST results should undergo an IGRA test (although sensitivity may decrease with increasing immunosuppression). In the case of discrepant results, any positivity (unless related to a documented BCG vaccination) should be considered for the treatment of LTBI. In those SOT candidates with negative results but a high-risk pre-transplant exposure history, consider thoracic imaging and/or LTBI therapy. Before initiation of treatment of LTBI, patients with positive immunological test results (TST and/or IGRA) should be evaluated in order to rule out active TB. If IGRA tests are unavailable, a second TST (7–10 days after the first test) should be performed in patients with a negative reaction, to exclude a boosting-related skin conversion.

Treatment of LTBI to prevent disease

Evaluate carefully to exclude active TB before initiating single-drug therapy for LTBI. The drug of choice is isoniazid supplemented with vitamin B6 for 9 months. Treatment should be considered pre-transplant to those on waiting lists or to recipients after transplantation who have one or more of the following conditions: (1) a TST (initial or after a booster effect) with a 5 mm induration or positive IGRA result; (2) a history of untreated TB; or (3) a history of contact with a patient with active TB. Careful monitoring for drug toxicity or interactions, particularly in patients with organ failure, should be performed.

Chemoprophylaxis/preventive therapy for LTBI need not be completed before transplant, but should be re-initiated as soon as the patient is stable after transplant. Treatment interruptions may require a reassessment for development of active TB and the duration may need to be extended.

When active TB cannot be ruled out, treatment should be considered with the standard four drugs. Treatment can be completed with isoniazid alone if cultures for MTBC are negative after 8 weeks.

Treatment of active TB

Pre-transplant treatment

Active TB under treatment is regarded as a relative contraindication for SOT in many centres other than emergency heart, lung, or liver transplant. Individuals developing severe anti-TB drug-induced liver injury may also require emergency transplantation. In general, patients should have at least completed the induction period (2 months).

Post-transplant treatment

In general, the same short-course treatment regimen (2 HRZE/4 RH) is recommended for transplant recipients as for other patients with TB. However, frequent interactions between rifamycins and immunosuppressants can complicate treatment and there is an increased frequency of adverse anti-TB drug events. A rifamycin-free anti-TB treatment regimen is therefore an important option in non-severe localized cases and in periods with high rejection rates to avoid drug interactions that may increase the risk of graft rejection.

Rifamycin-based regimens are recommended for severe localized or disseminated disease. When rifamycins are used, levels of immunosuppressive drugs should be closely monitored, and the dose of calcineurin inhibitors, mTOR, and steroids increased. Maintenance therapy with isoniazid and rifampicin/rifabutin is recommended for at least 9 months. In regimens that do not include rifamycins, maintenance therapy with isoniazid and ethambutol (or pyrazinamide) is recommended for 12–18 months; the incorporation of a third drug, such as pyrazinamide or levofloxacin, could reduce this to 12 months.

MDR-TB

Only a few case reports of MDR-TB in SOT recipients have been published. In non-SOT individuals with MDR-TB infection, treatment with second-line anti-TB therapy for 18–24 months achieved a 75% long-term success rate. If isoniazid and rifamycins cannot be used, induction should include four to six drugs, including injectables (e.g. streptomycin, amikacin, kanamycin, or capreomycin), linezolid/other second-line drugs, for up to 2 years after culture conversion.

Non-tuberculous mycobacteria

In SOT recipients, the incidence of NTM infections is highest in heart and lung transplants (0.24–2.8% and 0.46–2.3%, respectively). Pleuropulmonary NTM disease is the most common manifestation in lung transplant recipients, but most other SOT patients manifest with cutaneous lesions of the extremities (nodular/ulcerative), tenosynovitis, or arthritis. Over half exhibit dissemination with involvement of non-contiguous areas. NTM infections generally occur late, up to 10 years after SOT, and the causative agents vary with type of transplant. Failure to respond to standard antimicrobials may provide the first clue.

Diagnostic principles

Isolation of an NTM organism from a normally sterile body site (e.g. blood, CSF) provides conclusive proof of invasive disease. Local disease is diagnosed when skin, soft tissue, and lymph node lesions showing granulomata on biopsy yield an NTM species on culture. Diagnosis of significant lung infection is established when:

- clinical presentation is compatible *and*
- radiographic images are consistent with NTM *and*
- other diagnoses have been excluded *and*
- NTM organisms are recovered from respiratory specimens (one BAL/ two consecutive sputa) or from pulmonary tissue.

Treatment principles

(➲ See 'Non-tuberculous mycobacteria (NTM)' Chapter 14.)

Treatment may require a combination of antimicrobials, surgical excision, and/or reduction of immunosuppressants.

Prevention of infection

Antimicrobial prophylaxis

Antimicrobial prophylaxis has significantly altered the incidence and severity of post-transplant infections. Six general preventive strategies are used:

1. *Vaccination:* ➲ see Table 7.3 p.119–120.
2. *Surgical prophylaxis:* perioperative antibiotics according to local guidelines.
3. *Universal prophylaxis:* provides antimicrobial therapy to all transplant recipients for a defined time period e.g. TMP–SMX for *Pneumocystis jirovecii*.
4. *Pre-emptive or pre-symptomatic therapy:* utilizes a sensitive, quantitative assay (e.g. molecular, antigen detection) to monitor patients for the presence of a specific disease at predetermined intervals to detect early infection prior to the emergence of invasive disease. Positive assays initiate therapy. Pre-emptive therapy incurs extra costs for monitoring and coordination of outpatient care while reducing drug costs and drug toxicities.
5. *Targeted prophylaxis:* the use of prophylaxis in specific subgroups of transplant recipients who are deemed to be at particular risk following specific individualized assessment. For example, individuals considered to be over-immunosuppressed based on qualitative assays or intensification of immunosuppression for graft rejection.
6. *Educated avoidance:* includes lifestyle changes that may limit exposure to potential pathogens (wearing masks or gloves while gardening, avoiding attics or basements with moulds, and using filtered water supplies).

Three advances in prophylaxis have significantly altered transplant medicine: anti-*Pneumocystis jirovecii*, antifungal, and anti-CMV agents.

Pneumocystis jirovecii prophylaxis

(➲ See 'Atypical fungi' Chapter 13.)

TMP–SMX is given at most centres to prevent *Pneumocystis jirovecii*. It also provides prophylaxis for *Toxoplasma gondii*, *Cystoisospora belli* (previously known as *Isospora belli*), *Cyclospora cayetanensis*, many *Nocardia* and *Listeria* species, and common urinary, respiratory, and GI pathogens. The duration varies between different centres from 3 months to lifelong therapy. Low-dose TMP–SMX is well tolerated and should be used in the absence of specific data demonstrating allergy or interstitial nephritis. Alternative anti-pneumocystis prophylactic strategies (e.g. dapsone) lack this breadth of protection.

Antifungal prophylaxis

The use of antifungal prophylaxis forms part of the strategy for the prevention of invasive fungal disease. Other key measures include correct identification of patients at increased risk of fungal infection, optimization of surgical procedures, optimal manipulation of immunosuppression, and environmental control of certain filamentous fungi.

Table 7.8 Antifungal prophylaxis in SOT

Transplant type	Target population	Antifungal drug and alternatives	Duration
Kidney	No prophylaxis		
Liver	**High-risk liver transplant recipients**	If one major or two minor criteria:	2–4 weeks or until
	High-risk criteria	Micafungin or caspofungin or Lip-	resolution of risk
	Major: re-transplantation, fulminant hepatic failure, MELD ≥30,	AB IV or AB lipid complex IV or	factors
	renal failure requiring replacement therapy.	anidulafungin	
	Minor: MELD score 20–30, split, living-donor,		
	choledochojejunostomy (Roux-en-Y), high transfusion requirement		
	(≥40 units of cellular blood products), renal failure not requiring		
	replacement therapy (CrCl <50 mL/min), early reintervention,		
	multifocal colonization/infection by *Candida* spp.		
Pancreas	All recipients	Fluconazole	1–2 weeks
Pancreas-kidney	**High-risk pancreas transplant recipients**	Caspofungin or micafungin or	Determined by the
	High-risk criteria	anidulafungin or Lip-AB IV	presence of risk factors
	Enteric drainage		
	Haemodialysis, CrCL <50 mL/min		
	Acute rejection and poor initial allograft function		
	Laparotomy after transplantation, vascular thrombosis		
	Post-perfusion pancreatitis anastomotic problems		

(Continued)

Table 7.8 Contd.

Transplant type	Target population	Antifungal drug and alternatives	Duration
Intestinal	All recipients	Fluconazole	3–4 weeks or until healing of anastomosis and absence of rejection
	High-risk intestinal transplant recipients	Lip-AB IV or caspofungin or micafungin or anidulafungin or AB lipid complex	
	High-risk criteria		
	Acute rejection and poor initial allograft function		
	Haemodialysis		
	Laparotomy after transplantation, anastomotic problems		
Lung/lung-heart	All recipients or targeted prophylaxis for high-risk recipients	Nebulized Lip-AB until resolution of bronchial suture	Nebulized Lip-AB: indefinite or for a minimum of 12 months
	High-risk criteria	Voriconazole	Targeted prophylaxis determined by the presence of risk factors
	Induction with alemtuzumab		
	Thymoglobulin®		
	Acute rejection		
	Single-lung transplant		
	Aspergillus spp. Colonization pre or during first year post transplant		
	Acquired hypogammaglobulinaemia (IgG <400 mg/dL)		
Heart	**High-risk heart transplant recipients**	Itraconazole or voriconazole or posaconazole or echinocandins	At least 3 months
	High-risk criteria		
	Acute rejection haemodialysis		
	Re-exploration after transplantation		
	Aspergillus spp. heavy colonization of air		

CrCl, creatinine clearance; MELD, Model for End Stage Liver Disease.
Adapted from Gavalda et al. Invasive fungal infections in solid organ transplant recipients. *Clinical Microbiology and Infection* Sept 2014: 20(7):27–48. Copyright © 2014 European Society of Clinical Microbiology and Infectious Diseases. Open Access.

Due to a lack of clinical trials and to epidemiological differences in invasive fungal infection in different transplant programmes, there are no definitive recommendations on prophylaxis. The selection of universal versus targeted prophylaxis is based on the type of transplant and one must bear in mind the effectiveness, safety, side effects, and drug interactions of the antifungal agent selected (Table 7.8).

Invasive candidiasis is the most frequent infection in SOT, but invasive aspergillosis carries a higher morbidity/mortality, so in certain SOT populations, prevention strategies for both of these infections must be combined.

Prevention of NTM disease in lung transplant patients

Patients with cystic fibrosis or chronic lung diseases who may become SOT candidates and who are colonized with rapidly growing mycobacteria should be considered for post-transplant chemoprophylaxis to prevent surgical site infections. Patients infected or colonized with *Mycobacterium avium* complex (MAC) should be considered for multidrug MAC therapy prior to lung transplantation.

Immunization: general points

(For specific recommendations, ➔ see Table 7.3 p.119–120.)

- Vaccination should be withheld from SOT recipients during intensified immunosuppression, including the first 2-month post-transplant period, because of the likelihood of inadequate response. However, the inactivated influenza vaccine can be administered ≥1 month after transplant during a community influenza outbreak.
- Standard, age-appropriate inactivated vaccine series should be administered 2–6 months after SOT.
- Hepatitis B vaccine should be considered for chronic hepatitis B-infected recipients 2–6 months after liver transplant in an attempt to eliminate the lifelong requirement for hepatitis B immune globulin.
- Vaccination should not be withheld because of concern about transplant organ rejection

Cytomegalovirus prophylaxis

(➔ See 'Cytomegalovirus (CMV/HHV-5)' Chapter 11.)

Antiviral prophylaxis or pre-emptive therapy should be used for the prevention of CMV replication and disease after SOT. Risk is highest among:

- mismatched donor–recipient (donor positive/recipient negative)
- lung and intestinal transplant recipients
- those who have received lymphocyte-depleting antibody therapy (Thymoglobulin®, ATG, OKT®3, alemtuzumab).

In these patients, prophylaxis is the preferred strategy as any mistake in the essential surveillance for pre-emptive therapy could result in the development of CMV disease. CMV donor negative/recipient negative SOT patients do not require CMV prophylaxis but should receive CMV-negative or leucocyte-reduced blood products. Detecting CMV-specific cell-mediated immunity can identify patients at reduced risk of CMV replication and disease.

Drug choice

First-line choice is valganciclovir or ganciclovir. CMV immune globulin can be considered as an adjunct to prophylaxis in high-risk lung, heart/lung, heart, or pancreas SOT recipients.

Resistance to ganciclovir has been demonstrated in 5% of transplant recipients receiving primary prophylaxis. Duration depends on organ transplant. The minimum duration of antiviral prophylaxis should be 6–12 months for lung and intestinal transplantation and 3–6 months for D+/R– kidney, heart, and liver transplantation (Table 7.9).

Consider restarting prophylaxis (or pre-emptive strategy) for patients who have received lymphocyte-depleting antibodies for the treatment of rejection. Always maintain vigilance for late-onset CMV and treat accordingly.

Pre-emptive therapy

When a pre-emptive approach is used, monitoring of CMV viral load in peripheral blood by PCR should be done every 1–2 weeks for the first 3 months post SOT. More frequent testing (i.e. twice weekly) may be considered in patients at high risk (i.e. D+/R– patients, early post transplant, and following use of lymphocyte-depleting antibodies). If viraemia is detected, start valganciclovir or ganciclovir until clearance of viraemia, and not for <2 weeks. Then either switch to secondary prophylaxis or resume pre-emptive approach.

Table 7.9 Duration of CMV prophylaxis in SOT recipients by organ type

Transplanted organ	D+/R–	R+
Kidney	6 months	3 months
Pancreas; kidney/pancreas; liver; heart	3–6 months	3 months
Lung and heart/lung	>12 months	6–12 months
Small intestine	6–12 months	6–12 months

HSV/VZV prophylaxis should be considered in seropositive patients who are not already on CMV prophylaxis, at least during the first 1 month post SOT. Consider re-starting during periods of intensified immunosuppression (Zostavax® is contraindicated in these patient populations).

Acknowledgement

This chapter was kindly reviewed by Dr Richard Haynes, Consultant in Renal Medicine, at Oxford University Hospitals NHS Trust.

Further reading

1. Gavaldà J, Aguado JM, Manuel O, et al. A special issue on infections in solid organ transplant recipients. Clinical Microbiology and Infection 2014;20(Suppl 7):1–3.
2. Fishman JA, AST Infectious Diseases Community of Practice. Infection in solid organ transplant recipients. American Journal of Transplantation 2009;9(Suppl 4).S3–6.
3. Rubin LG, Levin MJ, Ljungman P, et al. 2013 IDSA clinical practice guideline for vaccination of the immunocompromised host. Clinical Infectious Diseases 2014;58(3):309–18.
4. Bumbacea D, Arend SM, Eyuboglu F, et al. The risk of tuberculosis in transplant candidates and recipients: a TBNET consensus statement. European Respiratory Journal 2012;40:990–1013.
5. Wright AJ, Fishman JA. Central nervous system syndromes in solid organ transplant recipients. Clinical Infectious Diseases 2014;59(7):1001–11.

Chapter 8

Infections in haematopoietic stem cell transplant recipients

Introduction

Haematopoietic stem cell transplantation (HSCT) has a central role in the treatment of a variety of benign and malignant diseases. The major causes of early morbidity and mortality are disease relapse, acute graft-versus-host disease (aGvHD), regimen-related toxicity, graft failure, and infection. Long-term survivors of HSCT are at risk of a variety of long-term adverse effects, including chronic GvHD (cGvHD), endocrine disturbances, disease relapse, second malignancy, and, again, infection. The incidence of and types of infection that can develop vary with time since transplantation, different sources of stem cells, different preparative regimens, different types of immunosuppression, comorbidities, and whether the individual experiences cGvHD.

Overview of haematopoietic stem cell transplant

HSCT involves the transplantation of multipotential haemopoietic stem cells by infusion in order to restore bone marrow function. HSCT is usually used in the treatment of haematological malignancy, benign causes of marrow failure, or in the treatment of congenital immune defects. Ablation of the native bone marrow is usually necessary prior to transplantation.

Stem cell sources

Traditional methods rely on harvest of bone marrow for the stem cell source. Possible sources for these stem cells include:

1. the patient's own cells (autologous)
2. an identical twin (syngeneic, HLA identical), or
3. a sibling, or related or unrelated donor (allogeneic; HLA identical, haploidentical, or mismatched).

Allogeneic mismatched/unrelated donors are being used more frequently now but carry an increased risk of GvHD and graft failure.

More recent methods include the use of granulocyte colony stimulating factor (G-CSF)-mobilized peripheral blood stem cells and umbilical cord blood (UCB) for transplantation (HLA identical, haploidentical, or mismatched).

- Peripheral blood stem cells provide improved myeloid and T-cell recovery (and therefore a reduced risk of early infections) but carry a greater risk for chronic GvHD and associated complications.
- UCB provides an alternative stem cell source for 70% of patients without a matched sibling donor. UCB transplants, once engrafted, have a lower rate of GvHD, and if GvHD develops, it responds better to treatment than GvHD associated with adult stem cell sources. However, UCB transplanted patients have prolonged engraftment, with delayed immune recovery from UCB-derived stem cells. This renders them transfusion dependent for long periods, and also makes them more prone to infections, especially viral (e.g. CMV).

Conditioning regimens

One of the main treatment benefits of allogeneic HSCT (AHSCT) is the effect of preparative chemoradiotherapy conditioning regimens in eradicating the underlying disease. Classical conditioning regimens are *myeloablative*—the commonest combinations being busulfan or total body irradiation together with cyclophosphamide. These produce more mucosal injury and longer durations of neutropenia than non-myeloablative regimens, and therefore higher risk of infections. The addition of T-cell-depleting agents (e.g. ATG or alemtuzumab) to conditioning regimens has been associated with a reduced incidence of GvHD and diminished graft rejection but may delay immune recovery and therefore increase the risk of infections. Increasingly *non-myeloablative* (reduced intensity conditioning) regimens are now being used. These use cytotoxic drugs or low-dose total body irradiation and have been associated with reduced non-relapse mortality, in part due to a reduction in bone marrow toxicity and reduced risk of GvHD, while retaining the beneficial effect of graft versus tumour (e.g. combination of fludarabine and busulfan).

Pre-transplant considerations

Screening for infection

This is important for detecting asymptomatic infection in the donor in order to exclude unsuitable donors. In the recipient, screening serves to identify infections with the potential to reactivate post transplant. It also helps define specific infection control policies and antimicrobial prophylaxis and therapy, which may be necessary after transplantation. All donors and recipients should have a thorough clinical evaluation for recent or past infectious disease exposures, and all recipients should have a chest X-ray. Table 8.1 outlines the pathogen-specific testing required 1–2 months prior to transplant. If the donor is living, a clinical/epidemiological and vaccination history should be taken and testing for TB considered.

Any cadaveric organs/perfusates should be cultured and blood products screened for HIV, HBV, HCV, and *Treponema pallidum*.

Malaria: donors who have travelled to a malaria-endemic area should defer donation for 1 year following their return. Former/current residents of endemic areas should defer donation for 3 years. If not feasible, the donor should be treated empirically for malaria prior to donation.

Contraindications to stem cell donation

- HIV infection.
- Acute CMV or EBV infection.
- Acute hepatitis A infection (determined by a positive hepatitis A IgM).
- Acute toxoplasmosis.
- Active TB (until it is well controlled).
- An acute tick-borne infection (e.g. Rocky Mountain spotted fever, babesiosis, anaplasmosis, ehrlichiosis, Q fever, or Colorado tick fever).
- Active or past history of Chagas disease.
- Acute or recent West Nile virus infection.

Management of current/recent recipient infections prior to transplant

- Bacterial infections should be treated until recovery, *prior* to transplantation. For more severe infections, including mycobacterial infections, extended treatment courses are often required and should be continued post transplant.
- Recipients with symptomatic viral infections (e.g. RSV, parainfluenza) should not be transplanted until there is full clinical resolution. CMV in particular has a high relapse rate post transplant and a high fatality rate if the patient is transplanted within 6 months of disease. (See 'Cytomegalovirus prophylaxis' p.142 for pre-emptive/prophylactic strategies post HSCT.)
- Recipients with invasive fungal infections (e.g. hepatosplenic candidiasis and aspergillosis) prior to transplant, should go straight onto secondary prophylaxis with low-dose antifungals after completion of a full treatment course. This should continue throughout the period of increased risk (i.e. while their neutrophil counts remain low).

Table 8.1 Pathogen-specific testing in pre-transplant screening

Pathogen-specific testing	Donor	Recipient (allogeneic or autologous)
CMV IgG	+	+
Hepatitis B (HBs, anti-HBs, anti-HB core) ± viral load	+	+
Hepatitis C IgG	+	+
Hepatitis C viral load	+	−
VZV IgG	+	+
HSV IgG	+	+
EBV (VCA IgG)	+	+ (especially allogeneic & T-cell depleted)
HIV-1 & -2 antibodies		
HTLV-1 & -2 antibodies		
RPR/VDRL/*T. pallidum* antibody	+	+
Toxoplasma gondii IgG	+	± (allogeneic only, especially T-cell depleted)
Screening for TB	±	+
MRSA nasal & VRE rectal culture	−	+
Travel to/residence in endemic areas		
Strongyloides stercoralis serology	+	+
Histoplasma capsulatum serology	−	±
Trypanosoma cruzi serology	+	±
Malaria film/rapid test ± PCR	+	+
West Nile virus antibodies	±	−

VCA, viral capsid antigen; VDRL, Venereal Disease Research Laboratory.

Immunizations prior to transplant

The HSCT donor should be up to date with routinely recommended vaccines based on age, vaccination history, and exposure history. However, administration of live vaccines (such as MMR and varicella (VAR)) to the donor should be avoided within 4 weeks of stem cell harvest. The same applies to HSCT candidates (if they are not already immunosuppressed); the interval prior to starting the conditioning regimen should be ≥4 weeks for live vaccines and ≥2 weeks for inactivated vaccines. Non-immune immunocompetent HSCT candidates aged ≥12 months should receive VAR (as a two-dose regimen if there is sufficient time) when the interval to start the conditioning regimen is ≥4 weeks.

Immune deficiency and infection during HSCT

Immune deficiency during and after HSCT results from destruction of the native marrow during conditioning and is then succeeded by the recovery of immune function following engraftment of the transplanted stem cells. This is best considered in three overlapping phases.

Phase 1 (0 to ~30 days, up to 45 days)

This is the pre-engraftment phase. It involves myeloablative conditioning leading to destruction of humoral and cell-mediated immunity. There is profound neutropenia lasting days to weeks. Approximate neutrophil recovery time is 2 weeks with G-CSF-mobilized peripheral blood stem cell grafts, 3 weeks with marrow grafts, and 4 weeks with UCB grafts. Myeloablative damage to natural protective barriers (mucosa, GI tract) also occurs, providing a source for bloodstream seeding of commensal GI tract pathogens. As a result, infectious complications in the immediate post-transplant period usually present as febrile neutropenia, with the severity of risk related to the depth and duration of neutropenia and the degree of mucosal damage induced.

Phase 2 (~30–100 days)

The stem cell infusion or transplant marks the beginning of phase 2; the immediate post-engraftment period where monocyte and T-cell immunity starts to recover (NK cells first, then CD8 T cells), but remains impaired. Immunological recovery continues beyond 100 days (into phase 3) and can take 18–36 months to fully replenish.

Phase 3 (beyond 100 days)

B cells and CD4 T cells take the longest to recover with slow restoration of repertoire during phase 3. Several studies have shown that CD4+ recovery is associated with diminished risk of infection and improved transplant outcomes. B-cell recovery is fastest after UCB grafts and is delayed by GvHD and its treatment (steroids). Infections seen at different phases reflect these changes in the immune repertoire (Figure 8.1).

For recipients of non-myeloablative grafts, infectious complications may be much less during phase 1, but the susceptibility to infections during phases 2 and 3 is largely similar, and driven primarily by the status of the underlying disease, a history of GvHD, and/or the need for ongoing immunosuppression.

This immune deficient state makes the HSCT recipient (especially if allogeneic) the perfect host for a variety of infections, some of which are already latent within the host and can reactivate (e.g. herpesviruses), but some of which may originate from the transplant or environment.

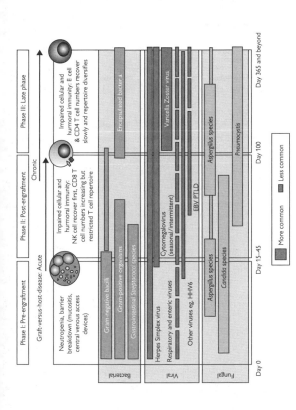

Fig 8.1 Common infections by time after transplantation. Reproduced with permission from Tomblyn M et al. Guidelines for preventing infectious complications among hematopoietic cell transplantation recipients: A global perspective. *Biology of Blood and Marrow Transplantation.* 2009; 15:1143.

Sources of infection

Host (endogenous)
- Reactivation of viruses.
- Barrier disruption causing invasive disease (mucositis/IV catheters).
- Colonization with resistant flora (VRE, yeasts).
- Reactivation of fungi (*Aspergillus*) or parasites (*Toxoplasma, Strongyloides*).

Environmental (exogenous)
- Inhalation of spores e.g. *Aspergillus* (need for positive pressure ventilation).
- Opportunistic pathogens (*Legionella, Listeria, Pneumocystis jirovecii, Cryptococcus neoformans*).

Transplant/blood products
- Viruses (CMV/HBV/HCV/HIV/HHV-6/HHV-7/TTV/parvovirus/HTLV-1/-2).
- Bacteria (stem cell contamination/TB).
- Unknown (e.g. variant Creutzfeldt–Jakob disease, pig retroviruses).

Clinical and investigative approach

Undifferentiated fever

>50% of HSCT patients will develop fever prior to engraftment and fever is the best indicator of infection in these patients. Infectious causes vary depending on the stage post transplant (➲ see Figure 8.1 p.151). In the early stages (prior to engraftment and up to 100 days, phases 1 and 2), the commonest causes are:

- systemic bacterial sepsis
- HSV and respiratory viruses
- mould infections (aspergillosis)
- chronic disseminated candidiasis
- catheter/line-associated infections.

Later on in phase 3 (>100 days), viruses such as CMV, EBV (➲ see 'EBV and post-transplant lymphoproliferative disease' p.167), adenovirus, and HHV-6 become significant. Sinopulmonary infection and mycobacterial infections, and other infections associated with chronic GvHD also become important. About a third of patients with NTM disease have a central venous catheter-related infection (bacteraemia, exit site, or tunnel infection), most of which are caused by the rapidly growing NTM (e.g. *Mycobacterium fortuitum, M. abscessus,* and *M. chelonae*).

There are several *non-infectious* causes of fever to consider. These include:
- steroids for conditioning-related toxicity (and other drugs)—any phase
- aGvHD (also predisposes to infection and can precipitate late bacteraemias, phase 2)
- tumour fever (e.g. in context of relapse, phase 2–3)
- cGvHD (phase 3)
- adrenal insufficiency (phase 3).

GvHD and EBV-associated lymphoproliferative disease must be carefully considered in the setting of persistent fever despite broad-spectrum antimicrobials and multiple negative tests for infection, in a patient with an HLA mismatch or unrelated donor.

Respiratory presentations

In addition to the more conventional factors to consider in the assessment of respiratory complaints, careful assessment in the HSCT recipient should include:
- time of onset of pulmonary disease (pre/post engraftment)
- pre-transplant serostatus (CMV/HIV/VZV/EBV)
- prior exposures (cats, birds, endemic fungi, mycobacteria)
- radiation exposure (timing/dose)
- drugs causing pulmonary or cardiac toxicity and/or predisposing to opportunistic infection
- prophylaxis.

All febrile HSCT recipients with respiratory symptoms should be treated empirically with broad-spectrum antibiotics, until a causative organism is identified or an alternative diagnosis is confirmed. The choice of empirical therapy should depend upon the risk for specific infections, whether the presentation is community or hospital acquired, and the local susceptibility patterns. Refer to local guidelines.

Antimicrobial prophylaxis is crucial to ascertain. For example, those taking co-trimoxazole are highly unlikely to have *Pneumocystis jirovecii* pneumonia, whereas in those with bilateral pulmonary infiltrates who are no longer taking this or who take a prophylactic agent without *P. jirovecii* cover, this becomes a much more likely differential. Similarly, those on aciclovir/valaciclovir prophylaxis are more prone to infection with CMV than those on valganciclovir.

In the unwell patient not responding to first-line antimicrobials, have a low threshold for performing a CT and bronchoscopy to obtain respiratory samples for bacterial culture (including *Legionella* spp.) and fungal culture (+ stain), viral PCR including CMV, *P. jirovecii* PCR/immunofluorescence, mycoplasma PCR, staining for AFB and mycobacterial culture ± galactomannan (depending on assay availability). In parallel, always send blood EDTA for CMV PCR, serum for CrAg and galactomannan, and urine for *Legionella* antigen.

Phase 1

Infections due to Gram-positive and Gram-negative bacteria occur in association with neutropenia. Mucositis due to the conditioning regimen contributes to aspiration risk. Pulmonary infection occurs in ~10% of HSCT recipients in phase 1.

Infectious causes:
- Bacterial pneumonia.
- Viral (including RSV, parainfluenza, CMV).
- Fungal (invasive aspergillosis; associated with the dip in neutrophil count).

Non-infectious causes are also important in this phase:
- Fluid overload.
- Conditioning-regimen related pneumonia/hypersensitivity drug reaction.
- ARDS (can be non-infective or associated with infection/sepsis).
- Pulmonary embolism/haemorrhage.
- Hyperacute GvHD (occurs in the first 14 days post transplant and is frequently associated with both skin involvement and non-cardiogenic pulmonary oedema).

Careful history and examination are required as chest X-rays can look very similar. Bilateral diffuse changes can be seen in most of the non-infectious causes, in fungal/viral/atypical bacterial infections, and in ARDS. Focal consolidation is more likely to be due to bacterial infection, mould infection, embolism, or haemorrhage. Viral pneumonias are often seasonal and associated with close contact, though parainfluenza occurs all year round. Steroids are a major risk factor in the progression of upper respiratory tract infection to lower tract involvement.

Phase 2

Infectious causes of pulmonary infection during phase 2:
- Bacterial pneumonia.

- Viral pneumonia (mainly RSV, parainfluenza, adenovirus, and CMV)— likely to cause diffuse infiltrates (Table 8.2).
- Fungal pneumonia (mainly *Aspergillus* spp.; localized nodular or diffuse X-ray changes).
- *P. jirovecii* pneumonia: bilateral diffuse X-ray changes.
- *Cryptococcus neoformans* pneumonia: presents as nodules, lobar infiltrates, adenopathy, or effusions. Often causes ARDS. Lumbar puncture is crucial to exclude CNS infection; treat as such if high CrAg titre or severe lung disease, even if lumbar puncture normal.
- *Nocardia* spp. (usually *N. asteroides*) pneumonia: suspect in any patient who presents with concurrent brain, soft tissue or cutaneous lesions, and focal/nodular lung consolidation.
- Other bacterial infections including *Legionella* spp., *Mycoplasma* spp., TB, NTM: likely to cause localized X-ray changes ± extrapulmonary features.
- Parasitic infections including disseminated toxoplasmosis and disseminated *Strongyloides* infection can involve the lungs and should also be considered (if exposure).

The differential also includes several other *non*-infectious causes:

- Idiopathic pneumonitis syndrome (seen with exposure to busulfan, high-dose cyclophosphamide, radiation, and non-myeloablative conditioning regimens; extensive opacities on imaging, tests for infection negative, often needs biopsy to confirm aetiology).
- Cryptogenic organizing pneumonia (associated with irradiation, CMV infection, and cGvHD; requires biopsy for confirmation).
- Bronchiolitis obliterans (seen in cGvHD and also after viral respiratory infections).
- Radiation pneumonitis (occurs acutely 4–12 weeks post radiation, ground-glass appearance on imaging. Also seen later at 6–12 months with evidence of scarring/dense consolidation/volume loss) (Table 8.2).
- Drug toxicity.
- Connective tissue disease (may be extrapulmonary manifestations/ autoantibodies but often needs biopsy to confirm type).
- Malignancy (underlying lymphoma).

Phase 3

During this phase, infections occur secondary to residual immunosuppression and immunosuppression associated with chronic GvHD and its treatment. The main respiratory infections seen in chronic GvHD include:

- late CMV pneumonitis (± disseminated disease)
- invasive aspergillosis
- pneumonia secondary to encapsulated bacteria such as *Streptococcus pneumoniae* (in those not receiving antibacterial prophylaxis or in whom prophylaxis has been stopped)
- VZV and EBV-related PTLD or lymphoma can also present with respiratory symptoms
- TB (➔ see 'Special considerations' p.166).

Radiographic changes in pulmonary infection

Table 8.2 Radiographic presentations of pulmonary complications, pre and post engraftment (*infectious causes in italics*)

| | Radiological appearances on chest X-ray and CT chest | | | | |
	Clear	Focal consolidation	Diffuse/ground glass	Nodular	Miliary
Pre engraftment (phase 1)	Early bron-chiolitis obliterans	*Bacterial/ aspiration pneumonia* Embolism Alveolar haemorrhage	Hyperacute GvHD *Respiratory viruses* *Atypical bacteria, e.g. Legionella* *Fungal pneumonia*	*Fungal pneumonia* *Nocardia* *Mycobacteria* Malignancy Embolism	*M. tuberculosis*
Post engraftment (phase 2/3)		*Bacterial pneumonia incl. NTM* Late radiation pneumonitis	*CMV* *Respiratory viruses* *P. jirovecii* *Cryptococcus* COP Pulmonary veno-occlusive disease Pulmonary oedema Idiopathic pneumonitis syndrome Acute radiation pneumonitis Late bronchiolitis obliterans Connective tissue disease	*CMV* COP	*M. tuberculosis* *VZV*

Invasive fungal infection

Always consider the HSCT recipient's risk profile for an invasive fungal infection due to the high morbidity and mortality associated with delayed diagnosis (see Table 8.3 for specific risk factors). Aspergillosis is far more common than mucormycosis, especially in the context of respiratory infiltrates. The majority occur *after* engraftment, corresponding to the period of aGvHD.

Table 8.3 Risk factors for invasive mould infections in HSCT recipients

Risk factors for invasive aspergillosis (IA)		Risk factors for mucormycosis in HSCT
In HSCT	General risk factors	
Prolonged engraftment e.g. UCB recipients	Haematological malignancies (effect of neutropenia)	Iron overload
Past history of IA pre HSCT	SOT (especially lung and liver)	Diabetes mellitus
HLA mismatched or unrelated donors	Severe liver disease	Chronic hyperglycaemia due to steroids
T-cell depleted grafts	COPD	Pre-exposure to *Aspergillus*-active drugs e.g. voriconazole/ echinocandins
GvHD and steroids	ITU patients	Colonization with *Zygomycetes*
Acute CMV or RSV infection	Influenza	
Active leukaemia	Post surgery	
Secondary graft failure	Chronic granulomatous disease (*A. tanneri*)	
Colonization with *Aspergillus* spp.		

Source: data from Kontoyiannis D.P. Antifungal prophylaxis in hematopoietic stem cell transplant recipients: the unfinished tale of imperfect success. *Bone Marrow Transplantation*. 46(2) 165–73. Copyright © 2011 Nature Publishing Group.

Gastrointestinal presentations

Diarrhoea

A very common presentation in HSCT patients. Stool should always be sent for microscopy, culture, and sensitivity, *C. difficile* toxin, ova, cysts and parasites ± viral PCR (depending on the exposure history/time of year/ phase post transplant).

Phase 1

- Bacterial gastroenteritis, especially:
  - *C. difficile*: can present atypically (normal leucocyte count, lack of pseudomembranes). Always consider if concomitant abdominal pain/ tenderness. GvHD can also complicate this.
  - *C. septicum* (rare).
- Neutropenic enterocolitis (typhlitis).
- Viral gastroenteritis: enteroviruses, norovirus (summer); rotavirus (winter and spring).

Phase 2

As for phase 1 plus:

- Adenovirus; can reactivate or be acquired *de novo*. Can cause diarrhoea and in severe cases a haemorrhagic colitis ± other organ involvement. Risk factors include severe GvHD requiring high-dose glucocorticoids, T-cell depletion, alemtuzumab or ATG, and matched unrelated donor/haploidentical or UCB grafts.
- *Cryptosporidium parvum* (rare).

Phase 3

As for phase 1 and 2 plus:

- CMV; can occur alone or concomitantly with GvHD. Colonic biopsies should therefore be carefully evaluated for both.
- EBV; late manifestations of EBV may include GI tract involvement with a risk of bleeding and perforation.

Note: diarrhoea is much less commonly a manifestation of cGvHD compared with aGvHD. Infectious aetiologies should therefore be thoroughly investigated.

While infections need to be excluded, there are several non-infectious causes that can occur at any phase, including:

- drug toxicity (particularly during phase 1), e.g. oral magnesium (frequently given to counteract the hypomagnesaemia induced by calcineurin inhibitors)
- mucosal injury secondary to conditioning regimen
- bleeding
- infarction
- GvHD (acute in phase 1 and 2, and the commonest and most important cause of diarrhoea in phase 2, usually occurring with a rash ± other organ involvement; acute or chronic in phase 3). Colonoscopy and biopsy may be necessary to evaluate this if diarrhoea is persistent and stool cultures/PCR are negative for infection.

Hepatitis

This can be caused by drug toxicity during any phase, but especially during the phase 1 conditioning regimen and by aGvHD or cGvHD. Hepatic sinusoidal obstructive syndrome (or hepatic veno-occlusive disease) can also occur during phases 1 and 2 and should be ruled out.

Infectious causes of hepatitis to consider include the following:

Phase 1

- Bacterial sepsis.
- HSV.
- Chronic disseminated candidiasis.

Phase 2

- Viruses: acute infection with hepatitis A or E (if exposure history); chronic infection with HBV, HCV, HEV, EBV, HSV, CMV, HHV-6—all representing viral reactivation in the context of immunosuppression.
- Bacterial sepsis.
- *P. jirovecii*.
- Chronic disseminated (hepatosplenic) candidiasis.

Phase 3
- Viruses as for phase 2 plus VZV.

As for immunocompetent patients, consider rarer causes in patients with an exposure history: e.g. leptospirosis, Q fever, and syphilis.

Oesophagitis

This can be caused by drugs during any phase, by *Candida* spp. and HSV during phase 1 and by *Candida* spp., HSV, and CMV during phase 2. Empirical treatment with antifungals is reasonable in the setting of clinically apparent oropharyngeal candidiasis (fluconazole unless oral swabs have cultured fluconazole resistant non-albicans *Candida*, in which case voriconazole or an echinocandin may be more appropriate). However, if no obvious cause after a full examination (with no clinical evidence of HSV/CMV reactivation elsewhere) and/or if no response to antifungals, endoscopic evaluation with biopsies sent for histology, viral PCR, and culture (with full fungal sensitivities if fungal) may be necessary.

Neurological presentations

Infections account for up to 40% of CNS lesions in HSCT patients, carry a high mortality, and may manifest subtly due to a blunted inflammatory response. Typical presentations include seizures or an altered Glasgow Coma Scale score, and fever may be absent. Seizures are less frequent than in immunocompetent counterparts and some SOT patients. Immunosuppressive drug toxicity and metabolic disturbances are still more common causes of CNS disturbance than infection and so non-infectious causes must always be considered in HSCT recipients with neurological symptoms and/or signs (Table 8.4). General systemic sepsis from an occult source should also always be in the differential.

Diagnostic approach

A thorough general clinical examination, in addition to neurological examination, should attempt to demonstrate signs of a possible metastatic infection, e.g. pneumonia, cardiac murmur, sinusitis, or skin lesions. Any skin lesions should be biopsied for culture and histopathology. Due to the non-specificity of clinical presentation, early brain imaging ± lumbar puncture in the first 24–48 hours are key if the cause is not apparent and the patient has persistent CNS symptoms or signs. Brain imaging appearances help to direct further diagnostic investigations. A brain biopsy may be necessary if the cause is not apparent on initial investigation. Focal brain abscesses often require physical drainage/debridement in addition to targeted antimicrobial therapy. See Figure 8.2. for a suggested approach to diagnosis and management of CNS lesions.

Causative organisms

Meningoencephalitis is predominantly due to viruses (largely the herpesviruses) and less frequently due to *Listeria monocytogenes, Toxoplasma gondii, and Cryptococcus* spp. Brain abscesses may be caused by mycelial fungi and by bacteria (NB *Nocardia* spp.). Table 8.5 outlines the key clinical/imaging features of these, and the time interval post transplant at which these tend to occur. This information can be valuable in the diagnostic work-up of a CNS presentation and can facilitate treatment decisions.

Table 8.4 Non-infectious neurological complications post HSCT

Phase post HSCT	Phase 1	Phase 2	Phase 3
Non-infectious causes of CNS disturbance	Drug toxicity	Drug toxicity—e.g. fludarabine causes delayed progressive cortical damage → encephalopathy	Leucoencephalopathy (immunosuppression related): always check TAC/CIC levels. Lesions reversible once drug reduced/stopped
	Subdural haematoma	Tumour relapse	Tumour relapse
	Infarcts		Posterior reverse encephalopathy syndrome (PRES): associated with calcineurin inhibitors (visual changes, altered sensorium)
			Central pontine myelinolysis

CIC ciclosporin; TAC tacrolimus.

Dermatological presentations

Drugs are the most common culprits of skin rash in HSCT recipients but there are a number of infections that can involve the skin/soft tissue and can often provide important clues to the aetiology of systemic disease (Table 8.6).

Positive blood culture

Bacteraemia is most common during the pre-engraftment period (phase 1) when patients are neutropenic. The associated mortality is high if appropriate treatment is delayed. In the setting of a confirmed bacteraemia antimicrobial therapy can be targeted in addition to re-culturing and the pursuit of a persistent focus/dual pathology. Therapy should be broadened if there is either no clinical improvement or a deterioration in the patient's condition.

The commonest organisms isolated from blood cultures are:

Phase 1
Bacteria: (*S. aureus*, coagulase-negative staphylococci, Gram-negative organisms including *Escherichia coli*, *Klebsiella* spp.). Fungi: *Candida* spp.

Phase 2
As for phase 1.

Phase 3
Encapsulated bacteria (e.g. *S. pneumoniae*, *Neisseria meningitides*), staphylococci, Gram-negative organisms including *Pseudomonas* spp.

Table 8.5 Key features of CNS infections at different phases post HSCT

CNS infections	Phase post HSCT	Clinical presentation/imaging[a]	Treatment
Bacteria			
Nocardia spp.	Usually 3 (2–6 months, after prolonged immunosuppression)	Brain abscess in AHSCT: multiple, often loculated, ring-enhancing. *N. asteroides*: pulmonary disease with CNS dissemination. *N. brasiliensis*: cutaneous lesions	Co-trimoxazole + meropenem ± surgery
Listeria spp.	Usually 3(> 100 days)	Meningoencephalitis, frequently + bacteraemia ± brain abscess (rhomboencephalitis rare). PCP prophylaxis (co-trimoxazole) usually protects against this	Ampicillin + gentamicin (3 weeks)
Staphylococcus aureus and Gram negatives (e.g. *Klebsiella* spp., *Pseudomonas* spp.)	1–3	Brain abscess, solitary or multiple. Usually associated with bacteraemia from a primary source (*S. aureus* abscess often associated with endocarditis)	6–12 weeks of systemic antimicrobials. Consider surgery if solitary/large
Viruses			
HSV	1	Early meningoencephalitis. No more likely than in immunocompetent	Aciclovir (3 weeks)
HHV-6(HHV-7)	1–2 (Reactivation with viraemia occurs in first 2–4 weeks ~50% of cases of encephalitis occur in first 4 weeks	Meningoencephalitis (rare) (hippocampus/limbic system → memory loss sequelae) Fever up to 40°C CSF often <5 cells/μL, raised CSF protein CT/MRI normal or asymmetric non-enhancing temporal lobes. HHV-6 DNA detected in CSF & peripheral blood	Ganciclovir/foscarnet (at least 21 days) Treat until HHV-6 PCR undetectable in peripheral blood Repeat lumbar puncture for HHV-6 PCR/other infective causes if no improvement

(Continued)

Table 8.5 Contd.

CNS infections	Phase post HSCT	Clinical presentation/imaging[a]	Treatment
CMV	2–3 (Usually ~150–300 days)	(1) Ventriculitis (rare). Rapidly progressive, periventricular flare & subependymal lesions on MRI. CSF pleocytosis + CMV DNA (2) Myelitis (3) Polyradiculopathy Occurs in delayed immune reconstitution, haploidentical, T-cell depletion, GvHD, recurrent CMV viraemia & ganciclovir-resistant CMV infection	Ganciclovir Alternatives: valganciclovir/foscarnet/cidofovir Continue until CMV PCR negative in CSF & serum & clinical resolution. Then secondary prophylaxis: valganciclovir
EBV	2–3 (usually late, but seen in phase 2 in T-cell deficient)	PTLD (⊙ see 'EBV and post-transplant lymphoproliferative disease' p.167) Can also cause seizures/aseptic meningitis	Reduce immunosuppression± Rituximab
VZV	2–3 (Usually phase 3)	Meningoencephalitis: associated with chronic GvHD Also seen after discontinuation of aciclovir prophylaxis	
JC virus	3 (>6 months to years)	PML. Infrequent in transplant recipients, insidious presentation, occurs in those with very low CD4 counts (& rituximab/fludarabine). Imaging: multifocal, asymmetric, spares grey matter, no oedema/enhancement. CSF analysis usually normal but JC virus PCR positive in 70–90%	No effective treatment in transplant setting Very poor prognosis
Fungi			
Moulds Aspergillus (A. fumigatus most common)	1–2	Early brain abscess (dissemination from lungs): predilection for frontoparietal lobes). Vascular invasion can → infarcts/bleed Rapidly progressive change in mental status; seizures > focal neurological signs/meningism	Voriconazole Consider adding echinocandin

Organism		Clinical features	Treatment
Yeasts			
Cryptococcus neoformans	2–3 (usually >100 days)	Late meningoencephalitis (leptomeningeal involvement); subacute onset with headache and fever. Raised CSF opening pressure and positive CSF CrAg in virtually all, moderate pleocytosis, positive CSF culture in 90%	Liposomal amphotericin B + flucytosine
Candida spp.	1		Fluconazole
Dematiaceous fungi e.g. Dactylaria	1–3 Usually ~3 months. NB Can occur as late as 2 years	Increasing cause of brain abscess (single or multiple, ring-enhancing). Concomitant pulmonary/cutaneous involvement	Surgical resection plus itraconazole (or voriconazole/posaconazole)
Zygomycetes e.g. Mucor spp. Rhizopus spp. Rhizomucor spp. Cunninghamella spp.	1–3	Usually rhinocerebral	Liposomal amphotericin B + surgical debridement + reduction of immunosuppressants where possible
Protozoa			
Toxoplasma gondii	1–2 (usually first 3 months)	Brain abscess (multiple, periventricular, ± ring-enhancing) Meningoencephalitis Myocardium & lungs also frequently involved. Risk factors: positive serology; no co-trimoxazole prophylaxis; severe GvHD; high-dose steroids; T cell depleting agents, e.g. ATG[b]	Pyrimethamine + sulfadiazine: minimum 6 weeks after clinical resolution, then suppress Disseminated disease very high mortality in HSCT recipients: early diagnosis and Rx are crucial

[a] Abnormal enhancement may be lacking in neutropenic HSCT recipients due to the dampened inflammatory response; serology can also be unpredictable. [b] *T. gondii* can also cause: chorioretinitis/GBS/haemophagocytic syndrome/graft failure/cutaneous infection.

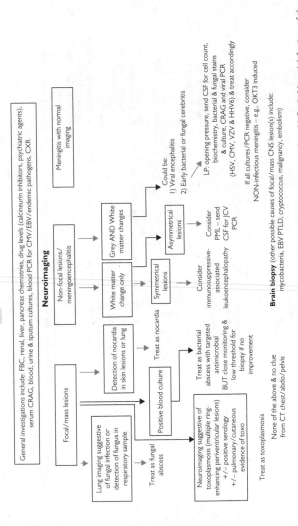

Fig 8.2 An approach to diagnosis and management of CNS lesions in HSCT recipients. Adapted with permission from N. Singh, H. N. et al. Infections of the central nervous system in transplant recipients. *Transplant Infectious Diseases.* 2(3), 101–111. Copyright © 2000 John Wiley & Sons. All rights reserved.

Table 8.6 Infectious causes of rash in HSCT recipients

Infectious causes of rash	Nature of rash		
Phase post HSCT	Maculopapular	Vesicular	Nodular
1	*Candida* Acute GvHD Drug toxicity	HSV Drug toxicity	Mould *Nocardia*
2	As above + HHV-6	VZV Drug toxicity	Mould NTM
3	MouldDrug toxicity Chronic GvHD	Drug toxicity	

Unexpected bone marrow suppression

- Phase 1/2: consider CMV, HHV-6, graft failure, drug toxicity, aGvHD.
- Phase 3: as for 1/2 *plus* parvovirus infection and cGvHD.

Special considerations

Graft-versus-host disease

GvHD is a syndrome in which transplanted immunocompetent donor cells recognize and attack host tissues in a stem cell recipient. Features occurring within 100 days of HSCT are classified as acute (aGvHD) and those occurring beyond 100 days as chronic (cGvHD). There is a considerable overlap between the two. GvHD remains a significant cause of morbidity and mortality in AHSCT recipients.

Acute GvHD

The incidence of aGvHD ranges from 10% to 80% with symptoms usually developing 2–3 weeks post transplant.

Risk factors for aGvHD include:

• degree of HLA mismatch
• older age
• previous donor alloimmunization
• nature of GvHD prophylaxis.

The diagnosis is often made clinically in patients who present with a classic maculopapular rash, abdominal pain with diarrhoea, and a rising serum bilirubin concentration within 2–3 weeks following HSCT. However, in many cases, the diagnosis is less straightforward and histological confirmation may be necessary. aGvHD is graded based on the degree of organ involvement; skin (surface area of skin rash), liver (serum bilirubin), GI tract (volume of diarrhoea) and assessment of clinical status. The stages of individual organ involvement are combined to produce an overall grade, which predicts prognosis:

• Grade I (A): mild disease (skin only, no liver or gut involvement)
• Grade II (B): moderate
• Grade III (C): severe
• Grade IV (D): life-threatening.

Chronic GvHD

cGvHD affects ~30–70% of AHSCT recipients surviving beyond 100 days, with a median onset of 4–6 months following HSCT. Risk factors include degree of HLA mismatch, age of recipient, and prior aGvHD. It remains the leading cause of late death in HSCT survivors, although it is associated with reduced relapse rate in patients transplanted for leukaemia. cGvHD commonly affects the skin (similar to lichen planus/cutaneous features of scleroderma), eyes, mouth, liver, GI tract, lungs, and genitalia. It is classified similarly to aGvHD, incorporating presence or absence of lung involvement. The latter can result in bronchiolitis obliterans from a combination of restrictive and obstructive lung disease. This can present similarly to infections (e.g. CMV, toxoplasmosis), interstitial lung disease, granulomatous disease (e.g. sarcoidosis), and diffuse alveolar haemorrhage. In many cases, histological confirmation is often necessary.

Corticosteroids remain the mainstay of treatment for both aGvHD and cGvHD, either alone or in combination with other immunosuppressants, and often continue for 2–3 years. GvHD and its therapy, leading to delayed immune reconstitution, are major risk factors for infection in HSCT recipients, especially with:

- herpesvirus infections: VZV and CMV
- invasive aspergillosis and other moulds
- *Pneumocystis jirovecii*
- encapsulated bacteria.

Some patients may suffer GvHD together with one or sometimes more infections simultaneously, each with overlapping clinical presentations. This can make diagnosis and treatment of all contributing insults challenging; the clinician must always consider the possibility of multiple pathologies in the most unwell HSCT recipients who have a slow response to one line of therapy.

EBV and post-transplant lymphoproliferative disease

EBV reactivation may originate from B cells from the donor and/or recipient. While most patients with EBV reactivation remain asymptomatic, a spectrum of virus-related lymphoproliferative disease can occur in HSCT recipients:

- An infectious mononucleosis-like acute illness: 2–8 weeks after induction, characterized by polyclonal B-cell proliferation without features of malignant transformation.
- As above but with features of early malignant transformation, e.g. cytogenetic abnormalities.
- PTLD: a more severe but heterogeneous clinical presentation with fever, lymphadenopathy, and/or extranodal monoclonal B-cell proliferation in various organs (liver, GI tract, lungs, central nervous system, bone marrow). The spectrum of disease ranges from nodular lymphoid lesions to widely disseminated high-grade B-cell lymphomas (Box 8.1). In the early stages it often presents non-specifically as fever/malaise and can adopt either an indolent or fulminant course. Early PTLD occurs within the first year of HSCT in EBV-seropositive recipients; late disease occurs beyond 5 years in EBV-seronegative recipients. The key differentials are infection and GvHD.

Box 8.1 Spectrum of PTLD

- Early lesions
  - Plasmacytic hyperplasia.
  - Infectious mononucleosis-like lesion.
- Polymorphic PTLD (lymphomatoid granulomatosis)
- Monomorphic PTLD (according to lymphoma they resemble)
  - B-cell neoplasms:
    —Diffuse large B-cell lymphoma.
    —Burkitt's lymphoma.
    —Plasma cell myeloma.
    —Plasmacytoma-like lesion.
    —Other.
  - T-cell neoplasms:
    —Peripheral T-cell lymphoma.
    —Hepatosplenic T-cell lymphoma.
    —Other.
- Classical Hodgkin lymphoma-type PTLD.

Risk factors for PTLD
- Unrelated/HLA mismatched/UCB transplants.
- T-cell depletion—e.g. ATG, alemtuzumab, anti-CD3.
- Chronic GvHD >1 year.
- EBV-positive donor, EBV-negative recipient.
- Prior EBV reactivation.
- Previous splenectomy.

Diagnosis and monitoring
Patients with risk factors for PTLD should get quantitative EBV DNA monitoring from day 0 to 3 months post HSCT. Those with chronic GvHD get continued monitoring for as long as immunosuppression continues. Viral load should be considered a guide only as it has a poor sensitivity and specificity for PTLD; rather it is a reflection of the extent of immunosuppression. Staging CT and biopsy of any lymphoid tissue lesions for histology (± EBV PCR) is fundamental to early diagnosis, especially as the main differentials—infection and GvHD—can also be life-threatening and may call for entirely different treatments.

Prevention and treatment
Recommendations are to intervene when EBV DNA reaches 1000–10,000 copies/mL, even without clinical evidence of PTLD and especially if there are two or more persistent titres of >10,000 copies/mL.

Management includes a combination of reducing the level of immunosuppression (where possible) and rituximab weekly infusions until DNA becomes undetectable by PCR. Other treatments that may be used include infusion of donor-derived EBV-specific T-cell lines, IFN-alfa-2b, and combination chemotherapy, particularly in rituximab-resistant disease.

It is especially important to remember to continue aciclovir and co-trimoxazole prophylaxis in patients receiving rituximab therapy due to the very high incidence of opportunistic infections.

Tuberculosis
(➜ See 'Tuberculosis in SOT' p.134 and ➜ Chapter 14.)
The magnitude of the TB risk in HSCT recipients is strongly associated with the epidemiology of TB in the general population to which the patient belongs. Recipients of AHSCT, particularly matched unrelated grafts, are at higher risk of TB than recipients of autologous HSCT. The risk of death from or with TB after HSCT is high (up to 50%).

Clinical spectrum
TB after HSCT is predominantly pulmonary with a wide spectrum of radiographic features. TB is generally a late complication, occurring beyond day 100. Earlier disease often manifests as a cryptic febrile illness. aGvHD, cGvHD, and the intensity of immunosuppressives are all independent risk factors.

Diagnosis of latent TB infection and active TB
Assessment for latent TB or active TB should be performed in candidates for HSCT with possible exposure risk (e.g. in recipients from endemic regions), using IGRA ± TST and a chest X-ray. Prior/recent chemotherapy, immunosuppressive therapy, or chronic renal failure may reduce TST

responses and render an IGRA falsely negative, so using a combination of both assays may result in a higher sensitivity.

Treatment of latent TB

All HSCT candidates with a positive TST or IGRA test result after targeted screening should receive preventive chemotherapy to reduce the risk for the development of TB. Given interactions with calcineurin inhibitors, rifampicin-free regimens may be preferred. Transplant patients are monitored closely during the first year and any new unexplained symptoms or signs should be analysed without delay. In this setting, the diagnostic approach must be aimed at direct detection of bacilli, and immunodiagnostic tests are not useful.

Donors with TB

Haematopoietic stem cells are very unlikely to harbour live *Mycobacterium tuberculosis* bacilli, except perhaps in a person with disseminated TB at the time of harvest. For living donors, the benefit of prophylactic chemotherapy to reduce the risk of TB transmission to the recipient is uncertain.

Treatment of active TB in HSCT recipients

In general, the same short-course treatment regimen (2 HRZE/4 RH) is recommended for transplant recipients as for other patients with TB; however, a rifamycin-free regimen (e.g. using a fluoroquinolone instead) is an important option in non-severe cases where interaction with immunosuppressives may be problematic. The continuation phase should be extended to 7 months in patients with pulmonary TB and cavitation on the initial chest radiograph and/or positive sputum cultures at 2 months of treatment, as they have a higher risk of relapse. Some experts recommend a continuation phase of 7–10 months in CNS TB because rifampicin and ethambutol have reduced CNS penetration. If a rifamycin is used, the risk of rejection may be increased due to lowered levels of prednisolone or calcineurin inhibitors. Consequently, steroid dosage should be increased by ~50%, and levels of ciclosporin, tacrolimus, and rapamycin should be carefully monitored and dosage adjusted accordingly. In general, patients awaiting HSCT who have active TB should have at least completed the induction period (2 months) if not the full treatment, prior to transplantation.

Cytomegalovirus (CMV)

(➲ See 'Cytomegalovirus prophylaxis' p.142 and ➲ 'Cytomegalovirus (CMV/HHV-5)' p.244.)

CMV is one of the most important viral infections in HSCT recipients, with significant morbidity and mortality. Disease tends to occur following engraftment up to ~100 days post transplant, but can occur later in the presence of heavy immunosuppression and/or GvHD. Where valganciclovir prophylaxis is used, late-onset CMV is now increasingly seen. Active CMV replication can also occur before or at the time of transplantation. In this situation, an antiviral should be started (IV ganciclovir, oral valganciclovir, or IV foscarnet) and the conditioning regimen should be delayed until the CMV infection is controlled (i.e. until evidence of decline of CMV viral load in the absence of CMV disease). The conditioning regimen may then be started during antiviral therapy. However, ganciclovir/valganciclovir should be switched to foscarnet at least 2 days prior to starting the conditioning regimen to prevent the myelosuppressive effects of these antivirals. Foscarnet may be stopped after 2 weeks if CMV PCR becomes undetectable, if there is no evidence of CMV disease, and if the patient does not fulfil the criteria for secondary prophylaxis. However, close monitoring should continue and treatment resumed at the first evidence of CMV reactivation or CMV disease. Table 8.7 shows the risk factors for CMV disease during the subsequent different phases post transplant and its clinical manifestations. The commonest presentations are with pneumonia and GI disease, though fever alone is common in seronegative patients, which can make diagnosis difficult.

Prevention strategies include both pre-emptive and prophylactic therapy, the former being used more commonly in this population due to risks of drug toxicity. Valganciclovir prophylaxis has not been found to be superior to a pre-emptive strategy in preventing CMV infection post HSCT; however, it has been associated with an increase in the use of haematopoietic growth factors. Table 8.8 outlines and compares prophylactic and pre-emptive strategies.

CMV treatment
(→ See Cytomegalovirus prophylaxis' p.142 and → 'Cytomegalovirus (CMV/HHV-5)' p.244.)

If the patient is CMV IgG-negative prior to transplant, any detectable CMV viral load post transplant is significant as this indicates a primary infection. If the patient is CMV IgG-positive prior to transplant, an increase of >1 log is considered significant and warrants treatment.

Table 8.7 Risk factors for CMV infection and end-organ disease in HSCT

Stage post HSCT	CMV risk factors	CMV presentation
Phase 1	CMV-positive recipient (& seronegative donor)	Infection or 'CMV syndrome': fever + leucopenia + thrombocytopenia without end-organ disease
	Increased age	(End-organ disease rare in first 30 days)
	Matched unrelated donor/ haploidentical/UCB transplant	
	T-cell depleting conditioning regimen: fludarabine/ATG/ Campath®/total body irradiation	
Phase 2	As above + GvHD	Infection or 'CMV syndrome':
	Delay of T cell recovery	Pneumonia (rare but most common end-organ disease)
Phase 3	Steroid use—GvHD	Infection or 'CMV syndrome':
	Delay of T-cell recovery	Pneumonia
	Non-myeloablative conditioning	GI disease (colitis/oesophagitis/ enteritis)
	CMV reactivation PRE day 100	CNS disease (ventriculitis), retinitis
		Other: myocarditis/ haemophagocytic syndrome/ adrenal gland involvement/cystitis/ nephritis

D = donor; R = recipient. Order of risk: D−/R+ > D+/R+ > D+/R−.

Table 8.8 CMV prevention strategies: pre-emptive versus prophylactic

Prevention strategy	Pre-emptive	Prophylactic
Description	Monitor weekly for CMV viraemia by PCR for 3-6 months post HSCT (longer in patients at risk for late-onset disease[a]): Start treatment on first sign of reactivation (identification of CMV viraemia—variable definitions used: copies/mL vs IU/mL) Continue until cleared and not less than 2 weeks Then switch to secondary prophylaxis or resume pre-emptive approach[b]	Start antiviral therapy immediately post engraftment
First-choice drug[c]	Valganciclovir or ganciclovir	Valganciclovir
Alternative	Foscarnet or cidofovir (+ probenecid)	Ganciclovir Foscarnet Cidofovir every other week (+ probenecid)
Advantages	Effective, targeted treatment Reduced risk of drug toxicity Less costly Reduced risk of late-onset CMV disease	Highly effective Activity against other herpes viruses
Disadvantages	Requirement for close virological monitoring Can miss cases/miss treatment window	High risk of neutropenia High risk of invasive fungal disease High risk of late CMV disease Delayed recovery of CMV-specific T cell function Overtreatment Potential for drug resistance

[a] Risk factors for late onset CMV disease: chronic GvHD; high dose steroids; T cell depleted or UCBT recipients; CD4 <100 cells/μL. [b] Secondary prophylaxis should be considered in patients recently treated with high dose immunosuppression (e.g. lymphocyte depleting antibodies); those with severe CMV disease; or those with >1 episode of CMV disease [c] IV ganciclovir is preferred in life threatening disease, very high viral loads, and if inadequate GI absorption.

CMV Treatment is with:

- valganciclovir orally or ganciclovir IV (may be preferred if life-threatening disease, very high viral loads, or if concern over GI absorption)
- adjunctive treatment with IV immunoglobulin (IVIG) or CMV-specific hyperimmune globulin should be considered in cases of life-threatening disease and is recommended in CMV pneumonitis due to its poor outcome.

Alternative CMV-active drugs that can be used if the patient is intolerant or has disease resistant to (val)ganciclovir include foscarnet and cidofovir. Ganciclovir resistance can occur and should be considered in the context of prolonged antiviral treatment or high-level immunosuppression, if the viral load does not fall after 2 weeks of appropriate therapy. CMV genotype testing to the *UL97* and *UL54* genes can confirm resistance. CMV *UL97* mutations are susceptible to foscarnet and cidofovir (and high-dose ganciclovir with certain mutations). Some units use a combination of ganciclovir and foscarnet (half dose of each) in patients who have resistance to or side effects from ganciclovir, or in patients who are already bone marrow suppressed. CMV *UL54* mutations may confer cross-resistance to all three drugs and here alternative treatments may be warranted. Newer agents include maribair, brincidofovir, and letermovir, currently in trials/available for compassionate use. Duration may vary but in principle, treatment should continue until CMV PCR has become undetectable, clinical disease has resolved, and at least 2–3 weeks of treatment have elapsed.

Chronic hepatitis B infection in HSCT

Figure 8.3 summarizes the natural course of chronic hepatitis B infection in transplant recipients. In the non-replicative (immune control) phase, most HSCT patients have a normal alanine aminotransferase (ALT), low or undetectable HBV DNA, and they can be either HBs positive or negative; those who are negative should have detectable HB core (HBc) antibody.

There is a high incidence of reactivation and subsequent HBV-related hepatitis, not only in HBsAg-positive patients (32–50%), but also in HBsAg-negative–anti-HBc-positive patients (3–50%). In the latter group, low titre anti-HBs (<10 mIU/mL) is a predictor of reappearance of HBsAg, and this risk can persist for many years after HSCT because of the long delay in reconstitution of the recipient's immune response to HBV. All HSCT recipients should therefore be screened for hepatitis B prior to transplant and screening should include a combination of testing for HBs, anti-HBs, anti-HB core and hepatitis B viral DNA, to ensure that HBs-negative (and/or DNA-negative) infected patients are identified. It is recommended that antiviral prophylaxis is offered to all HSCT patients with detectable HBV DNA, even if they are HBsAb positive. The choice of therapy is dictated by both the HBV DNA level and the duration of immunosuppression and therefore antiviral therapy required. Figure 8.4 outlines an approach to prophylaxis against HBV reactivation in immunosuppressed patients, including HSCT recipients.

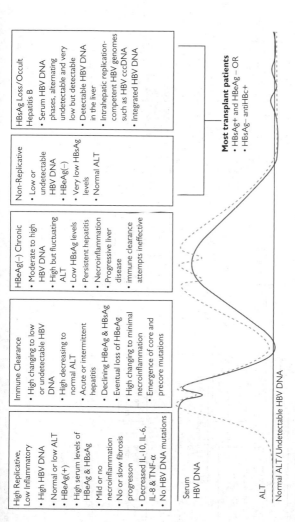

High Replicative, Low Inflammatory
- High HBV DNA
- Normal or low ALT
- HBeAg(+)
- High serum levels of HBeAg & HBsAg
- Mild or no necroinflammation
- No or slow fibrosis progression
- Decreased IL-10, IL-6, IL-8 & TNF-α
- No HBV DNA mutations

Immune Clearance
- High changing to low or undetectable HBV DNA
- High decreasing to normal ALT
- Acute or intermittent hepatitis
- Declining HBeAg & HBsAg
- Eventual loss of HBeAg
- High changing to minimal necroinflammation
- Emergence of core and precore mutations

HBeAg(−) Chronic
- Moderate to high HBV DNA
- High but fluctuating ALT
- Low HBsAg levels
- Persistent hepatitis
- Necroinflammation
- Progressive liver disease
- immune clearance attempts ineffective

Non-Replicative
- Low or undetectable HBV DNA
- HBeAg(−)
- Very low HBsAg levels
- Normal ALT

HBsAg Loss/Occult Hepatitis B
- Serum HBV DNA phases, alternating undetectable and very low but detectable
- Detectable HBV DNA in the liver
- Intrahepatic replication-competent HBV genomes such as HBV cccDNA
- Integrated HBV DNA

Most transplant patients
- HBsAg+ and HBeAg − OR
- HBsAg− antiHBc+

Serum HBV DNA

ALT

Normal ALT/Undetectable HBV DNA

Fig 8.3 The five major phases of chronic hepatitis B infection. Adapted with permission from Gish et al. Chronic hepatitis B. Virology, natural history, current management and a glimpse at future opportunities. *Antiviral Research*. 2015. 121, p. 47–58. ♾ http://dx.doi.org/10.1016/j.antiviral.2015.06.008

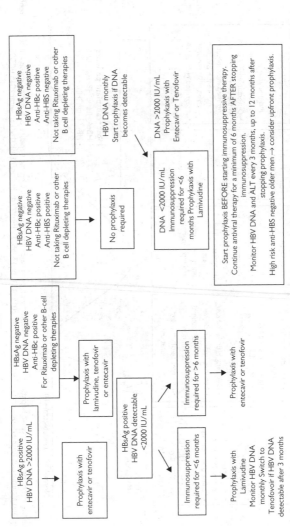

Fig 8.4 Approach to HBV prophylaxis in immunosuppressed patients. Source: data from National Clinical Guideline Centre (NICE). (2013) *Hepatitis B (chronic): Diagnosis and Management of chronic Hepatitis B in children, young people and adults*. London, UK: NICE. Copyright © 2013 National Clinical Guideline Centre. Available at: ℗ https://www.nice.org.uk/guidance/cg165/evidence/full-guideline-pdf-190175005.

HBsAg positive
HBV DNA >2000 IU/mL

↓

Prophylaxis with entecavir or tenofovir

HBsAg negative
HBV DNA negative
Anti-HBc positive
For Rituximab or other B-cell depleting therapies

↓

Prophylaxis with lamivudine, tenofovir or entecavir

HBsAg positive
HBV DNA detectable <2000 IU/mL

→ Immunosuppression required for >6 months → Prophylaxis with entecavir or tenofovir

→ Immunosuppression required for <6 months

Prophylaxis with Lamivudine
Monitor HBV DNA monthly Switch to Tenofovir if HBV DNA detectable after 3 months

---

HBsAg negative
HBV DNA negative
Anti-HBc positive
Anti-HBS positive
Not taking Rituximab or other B cell depleting therapies

↓

No prophylaxis required

DNA <2000 IU/mL
Immunosuppression required for <6 months Prophykaxis with Lamivudine

DNA >2000 IU/mL
Prophykaxis with Entecavir or Tenofovir

HBsAg negative
HBV DNA negative
Anti-HBc positive
Anti-HBS negative
Not taking Rituximab or other B cell depleting therapies

↓

HBV DNA monthly
Start rophylaxis if DNA becomes detectable

Start prophylaxis BEFORE starting immunosuppressive therapy.
Continue antiviral therapy for a minimum of 6 months AFTER stopping immunosuppression.
Monitor HBV DNA and ALT every 3 months, up to 12 months after stopping prophylaxis.
High risk anti-HBS negative older men → consider upfront prophylaxis.

Prevention of infection in HSCT

Donor selection

The key criterion in terms of donor selection is HLA match; this is critical for reducing the risk of complications that in turn increase the risk for infections following AHSCT (e.g. GvHD, graft failure, and delayed immune reconstitution).

Monitoring and prophylaxis are essential in the setting of CMV mismatch and if either donor or recipient is hepatitis B positive (see relevant sections for further details).

Pre-HSCT screening

➔ See 'Pre-transplant considerations' p.148.

Immunosuppression choice

It is crucial to strike a balance between sufficient immunosuppression (to prevent graft rejection and GvHD) but avoiding excessive immunosuppression or myelosuppression (and the increased risk of infection). In particular, steroids should be used carefully because of their profound effect on both innate and acquired immunity. When used, doses should be tapered as rapidly as possible to minimize the risk of infection. Avoidance or dose minimization of any myelosuppressive drugs should be ensured where possible.

Infection control measures

Patients and healthcare workers should be educated about the risk of and methods to prevent acquisition of potential nosocomial pathogens.

Protective isolation and room ventilation

All AHSCT recipients, especially during the early phases after HSCT, should ideally be placed in single protective environment rooms with the following features:

- ≥12 air exchanges per hour.
- High-efficiency particulate air (HEPA) filters.
- Directed airflow (so that air intake occurs at one side of the room and air exhaust occurs at the opposite side).
- Positive air pressure differential between the patient's room and the hallway.
- Well-sealed rooms, continuous pressure monitoring.
- Self-closing doors to maintain constant pressure differentials.
- (The benefit of laminar flow remains controversial.)

When there is a shortage of such rooms, priority should be given to those patients with the highest risk of infection (e.g. expected prolonged neutropenia, current treatment for GvHD, or those admitted for their initial transplant admission). Portable HEPA filter units may be used in normal rooms instead.

Construction or renovation

If construction or renovation occurs, intensified mould control measures should be put into place to minimize fungal spore counts in patient rooms. More intensive monitoring of clinical cases should also be performed at these times and AHSCT recipients should avoid construction areas and consider wearing respirator masks while outside of HEPA filtered areas.

Cleaning

HSCT units should be cleaned at least daily with special attention to dust control. Selection of furnishings should focus on creating and maintaining a dust-free environment.

Isolation and barrier precautions

At a minimum, standard precautions should be followed for all patient contacts. These include hand hygiene and appropriate personal protective equipment as for immunocompetent patients. Additional protective precautions (e.g. gloves and mask) are used in an attempt to further reduce the risk of transmission of respiratory viruses from healthcare workers and visitors to HSCT recipients. Some centres adopt these during respiratory outbreaks or during respiratory virus season, others all year round.

For further organism-specific guidance in the setting of a HSCT recipient, refer to 2009 guidelines (➲ see 'Further reading' p.182).

Care of intravascular catheters

Healthcare workers should follow established protocols for this.

Chlorhexidine bathing

Bathing patients daily with chlorhexidine gluconate has been shown to be an effective method of decreasing both hospital-acquired infections and colonization with drug-resistant organisms, primarily in the ICU setting. Benefit has also been shown in HSCT recipients.

Immunomodulation with colony stimulating factors

G-CSF and GM-CSF shorten time to engraftment, especially when the stem cell content of the graft is suboptimal after autologous HSCT. In a meta-analysis, colony stimulating factors were associated with a small reduction in the risk of documented infections but did not affect infection-related mortality or treatment-related mortality. At least one trial in AHSCT recipients suggested decreased survival in patients who received G-CSF. Thus, the use of growth factors is controversial in the setting of AHSCT.

Blood products

CMV-safe blood products (leucocyte filtered or from CMV-seronegative donors) should be used in CMV-seronegative AHSCT recipients whose allografts came from CMV-seronegative donors. Transfusion of red blood cells should be minimized when possible, due to the potential effect of iron overload. Several retrospective studies suggest iron overload may be associated with increased risk for post-transplant fungal and bacterial infection, as well as increasing the likelihood of aGvHD.

Intravenous immunoglobulin (IVIG)

Routine use of IVIG has not been found to be effective in preventing infections or other HSCT complications or in prolonging survival. Some centres check IgG levels in AHCT recipients with bacteraemia or recurrent sinopulmonary infections and administer IVIG to patients with levels below a threshold (e.g. ~400 mg/dL).

Antimicrobial prophylaxis

There are a number of recommended prophylactic antimicrobials to start routinely in HSCT recipients at the time of conditioning to protect against reactivation of latent infection and potential new exposures. These may vary slightly across institutions and it is always important to take into account both the specific susceptibilities of the particular HSCT candidate and the local epidemiology of infection. A suggested regimen based on the best available evidence and addressing the specific risks of different HSCT candidates is summarized in Table 8.9.

Antimicrobial prophylaxis should be started at the time of stem cell infusion and continued until either recovery from neutropenia or initiation of therapeutic antibiotics for febrile neutropenia. In general, the prophylaxis should not be continued after recovery from neutropenia.

Two exceptions to this are as follows:

TMP–SMX for Pneumocystis jirovecii

Generally started after engraftment and continued for as long as immuno-suppressive therapy is given (there is concern about myelosuppression during the first month post HSCT and the risk of *P. jirovecii* is low during this initial period).

Chronic GvHD

Prolonged antibiotic prophylaxis (with penicillin) is recommended for preventing infection with *S. pneumoniae* in AHSCT recipients with chronic GvHD, and in these patients is continued for as long as active treatment for GvHD is given (see Table 8.9)

Immunization in HSCT recipients

- Do not administer live vaccines to HSCT patients with active GvHD or ongoing immunosuppression.
- Avoid period of neutropenia.
- Avoid intramuscular injection if platelets are <50.
- Discount any 'during chemotherapy' doses in considering long-term protection.

Vaccinations considered 'optional' for HSCT recipients due to limited data on safety and efficacy and where the risk–benefit balance should be considered on a case-by-case basis, include hepatitis A, yellow fever, rabies, tick-borne encephalitis, and Japanese B encephalitis. Cholera, typhoid (oral live and intramuscular vaccines), and BCG are *not* recommended for HSCT recipients (Table 8.10).

Post-exposure prophylaxis in HSCT

Specific contacts or exposures post HSCT may warrant post-exposure therapy to reduce the risk of clinical disease (see Table 8.11).

Acknowledgement

This chapter was kindly reviewed by Dr Bhuvan Kishore, Consultant in Haematology, at University Hospitals Birmingham NHS Foundation Trust.

Table 8.9 Currently recommended antimicrobial prophylaxis regimens in HSCT recipients

Patient group/indication	Target pathogen	Antibacterial first choice	Alternative	Duration
All HSCT recipients with anticipated neutropenia of ≥7 days (those given myeloablative regimen) Autologous recipients with significant mucosal injury	Most common Gram-negative bacteria	Ciprofloxacin or levofloxacin	Azithromycin	Start at time of stem cell infusion and continue until recovery from neutropenia or start of empirical treatment for febrile neutropenia
Only allogeneic recipients with cGvHD or low IgG levels	Streptococcus pneumoniae	Penicillin	Macrolides, fluoroquinolones or second-generation cephalosporins	Continue as long as receiving active immunosuppression (beyond 100 days)
HSCT recipients or candidates with a positive TST or IGRA and no history of appropriate TB treatment and no clinical evidence of active TB disease or exposure to smear-positive patient	Mycobacterium tuberculosis	Isoniazid + pyridoxine	Rifampicin (but potential for significant interaction with immunosuppressants)	Start at completion of conditioning regimen (to avoid problematic drug interactions) & continue isoniazid for 9 months
Seropositive HSCT recipients: prevention of early reactivation (regardless of donor status)	HSV	Aciclovir	Valaciclovir	Start at beginning of conditioning & continue until engraftment or until mucositis resolves
Seropositive HSCT recipients: prevention of late reactivation	HSV	Aciclovir	Valaciclovir	Continue for 1 year after HSCT*
Prevention of disease reactivation	VZV	Aciclovir	Valaciclovir	Continue for 1 year after HSCT

CMV is covered in a more detailed separate table (see Table 8.8)

Recipients	Organism	Prophylaxis	Alternative	Timing
All recipients who have had/will have: Neutropenia & mucosal damage, or Graft manipulation, or Purine analogues But no other risk factors for invasive mould infection	Candida albicans (± non-albicans Candida less common)	Fluconazole	Echinocandin, e.g. micafungin Itraconazole/voriconazole/posaconazole	From start of conditioning until engraftment, or until 7 days after neutrophils >1000 cells/μL (continue 75 days in allo) Restart in patients with secondary graft failure
Allogeneic recipients with high risk for invasive mould infection[b]	Aspergillus(± Zygomycetes)	Posaconazole	Voriconazole/itraconazole (NB No mucor cover)	As above
Patients with specific risk for mucormycosis	Zygomycetes spp.	Posaconazole	Liposomal amphotericin B	As above
All allogeneic recipients	P. jirovecii	Trimethoprim–sulfamethoxazole[c]	Dapsone/ atovaquone(nebulized pentamidine)	Start at engraftment and continue for at least 6 months (>1 year in those on continued immunosuppression, with cGvHD or low CD4 counts <100 cells/μL)
Autologous recipients with underling haem malignancy/intense conditioning regimen/graft manipulation or purine analogues				
Other circumstances				
Immunocompromised recipients travelling to developing countries (see Chapter 10)		Ciprofloxacin		Continue for the duration of stay

[a] In AHSCT recipients consider aciclovir prophylaxis for >1 year if GvHD is present/ongoing immunosuppression/CD4 counts <100/μL to prevent VZV (zostavax is contraindicated in these populations). [b] Factors associated with high risk for IMI: prolonged engraftment; past history of invasive aspergillosis pre HSCT; haploidentical/T cell depleted/concurrent GvHD and steroids/active CMV infection or RSV/active leukaemia/re transplantation/secondary graft failure/colonization with fungi. [c] Also protects against Toxoplasma gondii reactivation in seropositive AHSCT recipients.

Table 8.10 Currently recommended immunizations for autologous and AHSCT recipients

Vaccine	Recommended for use after HSCT (quality of evidence[a])	Time post HSCT to initiate vaccine	No. of doses[b]
Pneumococcal conjugate (PCV13)	Yes (BI)	3–6 months	3[c], then single dose of polysaccharide PPVS23 at 12 months. NB if chronic GvHD give fourth dose of PCV13 instead
Tetanus, diphtheria, acellular pertussis[d]	Yes Tetanus–diphtheria: (BII) Pertussis (CIII)	6 months	3[d]
Inactivated polio	Yes (BII)	6–12 months	3
Haemophilus influenzae conjugate	Yes (BII)	6–12 months	3
Meningococcal C conjugate	Yes, for those aged 11–18 years (BII)	6–12 months	2, then booster at 16–18 years if received initial doses <15 years
Recombinant hepatitis B	Yes (BII)	6–12 months	3[e]
Inactivated influenza	Yearly (AII)	6 months4 if community outbreak	12 if aged 6 months–8 years
MMR[f] (live)	All children and seronegative adults. Measles: BII; mumps: CIII; rubella: BIII EIII (<24 months post HCT, active GvHD, on immune suppression)	24 months	1–2[g]
Varicella (Varivax®, live)	Varicella-seronegative patients (CIII): (>24 months, without active GvHD or on immunosuppression (NB Limited data regarding efficacy)	≥24 months	2 at 24 months(8–11 months after last dose of IVIG)

DtaP, diphtheria tetanus pertussis vaccine; HCT, haematopoietic cell transplant; PCV, pneumococcal conjugate vaccine; Tdap, tetanus toxoid reduced diphtheria toxoid reduced acellular pertussis vaccine.

[a] Evidence based rating system used in the HSCT guidelines: *Strength of recommendation* comprised of categories A–E: A—should always be offered; B—should generally be offered;

Table 8.10 *Contd.*

C—optional; **D**—should generally not be offered; **E**—should never be offered. *Quality of evidence supporting the recommendation*: **I**—evidence from at least one well executed randomized, controlled trial; **II**—evidence from at least one well designed clinical trial without randomization; cohort or case controlled analytic studies (preferably from more than one centre); multiple time series studies; or dramatic results from uncontrolled experiments; **III**—evidence from opinions of respected authorities based on clinical experience, descriptive studies, or reports of expert committees.

[b] As a general guideline, a minimum of 1 month between doses may be reasonable. [c] Following the primary series of 3 PCV doses, a dose of the 23 valent polysaccharide pneumococcal vaccine (PPSV23) to broaden the immune response might be given (BII). For patients with chronic GvHD who are likely to respond poorly to PPSV23, a fourth dose of the PCV should be considered instead of PPSV23 (CIII). [d] Three doses of tetanus/diphtheria–containing vaccine should be administered 6 months after HSCT. For children aged <7 years, 3 doses of DTaP should be administered. For patients aged ≥7 years, administration of 3 doses of DTaP should be considered. Alternatively, a dose of Tdap vaccine should be administered followed by either 2 doses of diphtheria toxoid combined with tetanus toxoid (DT) or 2 doses of Td vaccine. [e] If a post vaccination anti HBs concentration of ≥10 mIU/mL is not attained, a second 3 dose series of HepB vaccine should be administered (standard dose for children, high dose (40 mcg) for adolescents and adults). Significant improvement of the recipient response to hepatitis B vaccine post transplant can be expected only if the donor receives more than one hepatitis vaccine dose before donation. [f] A 2 dose series of MMR (measles, mumps, and rubella combination) vaccine should be administered to measles seronegative adolescents, adults, and children 24 months after HSCT in patients with neither chronic GvHD nor ongoing immunosuppression and 8–11 months (or earlier if there is a measles outbreak) after the last dose of IVIG. [g] Also consider administration of 3 doses of HPV vaccine 6–12 months after HSCT for female patients aged 11–26 years and HPV 4 vaccine for males aged 11–26 years (CIII)

Adapted with permission from Rubin et al. 2013 IDSA Clinical Practice Guideline for Vaccination of the Immunocompromised Host. *Clinical Infectious Diseases*. 58(3) 44–100. Copyright © 2013 Oxford University Press.

Table 8.11 Post-exposure prophylaxis in HSCT recipients

HSCT patient group	Target pathogen	Antimicrobial	Duration
Household contacts of person with invasive Hib disease[a]	H. influenzae	Rifampicin (or alternative if interference with other prophylactic agents, e.g. azoles)	4 days
Post-exposure prophylaxis (regardless of vaccination status)	Bordetella pertussis	Azithromycin or alternative macrolide or trimethoprim–sulfamethoxazole	4 days
Exposure to zoster or varicella or vaccinee who develops a rash: <24 months post HCT or >24 months or immunosuppressed or cGvHD	VZV	Varicella zoster IgG or (if IgG unavailable) valaciclovir	Ideally administer within 96 hours after close contact
Prevention of Strongyloides hyperinfection in HSCT recipients who show: Positive screening tests for Strongyloides spp. or	Strongyloides stercoralis	Ivermectin or albendazole	Repeat 2-day course after 2 weeks
Unexplained eosinophilia & travel history/ residence associated with Strongyloides spp. exposure			

[a] NB If all household contacts <4 years old are vaccinated then this is not necessary.
Source: data from Tomblyn M. et al. Guidelines for Preventing Infectious Complications among Hematopoietic Cell Transplant Recipients: A Global Perspective. Biology of Blood and Marrow Transplantation. 15(10) 1143–1238. Copyright © Elsevier. All rights reserved.

Further reading

1. Arnaout K, Patel N, Jain M, et al. Complications of haematopoietic stem cell transplant recipients. Cancer Investigation 2014;32:49–62.
2. Tomblyn M, Chiller T, Einsele H, et al. Guidelines for preventing infectious complications among hematopoietic cell transplantation recipients: a global perspective. Biology of Blood Marrow Transplantation 2009;15:1143–238.
3. Kontoyiannis DP. Antifungal prophylaxis in hematopoietic stem cell transplant recipients: the unfinished tale of imperfect success; Blood Marrow Transplantation 2011;46:165–73.
4. Bumbacea D, Arend SM, Eyuboglu F, et al. The risk of tuberculosis in transplant candidates and recipients: a TBNET consensus statement. European Respiratory Journal 2012;40:990–1013.
5. Engelhard D, Akova M, Boeckh MJ, et al. Bacterial infection prevention after hematopoietic cell transplantation. Blood Marrow Transplantation 2009;44:467–70.
6. National Comprehensive Cancer Network®. Guidelines on Prevention and Treatment of Cancer-related Infections: ℬ http://www.nccn.org
7. Rubin LG, Levin MJ, Ljungman P, et al. 2013 IDSA clinical practice guideline for vaccination of the immunocompromised host. Clinical Infectious Diseases 2014;58(3):309–18.

Medical conditions associated with immunocompromise

Introduction

In addition to conditions more usually associated with immunodeficiency (e.g. HIV, stem cell or SOT), several common conditions are known to be associated with defective immune function. This may be the result of pathological processes causing mainly structural damage (e.g. COPD, other chronic chest diseases), multisystem disease (e.g. diabetes), or chronic organ failure (e.g. renal and hepatic failure). The degree of immune paresis tends to mirror the progression of the underlying disease. In general, the precise mechanisms of immune dysfunction in many of these conditions are unclear, but the result is usually a broad impairment in immune function.

Acute insults to the body (such as trauma or critical illness) similarly result in an impaired ability to defend against infection; a fact that may be overlooked when concentrating on more immediate management priorities. However, infection is a leading cause of secondary complications in these patients. Physiological states such as pregnancy and the extremes of age result in immune function that may be significantly impaired when compared to the 'normal' host.

The approach to these conditions from an infection point of view must take account of the following:

• *Degree of immune compromise* may vary from relatively mild to severe.
• *Exposure to infection* is often much higher (e.g. repeated vascular access in renal dialysis).
• *Diagnosis may be challenging* as clinical features may be blunted, delayed, or absent.
• *Response to treatment* is often slow or poor.
• *Treatment options may be complicated* by underlying disease (e.g. use of drugs and dosing in renal and hepatic failure).
• *Morbidity and mortality* due to infection are often significantly higher than the background population.

These patients represent a challenge to the physician greatly in excess of patients with intact immune function; and they are *common*.

Mechanisms of immunosuppression

Immune defence is a complex and interconnected system; the effects of multisystem medical conditions on its function are diverse and poorly understood. Although separating specific associations between arms of immunity and specific medical conditions is problematic, broad associations include those listed in Table 9.1.

Table 9.1 Associations between medical conditions and defects in arms of the immune system

Arm of immune system	Medical conditions causing immune suppression	
Acute-phase proteins/ complement	• Congenital/acquired complement deficiency • Early HSCT • Diabetes mellitus • Liver failure	• Renal failure • Malnutrition • Major trauma • Alcoholism
Neutrophil/phagocytic function	• Diabetes mellitus • Liver failure • Pregnancy • Alcoholism • Leukaemia • Aplastic anaemia	• Down syndrome • Total body irradiation • Drugs (cytotoxic chemotherapy, methotrexate, azathioprine)
Cell mediated/ lymphocytic function	• HIV infection • SOT • HSCT • Diabetes mellitus • Primary T-cell deficiency syndromes • Thymic aplasia (Di George syndrome) • Renal failure • Pregnancy • Old age	• Malnutrition • Alcoholism • Drugs (corticosteroids, ciclosporin, methotrexate, cyclophosphamide, azathioprine, mycophenolate, biologics: rituximab, etanercept, infliximab) • Down syndrome
Adaptive immunity/ antibody	• Splenectomy and hyposplenism • Prematurity • Primary antibody deficiency syndromes • Prolonged critical illness • Major trauma	• Myeloma • Chronic lymphocytic leukaemia • Nephrotic syndrome • Protein-losing enteropathy • Dystrophia myotonica • Down syndrome

Diabetes and other endocrine disorders

Diabetes

Hyperglycaemia has wide-ranging negative effects on the immune system; precise mechanisms are unclear but innate and cellular immunity are affected, complement levels are depressed, and both cytokine production and clearance are poorly regulated. Neutrophil function appears particularly affected, as is macrophage and T-cell activity. Antibody production and function are largely intact and diabetics respond to vaccination as well as non-diabetics. Other consequences of diabetes act synergistically with infection to increase severity of illness (e.g. peripheral vascular disease, neuropathy). Infection is the precipitant or a complication of diabetic keto-acidosis in 75% of cases. Sepsis occurs with increased frequency and severity in people with diabetes, accompanied by higher mortality. Frequent hospitalization and antibiotic use make resistant organisms more likely.

Major presentations

Urinary tract infection/pyelonephritis
Glycosuria results in increased bacterial and candidal colonization and enhanced growth rate in the urinary tract.

Skin, soft tissue, and bone
Large vessel disease leads to limb ischaemia and necrosis, providing favourable circumstances for infection (particularly microaerophilic and anaerobic bacteria). Small vessel disease results in poor skin perfusion and neuropathy, contributing to pressure sores/ulcers and persistent superficial colonization with pathogenic organisms (e.g. *Staphylococcus aureus*, *Candida* spp.) Cannulation of the feet/legs should be avoided.

Superficial fungal infections
Impaired neutrophil function leads to increased susceptibility to fungal infection (e.g. candidiasis, onychomycosis, intertrigo); these can provide a portal of entry for the secondary bacterial infection.

Ulcers
Chronic skin defects due to vascular insufficiency and/or sensory neuropathy. They are usually chronically colonized and can be a source for infection of surrounding structures. Look for evidence of surrounding cellulitis or underlying deep tissue or bone infection. Infection usually caused by *S. aureus*, β-haemolytic streptococci, Enterobacteriaceae, or *Pseudomonas aeruginosa*. Antibiotic treatment or swabbing for culture of uninfected ulcers is of limited utility.

Cellulitis
Can occur either in association with ulcers or independently. Most common organisms are *S. aureus* (including MRSA) and β-haemolytic streptococci. Presents with redness, swelling, and pain associated with systemic symptoms of infection. Pain may be blunted by sensory neuropathy.

Soft tissue infection/necrotizing fasciitis
May be indolent or rapidly progressive with subcutaneous tissue necrosis (necrotizing fasciitis); this is a surgical emergency and urgent debridement

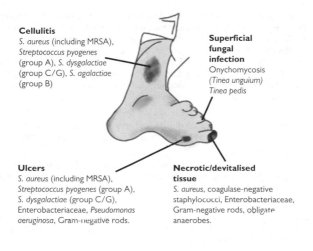

Cellulitis
S. aureus (including MRSA),
Streptococcus pyogenes
(group A), S. dysgalactiae
(group C/G), S. agalactiae
(group B)

**Superficial
fungal
infection**
Onychomycosis
(Tinea unguium)
Tinea pedis

Ulcers
S. aureus (including MRSA),
Streptococcus pyogenes (group A),
S. dysgalactiae (group C/G),
Enterobacteriaceae, Pseudomonas
aeruginosa, Gram-negative rods.

**Necrotic/devitalised
tissue**
S. aureus, coagulase-negative
staphylococci, Enterobacteriaceae,
Gram-negative rods, obligate
anaerobes.

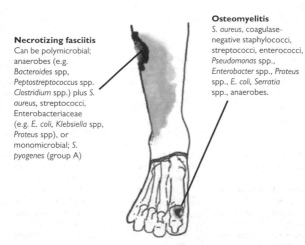

Osteomyelitis
S. aureus, coagulase-
negative staphylococci,
streptococci, enterococci,
Pseudomonas spp.,
Enterobacter spp., Proteus
spp., E. coli, Serratia
spp., anaerobes.

Necrotizing fasciitis
Can be polymicrobial;
anaerobes (e.g.
Bacteroides spp,
Peptostreptococcus spp.
Clostridium spp.) plus S.
aureus, streptococci,
Enterobacteriaceae
(e.g. E. coli, Klebsiella spp,
Proteus spp), or
monomicrobial; S.
pyogenes (group A)

Fig 9.1 Microbiology of diabetic foot infections.

is indicated in addition to antibiotics. Usually polymicrobial (synergistic); Gram-negative rods (Enterobacteriaceae), streptococci, *S. aureus* (including MRSA and PVL (Panton–Valentine leucocidin-producing strains), anaerobes (*Bacteroides, Peptostreptococcus*), or the classical group A (*Streptococcus pyogenes*) necrotizing fasciitis. Early necrotizing fasciitis is remarkable for the paucity of hard symptoms and signs. Pain is the most reliable and this may be attenuated by sensory neuropathy. Subcutaneous crepitus may be present if there are gas-forming organisms.

Pyomyositis

Bacterial infection of skeletal muscle leading to one or more intramuscular abscesses (majority caused by *S. aureus*). Found particularly in the tropics.

Necrotic or 'dead foot'

Culture yields multiple microbes, treatment is surgical. The presence of anaerobes signifies dead tissue. The presence of dead tissue should prompt surgery.

Osteomyelitis

Commonly *S. aureus* (including MRSA), coagulase-negative staphylococci, streptococci, enterococci, *Pseudomonas* spp., *Enterobacter* spp., *Proteus* spp., *Escherichia coli, Serratia* spp., and anaerobes.

Septic arthritis

Most commonly caused by *S. aureus* (including MRSA) followed by streptococci.

Abdominal

Increased risk of emphysematous cholecystitis (particularly in elderly diabetic men), ~50% will have gallstones. Major organisms are Gram-negative bacilli (*E. coli, Klebsiella* spp., *Enterobacter* spp., *Proteus* spp.), enterococci, and anaerobes (*Bacteroides* spp., *Clostridium, Fusobacterium* spp.). Leads to gallbladder empyema/perforation and septic shock.

Head and neck

Increased risk of soft tissue infections of the head and neck, two notable conditions:
- 'Malignant' otitis externa: caused by *Pseudomonas aeruginosa*, severe and life-threatening necrotizing infection extending into the base of skull (osteomyelitis) and CNS (cranial nerve lesions/neurological infection). Presents with yellow-green drainage from the ear, pain, and fever.
- Mucormycosis, or rhinopulmonary zygomycosis: caused by *Rhizopus* spp. (a saprophytic aerobic fungus (mould) found in soil), infection initiated by inhaled spores, and initially presents as acute sinusitis with rapid necrotizing infection of deeper structures causing cranial nerve defects and CNS infection. (➔ See 'Murcomycosis', p.315)

Tropical infection

➔ See Chapter 10.

Melioidosis-diabetes is a strong risk factor for diseases caused by *Burkholderia melioidosis*, endemic areas include Asia (particularly Southeast Asia) and northern Australia. Infection is acquired by exposure to soil and mud, particularly in rice paddies. (➔ See '*Burkholderia pseudomallei*', p.354)

Adrenal disease

Adrenal corticosteroids have wide-ranging effects on the body, including a major role in modulating immune response and physiological reactions to infection. Exact mechanisms are poorly understood, cellular immunity is particularly affected.

Adrenal insufficiency

Inadequate cortisol production profoundly affects the ability to mount an effective response to infection. Cortisol requirements are increased during infection and adrenal insufficiency may be unmasked by an infection causing life-threatening circulatory collapse. More commonly, secondary insufficiency due to long-term exogenous steroid use is a powerful risk factor for overwhelming sepsis if corticosteroid is not supplemented.

Cushing's syndrome/corticosteroid excess

Chronic corticosteroid excess causes depressed cellular immunity in a manner similar to long-term therapeutic use of exogenous corticosteroids. (➲ See 'Corticosteroids' p.35.)

Thyroid disease

Thyroid hormones have widespread effects on metabolism (including protein synthesis), and basic physiology, including immune function. Mechanisms are very poorly understood. Both hypothyroidism and hyperthyroidism are relatively immune-suppressed states.

Chronic liver disease

(➜ See Chapter 7 for infections relating to liver transplantation.)

The liver is a key immune organ; acute-phase proteins (including complement) that form the basis of the innate response are produced here and circulating endotoxin and cytokines are cleared by the liver. It also plays a vital role by clearing bacteria and toxins coming from the bowel via the portal circulation. Chronic liver disease results from repeated hepatic insults over a prolonged period of time leading to chronic inflammation and fibrosis. This has important deleterious effects on the liver as an immune organ. Production of complement and other acute-phase proteins is reduced; clearance of endotoxin cytokines is impaired. Damaged endothelium along the hepatic sinusoids along with depleted number and function of Kupffer cells prevent effective clearance of bacteria and toxins arriving from the bowel. Raised portal pressures result in porto-systemic shunting, allowing blood from the bowel to bypass the liver into the systemic circulation. Neutropenia occurs—this is thought to be mainly as a consequence of hypersplenism. Bowel mucosal integrity and immunity is impaired in chronic liver disease leading to increased gut translocation of bowel organisms. The situation is exacerbated by malnutrition and the accumulation of toxic nitrogenous compounds (e.g. ammonia) that have been shown to impair cellular immunity. In advanced liver disease, hepatic encephalopathy can result in depressed conscious states and impaired airway reflexes. (See Figure 9.2)

Many of the underlying causes of chronic liver disease are independent causes of immune dysfunction. These include chronic alcoholism (➜ see 'Alcoholism and substance misuse' p.213), hepatitis viruses, autoimmunity and its treatment, and haemochromatosis. Repeated hospitalization greatly increases the risk of acquiring resistant organisms. End-stage liver failure is a profoundly immunosuppressed state. ➜ see Chapter 7 for infections relating to liver transplantation.

Major presentations

Sepsis

Bloodstream infection leading to the systemic inflammatory response syndrome is common and can rapidly progress to multiorgan dysfunction and death (>30% of systemic infections in cirrhosis result in death). Renal failure complicates approximately one-third of presentations with sepsis in patients with cirrhosis. Common sources of infection in order frequency are: spontaneous bacterial peritonitis (SBP), urinary tract infection, pneumonia. Impaired cortisol synthesis results in adrenal insufficiency exacerbating circulatory compromise.

Variceal haemorrhage

Up to 45% of upper GI bleeds in patients with cirrhosis lead to bacteraemia or SBP. Bidirectional synergy exists between bleeding and infection; GI bleeding leads to increased infection and infection increases the risk of re-bleeding (potentially due to endotoxin-induced raised sinusoidal pressure). Antibiotic prophylaxis is indicated regardless of the presence ascites.

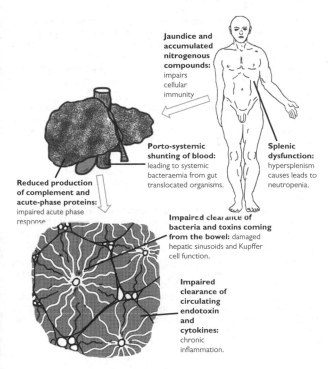

Jaundice and accumulated nitrogenous compounds: impairs cellular immunity

Splenic dysfunction: hypersplenism causes leads to neutropenia.

Porto-systemic shunting of blood: leading to systemic bacteraemia from gut translocated organisms.

Reduced production of complement and acute-phase proteins: impaired acute phase response

Impaired clearance of bacteria and toxins coming from the bowel: damaged hepatic sinusoids and Kupffer cell function.

Impaired clearance of circulating endotoxin and cytokines: chronic inflammation.

Fig 9.2 Mechanisms of immunosuppression in chronic liver disease.

Spontaneous bacterial peritonitis
Results from a combination of intraluminal bacterial overgrowth and damaged hepatic immune defence. In-hospital mortality rate from SBP is ~30%. The most common organisms are *Escherichia coli, Klebsiella* spp., other Gram-negative enteric bacteria, enterococci, and streptococci. There is a significant risk of recurrence following an episode of SBP; this is reduced by prophylactic antibiotics (usually quinolones), although this does result in increased rates of resistant organisms. Diagnosis is made by paracentesis. This procedure is indicated in all patients with ascites presenting with an illness compatible with infection. Polymorphonuclear cell count in ascitic fluid >250 cells/µL is considered diagnostic.

Other infections in chronic liver disease

Infections associated with iron overload
Defective iron processing in chronic liver disease results in an iron over-load state, this impairs cellular immunity. The growth of siderophilic

bacteria such as *E. coli, Listeria monocytogenes, Yersinia enterocolitica, Y. pseudotuberculosis* and *Vibrio* spp. are enhanced. *Vibrio vulnificus*, a mainly aquatic organism, is usually ingested in raw oysters or contaminates wounds exposed to the aquatic environment. It is particularly virulent in patients with chronic liver disease, and especially in untreated haemochromatosis.

Tuberculosis

Liver cirrhosis is a significant risk factor for clinical *Mycobacterium tuberculosis* disease. Incidence, virulence, and extrapulmonary involvement are all increased. Treatment is complicated by hepatotoxicity of antituberculosis drugs. (➔ See 'Tuberculosis (TB)', p.337).

Cryptococcal infection

Incidence of invasive disease caused by *Cryptococcus neoformans* is elevated in chronic liver disease. (➔ See '*Cryptococcus* spp', p.323).

Endocarditis

Increased risk due to recurrent bacteraemias, impaired immune clearance, and frequent invasive medical investigations. *S. aureus*, β-haemolytic streptococci, and enterococci are the main pathogens.

Enteric disease

Clostridium difficile disease occurs more frequently; likely due to recurrent courses of antibiotics, the use of long-term prophylactic antibiotics, and the use of proton pump inhibitors. (➔ See '*Clostridium difficile*', p.347)

Y. enterocolitica and *Y. pseudotuberculosis* are Gram-negative bacilli associated with a wide variety of domestic and wild animals. They cause diarrhoea and invasive disease in cirrhosis including hepatic abscesses and septicaemia. Invasive disease has a poor prognosis.

Chronic renal failure and dialysis

(➜ See Chapter 7 for infections relating to renal transplantation.)

Infection is the second most frequent cause of death in end-stage kidney disease. Exposure to infection is increased and immune function is globally suppressed. In addition, infection is harder to diagnose and more difficult to manage (fluid management, drugs, etc.). Immune suppression is multifactorial; uraemia impairs cellular immune response, chronic protein loss depletes acute-phase proteins. Renal replacement therapy contributes to increased exposure to infection and to the suppression of immune response. Haemodialysis causes nephrotic-range protein loss and exposure of blood to haemodialysis membranes activates acute-phase proteins contributing to the depletion of important components of the innate response such as complement. Recurrent vascular puncture and indwelling vascular catheters provide a regular portal of entry and favourable environment for pathogens. Although much reduced in many parts of the world, transmission of blood-borne viruses via dialysis equipment remains a significant threat. Peritoneal dialysis catheters are a source of infection, both at the entry site and in the peritoneum. Frequent attendance at hospitals and recurrent antibiotic use increase the occurrence of resistant organisms and nosocomial infections such as MRSA and *Clostridium difficile*. The prevalence of significant comorbidity in patients with renal disease (e.g. diabetes, vascular disease) contributes to poorer outcomes from infection. ➜ see Chapter 7 for infections relating to renal transplantation.

Infections associated with chronic renal failure (non-renal replacement related)

Sepsis

Common and severe in chronic kidney disease. Degree of immunosuppression mirrors severity of renal disease. Usually caused by common organisms (*Escherichia coli*, staphylococci, streptococci). Antibiotic use, dosing, and fluid management are also complicated by renal impairment.

Respiratory

Incidence of pneumonia in chronic kidney disease is increased up to three times, and up to five times in end-stage renal disease. Large pulmonary fluid shifts occur in haemodialysis resulting in a range of clinical signs. This makes diagnosis more complicated and may impair pulmonary defence mechanisms.

Urinary tract

Urinary tract infection presents in a similar manner to non-chronic kidney disease patients. Anuric patients can still get urinary tract infections, but it tends to present non-specifically with vague suprapubic pain and fever. Acquiring a microbiological sample is obviously more challenging. The significance of leucocytes in any residual urine is questionable, particularly in isolation. Pyocystis (large collection of pus in a non-functioning bladder) occurs in anuric dialysis patients and is important to exclude as a source of infection. Proximal infection of the upper urinary tract and kidneys also occurs, even if these are non-functional. The severely abnormal upper renal tract (e.g. adult polycystic kidney disease) is particularly prone to recurrent and severe infection.

Skin and soft tissue

Cellulitis and osteomyelitis are important causes of morbidity in chronic renal failure, particularly in association with vascular disease and diabetes. VZV reactivation (shingles) occurs with greater frequency in renal failure. Patients treated with that desferrioxamine for aluminium overload are particularly at risk of mucormycosis (an invasive and necrotizing soft tissue fungal infection caused by *Rhizopus* spp.). This infection is also found in association with diabetes so the combination of both conditions multiplies the risk (➔ see 'Diabetes' p.186) (➔ Also See 'Murcormycosis' p.315).

Tuberculosis

Chronic renal disease carries at least 30 times increased risk of clinical TB when compared to the background population. This is likely due to impaired cellular immunity leading to reactivation. These patients are mostly anergic and do not respond to tuberculin skin testing. IGRAs are the preferred method of screening for latent disease, (➔ see 'Tuberculosis (TB)', p.337).

Infections associated with renal replacement therapy

Haemodialysis

Frequent bacteraemias occur secondary to repeated vascular puncture. Causative organisms are usually *Staphylococcus aureus* (including MRSA), coagulase-negative staphylococci, *Clostridium* spp. and other skin commensals. Risk of *S. aureus* bacteraemia is increased by nasal carriage. Organisms can also contaminate dialysis fluids; these include *Aerobacter* spp., *Bacillus* spp., *Clostridium* spp., *Corynebacterium* spp., *E. coli*, *Enterobacter* spp., *Flavobacter* spp., *Klebsiella* spp., *Micrococcus* spp., environmental mycobacteria, *Pseudomonas* spp., *Staphylococcus* spp., *Streptococcus* spp., *Stenotrophomonas maltophila*, and *Xanthomonas* spp.

Peritoneal dialysis

Exit site and catheter

Most common organisms are *S. aureus*, coagulase-negative staphylococci, *Pseudomonas* spp., and *Clostridium* spp. Presents with purulent discharge. Erythema at the catheter site may represent infection or a localized skin reaction. Recurrence rates are high and staphylococcal infection may be difficult to treat without removing the catheter.

Peritonitis

Presents with abdominal pain, fever, and cloudy fluid on drainage and occurs roughly one episode per 24 patient-months. Usually caused by skin flora but the peritoneal catheter can erode into the bowel and cause feculent peritonitis (particularly if there is concomitant diverticulitis); this needs surgical intervention and is associated with significant mortality. Normal peritoneal fluid contains <8 white cells/μL. White cell count in dialysate rises with dwell time; a white cell count of >100/mL after a dwell time of at least 2 hours, with >50% neutrophils is strongly suggestive of infection. In peritonitis not associated with bowel perforation, intraperitoneal antibiotics can be added to dialysis fluid and are an effective treatment strategy.

Indwelling vascular lines

A common cause of bacteraemia and persistent infection. Usually *S. aureus*, *S. epidermidis*, or other coagulase-negative staphylococci. Site infection presents with purulent discharge and tenderness over tunnelled catheters. Adherence and formation of biofilms on catheters make staphylococcal infections difficult to treat with antibiotics alone. Ideal management includes removal of the line and allowing 24–48 hours of IV antibiotics before placing a new line in a different site, although this may not always be feasible. Line rescue strategies include prolonged IV antibiotic therapy (>2–4 weeks), guidewire catheter exchange, intraluminal antibiotics (line locks), and intraluminal thrombolytics to improve antibiotic access to bacteria in biofilms. Staphylococcal infection should prompt consideration of secondary or embolic sites of infection, e.g. endocarditis, osteomyelitis, spinal abscess, disc infection, and intracerebral abscesses. Obtaining cultures from all lumens and peripherally prior to treatment is vital to management (Figure 9.3).

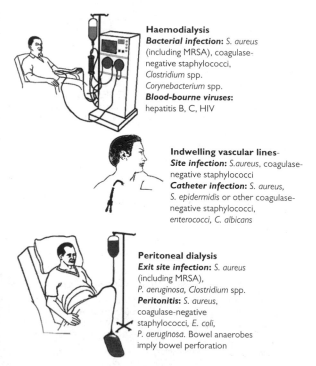

Haemodialysis
Bacterial infection: *S. aureus* (including MRSA), coagulase-negative staphylococci, *Clostridium* spp. *Corynebacterium* spp.
Blood-bourne viruses: hepatitis B, C, HIV

Indwelling vascular lines
Site infection: *S.aureus*, coagulase-negative staphylococci
Catheter infection: *S. aureus*, *S. epidermidis* or other coagulase-negative staphylococci, enterococci, *C. albicans*

Peritoneal dialysis
Exit site infection: *S. aureus* (including MRSA), *P. aeruginosa*, *Clostridium* spp.
Peritonitis: *S. aureus*, coagulase-negative staphylococci, *E. coli*, *P. aeruginosa*. Bowel anaerobes imply bowel perforation

Fig 9.3 Infections associated with renal replacement therapy.

Prevention of infection in chronic renal failure

General measures

Nutrition
- Malnutrition and protein catabolism are common and have important deleterious effects on immunity and wound healing.

Tuberculosis
- Patients should be screened with an IGRA for latent TB and offered treatment if positive.

Vaccination
- All routine vaccinations should be kept up to date, in addition, pneumococcal, influenza, and hepatitis B vaccination are indicated.

Nasal carriage
- Eradication of nasal staphylococcal carriage with intranasal mupirocin reduces rates of bacteraemia and other infections.

Screening for resistant organisms
- All patients should be regularly screened for resistant organisms. Patients colonized with MRSA should undergo a full MRSA eradication protocol (according to local guidelines) and should be isolated from other patients.

Haemodialysis
- Blood-borne viruses
- All patients should be screened for hepatitis B (HBsAg), C (hepatitis C antibody), and HIV (HIV antibody and p24 antigen). Patients who are infected should use a single machine that is not used by other patients.

Infection control
- Scrupulous hygiene of the patient, nursing staff, and dialysis unit. Meticulous dialysis fluid purification.

Peritoneal dialysis

Hygiene
- Encourage good personal hygiene of patient. Maintenance of dialysis fluid sterility.

Catheter site
- Topical mupirocin application to exit site reduces infection.

Indwelling vascular lines

Hygiene
- Sterile technique when accessing intravascular line.

Impregnated vascular catheters
- With antibiotics, silver, or other antimicrobials, reduces line infection rates, but these are expensive.

Line locks
- Intraluminal antibiotics following use.

Chronic lung disease

The lungs represent a major portal of entry for pathogens; every minute, anywhere between 5 and 12 L of air is brought into contact with an epithelial membrane roughly 100 m² and one cell thick. The lungs are protected by structural barriers, local and innate reaction, and adaptive immune responses (See figure 9.4). Chronic lung diseases interrupt these mechanisms resulting in recurrent and/or persistent infection and in the pathogenicity of organisms that are usually unable to infect the healthy lung (Table 9.2).

Chronic obstructive pulmonary disease (COPD)

Progressive parenchymal damage provides increasingly confluent areas of damaged alveoli that become chronically colonized. Innate lung defence is impaired (e.g. alveolar macrophage function). Smoking significantly damages the mucociliary clearance mechanism. Infectious exacerbations become frequent and multiple courses of antibiotics can drive the development of resistant organisms. This can result in a lung microbiome consisting of persistent and difficult to treat organisms.

Bronchiectasis (including cystic fibrosis)

Permanent dilatation of bronchi and bronchioles caused by cystic fibrosis, other congenital conditions (e.g. Kartagener's syndrome), or post infection (e.g. measles, pertussis, TB). Inability to clear mucus leads to persistent colonization of the lung and acute infective exacerbations. Organisms include *H. influenzae, S. pneumoniae, S. aureus, P. aeruginosa, B. cepacia, M. avium-intracellulare, S. maltophilia, Alcaligenes xylosoxidans,* and *B. gladioli.*

Table 9.2 Pathogens causing respiratory infection

Classical or usual pathogens	Unusual or opportunistic organisms (found in immunosuppressed patients or damaged lungs)
Streptococcus pneumoniae	**Bacteria**
Haemophilus influenzae	*Pseudomonas aeruginosa, Legionella* spp., *Staphylococcus aureus, Burkholderia pseudomallei, Burkholderia cepacia* complex, *Stenotrophomonas maltophilia, Mycobacterium tuberculosis, M. kansasii* and other non-tuberculous mycobacteria, *Nocardia* spp., *Rhodococcus equi, Actinomyces* spp.
Moraxella catarrhalis	
Adenoviruses	
Parainfluenza viruses	
RSV	
Mycoplasma pneumoniae	**Fungi**
Chlamydophila pneumoniae	*Pneumocystis jirovecii, Histoplasma capsulatum, Blastomyces dermatitidis, Coccidioides immitis/ posadasii, Paracoccidioides brasiliensis, Cryptococcus neoformans,* and *C. gattii, Aspergillus* spp., *Scedosporium* spp.
Influenza A & B	
	Viruses
	Varicella zoster, HSV

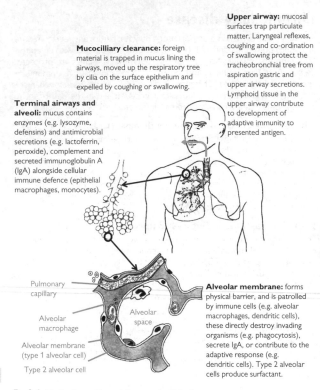

Upper airway: mucosal surfaces trap particulate matter. Laryngeal reflexes, coughing and co-ordination of swallowing protect the tracheobronchial tree from aspiration gastric and upper airway secretions. Lymphoid tissue in the upper airway contribute to development of adaptive immunity to presented antigen.

Mucocilliary clearance: foreign material is trapped in mucus lining the airways, moved up the respiratory tree by cilia on the surface epithelium and expelled by coughing or swallowing.

Terminal airways and alveoli: mucus contains enzymes (e.g. lysozyme, defensins) and antimicrobial secretions (e.g. lactoferrin, peroxide), complement and secreted immunoglobulin A (IgA) alongside cellular immune defence (epithelial macrophages, monocytes).

Pulmonary capillary

Alveolar macrophage

Alveolar membrane (type 1 alveolar cell)

Type 2 alveolar cell

Alveolar space

Alveolar membrane: forms physical barrier, and is patrolled by immune cells (e.g. alveolar macrophages, dendritic cells), these directly destroy invading organisms (e.g. phagocytosis), secrete IgA, or contribute to the adaptive response (e.g. dendritic cells). Type 2 alveolar cells produce surfactant.

Fig 9.4 Mechanisms of lung defense against infection.

Splenectomy and hyposplenism

The spleen is central to optimal immune function, in particular, clearing circulating microorganisms, phagocytosing senescent or damaged cells, and facilitating interaction between antigen-presenting cells and B lymphocytes or T lymphocytes. It has a key role in the development of natural antibodies (IgM) and opsonizing bacteria to facilitate phagocytosis (much of which also occurs in the spleen). Absent or impaired splenic function is caused by the removal of the spleen or conditions that damage its ability to function normally (functional hyposplenism). These patients are at risk of overwhelming post-splenectomy infections (OPSI), particularly caused by encapsulated bacteria (e.g. *Streptococcus pneumoniae* with its polysaccharide capsule, *Neisseria meningitidis*, and *Haemophilus influenzae* type b). Opsonization of bacteria is carried out by the attachment of complement, IgM, and/or other opsonizing molecules to the bacterial surface. These molecules then interact with receptors on phagocytic cells (e.g. macrophages) and facilitate phagocytosis. The surface of capsulated bacteria interferes with binding of complement and other opsonization molecules. These organisms are only effectively opsonized by IgM prior to the development of an adaptive IgG response. In the hyposplenic patient, the absence of IgM-producing memory B cells situated in the spleen results in ineffective opsonization and clearance of these bacteria. This renders them particularly susceptible to overwhelming sepsis.

Causes of splenectomy and functional asplenia

The most common cause worldwide of an absent spleen is surgical removal, either secondary to trauma or therapeutic splenectomy for haematological or immunological conditions. In economically developed countries, splenectomy is more commonly carried out for therapeutic reasons, rather than as a result of trauma surgery. This ratio is very likely to be reversed in countries with a much higher per capita incidence of major trauma. Sickle cell disease is the major cause of profound hyposplenism or autosplenectomy in regions of the world where this is common.

Trauma

Usually surgically removed in order to arrest major haemorrhage. While the spleen is relatively well protected from penetrating trauma when compared to other abdominal organs, it is particularly vulnerable to rupture if there is a rapid increase in intra-abdominal pressure during blunt force trauma.

Alcohol

Excessive alcohol use causes hyposplenism. Mechanisms are unclear but may involve a direct toxic effect of alcohol. There is some evidence that splenic function returns with abstinence (➜ see 'Alcoholism and substance misuse' p.213).

Haematological (non-malignant)

Sickle cell disease, autoimmune haemolytic anaemia, hereditary spherocytosis, thalassaemias, and G6PD deficiency.

Haematological malignancy

Acute leukaemias, chronic myeloid leukaemia, chronic lymphocytic leukaemia, polycythaemia rubra vera, essential thrombocythaemia, myelofibrosis, lymphomas, bone marrow transplantation, and GvHD.

Connective tissue disease
SLE and Felty's syndrome.

Gastrointestinal
Coeliac disease and inflammatory bowel disease.

Tropical
Malaria (and tropical splenomegaly syndrome), visceral leishmaniasis, schistosomiasis, and hydatid disease.

Other
Amyloidosis and sarcoidosis.

Post-splenectomy sepsis

The risk of overwhelming post-splenectomy sepsis appears highest in the first months post splenectomy, but lifetime risk remains four to five times higher than the general population. The reason for splenectomy also strongly affects the risk of sepsis, with splenectomy due to haematological or autoimmune conditions at the highest risk, presumably due to underlying disease and comorbidity. Encapsulated bacteria are the major cause of sepsis; in decreasing order of frequency: *S. pneumoniae*, *H. influenzae*, *N. meningitidis*. Other organisms particularly associated with splenectomy and hyposplenism are *Salmonella* spp., *Capnocytophagia canimorsus*, *Plasmodium* spp., *Babesia* spp., *Erlichia* spp., and *Bartonella bacilliformis*. *Escherichia coli* and *Klebsiella* spp. may also be of particular importance in infants.

Management of splenectomy/hyposplenism

Education
Education of patients, relatives, and carers is important; early assessment and treatment of any acute febrile illness is vital to preventing overwhelming sepsis. It is recommended the patient carries an alert card. Particular care should also be taken to avoid animal bites and to reduce the risk to travellers from malaria.

Antibiotic prophylaxis
This is standard practice in most parts of the world, although there is no firm evidence base for this. Duration, dose, and choice of antibiotic are similarly based on expert opinion but are usually oral penicillins or macrolides. Another strategy is for patient-controlled episodic antibiotics in response to a febrile illness. The use of prophylactic antibiotics immediately post splenectomy is almost universally recommended; this applies to both planned and unplanned splenectomy. Ongoing prophylaxis and prophylaxis in functional hyposplenism is less clear. UK guidelines recommend lifelong oral prophylaxis with penicillins or macrolides for patients considered at high risk of pneumococcal infection. Patients considered not to be at high risk may choose to discontinue prophylaxis after several years.

Vaccination
Vaccination is an important part of the post-splenectomy infection prevention strategy. UK guidelines recommend that all the patients should receive pneumococcal vaccination, *H. influenzae* type b conjugate vaccine,

and meningococcal conjugate vaccine (B, C) alongside yearly influenza immunization. The measurement of antibody titres in response to vaccination may help direct the need for and timing of repeated vaccination. In planned splenectomy, it is recommended to immunize at least 2 (but ideally 4–6) weeks prior to surgery. Emergency or unplanned splenectomy it is recommended to immunize at least 2 weeks post surgery and when sufficiently well. Antibody response to pneumococcal vaccine is poorer if it is given within 2 weeks of emergency splenectomy.

Prophylaxis post partial splenectomy and splenic embolization requires a clinical judgement as to the degree to which splenic function may have been affected.

Physiological states: pregnancy and the extremes of age

Pregnancy

(Infections in pregnancy and childbirth mainly affecting the fetus are not discussed here.)

Alterations in immune function in pregnancy are complex but likely result from modulation of maternal immunity (immune 'tolerance') to prevent 'rejection' of the fetus and placenta. While many aspects of immunity are intact in pregnancy, cellular immunity and immune regulation are somewhat impaired (particularly ↓CD4 lymphocytes and NK cells). Immune dysregulation may underlie the severity of the systemic inflammatory response to infections such as influenza. Certain infections have a particular affinity for the placenta (e.g. *Listeria*, malaria); this may be a result of local alterations in immune function in the placenta. Structural changes of pregnancy (e.g. reduced lung volumes/atelectasis and urinary stasis due to obstruction by the enlarging uterus) contribute to an increased susceptibility to infection. Biological demands of pregnancy result in a relative lack of physiological reserve in response to severe infection. Severe infection is the second highest cause of death in pregnancy worldwide; in the UK it is now the leading cause of death.

Bacterial sepsis

Bacterial infection in pregnancy may rapidly develop into septic shock, multiple organ dysfunction, and death. Early detection may be problematic as it may present insidiously. Physiological changes in pregnancy (e.g. ↑ heart rate, ↓ peripheral vascular resistance and arterial pressure, anaemia, ↓ mean urea and creatinine values due to ↑GFR, procoagulant state) may mask initial signs and/or contribute to the rapid development of organ dysfunction. The urogenital tract is the most frequent source of infection. Other sources include the respiratory tract, chorioamnionitis, septic abortion, post surgery (caesarean section wound), and episiotomy infection. Important causative organisms are *Escherichia coli*, *Streptococcus pyogenes* (group A β-haemolytic), *Staphylococcus aureus*, *S. pneumoniae*, *Listeria monocytogenes*, *Klebsiella pneumoniae*, *Pseudomonas aeruginosa*, and anaerobes (e.g. *Bacteroides* spp.).

Two organisms deserve special mention:

S. pyogenes (group A β-haemolytic)

Particularly associated with mortality in pregnancy and easily transmitted via the hands and close contact in households. Pregnant women presenting with a sore throat should have throat swabs to exclude group A streptococcal infection.

L. monocytogenes

Food-borne pathogen, with a predilection for the placenta. *Listeria* is an intracellular pathogen and requires an appropriate T-cell response to clear infection. This is particularly suppressed in the placenta. There is a ~20-fold increased risk in pregnancy, mainly in the third trimester.

Viral infection

Influenza

Increased risk of severe disease and mortality, particularly in the third trimester.

Hepatitis E virus (HEV)

Increased severity, with high mortality during the third trimester. Faecal–oral transmission. Presentation is with an acute hepatitis and can progress to fulminant liver failure. Highly endemic in Asia, Middle East, and Africa; although becoming more common in other parts of the world including the UK.

Herpes simplex virus (HSV)

Increase in reactivation, severity, and risk of disseminated disease (especially hepatitis, CNS infection). Around 15% of women with a previous history of genital HSV will have clinically recurrent disease at delivery.

Other viral infections

With limited evidence of increased severity in pregnancy include VZV and measles. Susceptibility to HIV transmission also appears increased in pregnancy.

Parasitic infection

Malaria

(Mainly *Plasmodium falciparum*.) Increased susceptibility, severity, and mortality. A major cause of maternal mortality in endemic regions. Malarial parasites are particularly trophic for placental tissue.

Infection in older people

Increased susceptibility to infection with increasing age is multifactorial. Contributory factors include comorbidity, polypharmacy (including immune-suppressant medication), impaired skin and mucosal barriers, malnutrition, and blunted physiological responses. The immune system changes with increasing age ('immunosenescence'), while many aspects appear intact, the ageing immune system becomes dysfunctional or less effectively regulated. Poor T-cell function results in reactivation of latent infections such as VZV (shingles) and TB, as well as a reduction in vaccine efficacy.

Presentations

Diagnosis of infection in the elderly can be challenging as classical signs may be absent. A senescent hypothalamic response can result in the absence of fever or in hypothermia. Conducting system disease and/or rate-limiting drugs may attenuate tachycardia. Laboratory markers of infection are usually delayed; profound sepsis can present with normal inflammatory markers. Physiological response to severe infection is diminished; abnormal cardiorespiratory function, vascular contractility, and reduced renal reserve result in the rapid development of tissue hypoxia and multiorgan dysfunction.

Severe infection commonly presents with falls, delirium, decreased conscious state, and/or 'functional' decline without more typical localizing features. Potential sources of infection are often multiple as there is a high prevalence in this population of chronic lung disease, skin ulcers, gallstones, diverticular disease, and urinary tract abnormality (prostate disease in men, uterine/vaginal prolapse in women). Multiple admissions, antibiotic treatment, and nursing home residence increase the risk of colonization and disease from resistant organisms (ESBL/CPE-producing organisms, MRSA, *Clostridium difficile*).

Specific infections

Pneumococcal pneumonia

Remains a leading cause of death in older people. Risk of community-acquired pneumococcal pneumonia rises with age along with case fatality rate. Comorbidity is a strong predictor of mortality in older patients with community-acquired pneumonia.

Influenza

Over 65-year-olds bear the greatest burden of severe influenza disease, >70% of influenza-related deaths are in this age group.

C.difficile-associated colitis

Altered gut microbiota with age, frequent exposure to antibiotics, gastric acid suppressants, institutionalization, and immune senescence likely underlie the greatly increased risk and severity of *C. difficile*-associated colitis in the elderly.

Urinary tract infection

The most common cause of infection in older adults. In men, urinary stasis due to prostatic disease is the major cause, while in women, uterine or vaginal prolapse plus atrophy of vaginal tissue due to postmenopausal lack of oestrogen is the main cause. Colonization of the urinary tract is common; as such, a positive urine dipstick does not signify infection in the absence of symptoms or signs. Asymptomatic bacteriuria should not be treated. *E. coli* remains the most common causative organism followed by *Enterobacter* spp., *Klebsiella* spp., *Proteus* spp., *P. aeruginosa*, and enterococci.

Prevention

Vaccination

Vaccination is a key prevention strategy in the elderly. Although immunological response is poorer than in younger adults, the benefit of vaccination is greater in this age group as they are at risk of more frequent and severe disease. In the UK, current recommendations are that all those >65 years old receive the pneumococcal vaccine and annual influenza vaccination. Reactivation of VZV infection is common in the elderly and immunization of those >65 years old against herpes zoster has been shown to reduce the incidence of disease and of post-herpetic neuralgia.

Antibiotic stewardship

Responsible and careful prescribing of antibiotics to reduce the selection of resistant organisms and complications such as *C. difficile* disease. There is no evidence to suggest that longer than standard durations of antibiotics are of any benefit in the elderly.

Infection control
Robust infection control procedures to prevent transmission of infection (e.g. resistant organisms, *C. difficile*).

Nutrition
Malnutrition is common in the elderly and adversely affects immunity and physiological response to infection. Encouraging normal balanced nutrition, with supplements if tolerated, is likely to be the best strategy.

Optimal management of comorbid conditions
E.g. diabetes, chronic lung disease, liver and renal disease.

Other prevention strategies
Aiming to prevent and/or reduce the frequency of infection, e.g. podiatry, urogynaecological or urological treatment, pressure care, prevention of constipation, etc.

Infection in the newborn

The immune system remains immature at birth. Placental transfer of immunoglobulin occurs throughout most of the second and third trimesters and is continued after birth via the colostrum. Infants are reliant on this passively acquired form of adaptive immunity until around 6 months when there is a trough in IgG levels while native immune function takes over. Cellular immunity is also immature at birth; neutrophil and T-cell function is markedly less effective than in the adult. Infants <3 months of age are at risk of overwhelming sepsis. As the infant immune system gains antigenic experience, there is considerable improvement in function by the first 3 months of life. Factors that influence immune function in the first months of life and the development of a functional immune system include the following:

Prematurity
This diminishes the effectiveness of innate and adaptive immunity (including the integrity of skin and mucosal barriers) further than babies born at term, reduces the degree of placental transfer of immunoglobulin, and prolongs the development of a fully functioning independent immune system.

Breastfeeding
Facilitates the transfer of antimicrobial components and breastmilk including IgA.

Nutrition
Malnutrition has deleterious effects on the effectiveness and maturation of the immune system.

Maternal health
Poor maternal health, malnutrition, and alcohol or substance misuse negatively affect the developing immune system.

Primary immunodeficiency
➲ See Chapter 3.

Key organisms in neonatal infection (<4 weeks from birth)

Early neonatal infection (<7 days)

This is largely caused by organisms with which the neonate is likely to have come into contact with during passage through the birth canal or from close contact with the mother; *Streptococcus agalactiae* (group B β-haemolytic streptococci), *E. coli, L. monocytogenes*, HSV, and VZV.

Later neonatal infections (7–28 days)

Later neonatal infections also include organisms acquired more environmentally as the naïve immune system of the infant encounters new organisms: *S. aureus, Klebsiella* spp., *Enterobacter* spp., *Enterococcus* spp. *P. aeruginosa, Candida* spp., RSV, enterovirus, and parechovirus.

Critical illness: intensive care, trauma, and burns

Intensive care

While infectious illness is a common cause for admission to the ICU, secondary infection is the foremost secondary complication of all admissions. Acute severe illness results in considerable immune activation and release of inflammatory cytokines. The systemic inflammatory response syndrome (SIRS) describes this systemic immunological response to an infectious or non-infectious insult. While mobilization of components of the innate immune system provide a rapid response to infection or other disease processes, poor regulation can lead to complications. These include impairment of vascular tone and circulatory shock, acute lung injury, and acute kidney injury. Prolonged critical illness (>10 days), can result in a state of immune dysfunction and susceptibility to infection known as the persistent inflammation, immunosuppression, and catabolism syndrome (PICS). It is characterized by a defective adaptive immune response, poor regulation of inflammation, protein loss, and metabolic dysfunction. This results in multiorgan failure and is associated with significant mortality.

Susceptibility to infection on ICU

Critically unwell patients are highly prone to infection for a number of reasons (Figure 9.5) including:

- *The underlying illness/condition precipitating ICU admission.*
- *Multiple invasive devices and catheters*: intravascular lines, urinary catheters, surgical drains, etc.
- *Mechanical ventilation and related lung injury*: endotracheal intubation bypasses important oro- and nasopharyngeal barriers to infection. Lower airway infection is caused by pooling of secretions and increased microaspiration, along with bacterial colonization and biofilm formation on tubes. Positive-pressure mechanical ventilation can result in lung injury (barotrauma, volutramua, and atelectotrauma) impairing lung defence mechanisms.
- *Pulmonary atelectasis and difficulty clearing secretions* due to prolonged dependence, weak respiratory muscles, and weakened cough. Clearance of secretions is decreased due to gravity and impaired mucociliary function.
- *Cardiovascular instability*: leading to abnormal tissue perfusion.
- *CNS depression*: either due to pathology or pharmacotherapy, depressing protective reflexes.
- *Pressure skin and soft tissue damage*: particularly to dependent areas.
- *Cross infection*: from other patients/healthcare staff.
- *Renal replacement therapy*: causing acute-phase protein depletion and as a potential source of infection.
- *Catabolic state*: hypoalbuminaemia, immuneparesis, and vascular leak.
- *Bowel translocation of bacteria*: particularly with damaged, poorly perfused, or oedematous bowel.

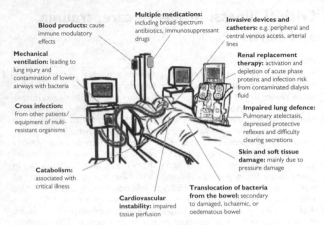

Blood products: cause immune modulatory effects

Multiple medications: including broad-spectrum antibiotics, immunosuppressant drugs

Invasive devices and catheters: e.g. peripheral and central venous access, arterial lines

Mechanical ventilation: leading to lung injury and contamination of lower airways with infection

Renal replacement therapy: activation and depletion of acute phase proteins and infection risk from contaminated dialysis fluid

Cross infection: from other patients/ equipment of multi-resistant organisms

Impaired lung defence: Pulmonary atelectasis, depressed protective reflexes and difficulty clearing secretions

Skin and soft tissue damage: mainly due to pressure damage

Catabolism: associated with critical illness

Translocation of bacteria from the bowel: secondary to damaged, ischaemic, or oedematous bowel

Cardiovascular instability: impaired tissue perfusion

Fig 9.5 Mechanisms of immunosuppression and susceptibility to infection in critical illness.

- *Transfusions of blood products*: causes NK cell, macrophage, and lymphocyte dysfunction, a condition known as transfusion-related immunomodulation (TRIM).
- *Multiple medications*: including immunosuppressant drugs.
- *Broad-spectrum antibiotic use*: predisposing to invasive fungal infection.

Specific ICU infections

Intravascular catheters

Infection of intravascular catheters may present with fever, cardiovascular instability and sepsis, catheter blockage, or positive blood cultures. Infection may be acquired by invasion of skin colonizers at the catheter site, intraluminal contamination during use, or seeding from other sites by haematogenous spread. The risk of infection increases with less than ideal circumstances of insertion, duration of catheterization (although there is no indication for routine line changing based on number of days), sites of insertion (femoral > internal jugular > subclavian), use for renal replacement or total parenteral nutrition, type of catheter material (including antibiotic impregnation), catheter care practices, and heavy skin colonization of the patient. Major organisms include coagulase-negative staphylococci, *Staphylococcus aureus*, enterococci, *Candida* spp., *Escherichia coli*, *Klebsiella* spp., *Pseudomonas* spp., *Enterobacter* spp., *Serratia* spp., and *Acinetobacter* spp. Treatment usually requires removal of catheter ± systemic antibiotics.

Ventilator-associated pneumonia (VAP)

Usually presents with fever, increasing volume and purulence of respiratory secretions, rising inflammatory markers, new radiographic pulmonary infiltrates, and increasing ventilator requirements/deterioration in a patient's respiratory performance. Critically unwell patients in the intensive care environment, particularly if ventilated, undergo a transformation in the microbiota colonizing the upper airways from typical upper airway organisms (e.g. α-haemolytic streptococci, non-haemolytic streptococci, coagulase-negative staphylococci, non-pathogenic *Neisseria* spp., and *Corynebacterium* spp.) to staphylococci and Gram-negative organisms. These organisms are the most likely to invade the lower airways and cause VAP. The major organisms are known as the 'ESKAPE' organisms: *Enterococcus faecium*, *S. aureus*, *Klebsiella pneumoniae*, *Acinetobacter baumannii*, *Pseudomonas aeruginosa*, and *Enterobacter* spp. as well as *E. coli*, *S. maltophilia*, and *Serratia marcescens*. Deep respiratory samples (BAL) are important in directing antimicrobial treatment.

Abdominal infection
Abdominal infection in the ICU usually involves the following:
• Perforated viscus: due to gastroduodenal perforation (associated with ulceration), perforation due to trauma, ischaemia, tumour, or diverticulum.
• Gut translocation: associated with ascites or oedematous bowel.
• Post-surgical infection: wound infection/anastomotic breakdown.
• Infection complicating intra-abdominal inflammatory conditions, e.g. pancreatitis and inflammatory bowel disease.

Main organisms are *E. coli*, *Klebsiella* spp., *Proteus* spp., *Enterococcus* spp., and anaerobes (e.g. *Bacteroides* spp., *Clostridium* spp., *Peptostreptococcus*, and *Pseudomonas* spp.).

C.difficile
Diarrhoea, abdominal pain, and distension should always prompt consideration of *C. difficile* colitis—associated with antibiotic use.

Urinary infection
Usually urinary catheter related. Organisms include *E. coli*, *Klebsiella* spp., *Proteus* spp., *Enterococcus* spp., *S. aureus*, *Pseudomonas* spp., and *Candida* spp.

Fungal infection
Colonization by fungi is common in the ICU. *Candida* spp. are frequently isolated from urine, sputum, and BAL specimens and do not necessarily represent disease. Major risk factors for invasive fungal infection include broad-spectrum antibiotic use, immune suppression, intravascular lines (especially if used for total parenteral nutrition), and abdominal surgery. Major fungal species include *Candida albicans*, other *Candida* spp. (e.g. *C. glabrata*, *C. rugosa*, *C. parapsilosis*, *C. tropicalis*, *C. krusei*, *C. auris*, and *C. dubliniensis*), and *Aspergillus* spp. Patients with candidaemia require the removal of intravascular catheters and other prosthetic material, and should be assessed by echocardiography for endocarditis and by ophthalmoscopy for eye involvement. Invasive infection by *Aspergillus* spp. is uncommon in the absence of immunosuppression—the lungs are most commonly involved. Invasive aspergillosis in the ICU is associated with significant mortality.

Multi-resistant organisms
MDR pathogens on ICU are an increasingly significant problem. Major organisms:
- Gram-positive bacteria: MRSA and VRE.
- Gram-negative bacteria: Enterobacteriaceae that produce ESBL and/or carbapenemases (CPE), carbapenem-resistant *Pseudomonas aeruginosa*, multi-resistant *Acinetobacter* (MRAB).
- Fungi: non-albicans species of *Candida* may be resistant to 'first-line' antifungal therapy (azoles), e.g. *C. glabrata*, *C. auris*, etc.

Other infections to consider in undiagnosed fever in the ICU
CNS infections, sinusitis (particularly if nasopharyngeal airway *in situ*), empyema, infective endocarditis, biliary infection, intra-abdominal abscess, myonecrosis, and thrombophlebitis. Always obtain a travel history.

Trauma

Infection and multiorgan failure are the major causes of late mortality in trauma (the third peak in the 'trimodal pattern of mortality' following trauma). Causative organisms depend on the nature of trauma and degree of wound contamination but may involve skin flora, environmental organisms, and bowel flora (e.g. in abdominal trauma). Tetanus caused by *Clostridium tetani* must always be considered in trauma as *C. tetani* is a ubiquitous environmental organism.

Trauma predisposes to infection in the following ways:
- *SIRS and immune paralysis*: major trauma initiates enormous immune activation and inflammation. The initial immune response can contribute to organ system damage and dysfunction. This is followed by a second phase of 'immune paralysis' where a compensatory anti-inflammatory response dampens inflammation. A reduction in protein synthesis and an increase in protein degradation deplete acute-phase proteins. Generalized immune activation leads to difficulty mounting an effective adaptive response.
- *Penetrating injury and disruption of mucosal barriers*: interruption of barrier integrity (skin, mucosal surfaces) provides a portal of entry for pathogens and may deliver pathogenic organisms deep into tissues or body cavities.
- *Haematomas/necrotic tissue*: provides a favourable environment for microbial growth and is poorly accessible to immune response.
- *Massive transfusion*: causes depression of cellular immunity (TRIM).
- *Hypotension*: leading to ischaemia and poor tissue perfusion; a favourable environment for microbial growth.
- *Prolonged ventilation*: ventilator-associated lung injury and increased access of organisms to lower airway.
- *Multiple invasive drains and catheters*.

Burns

Secondary infection is the most common cause of morbidity and mortality in burns patients. The loss of the barrier that is normal skin to invasion of environmental organisms leaves burns patients highly susceptible to local and systemic infection. Common causative organisms are *S. aureus* (including MRSA) and *P. aeruginosa*.

Malnutrition and deficiency illness

Malnutrition

Malnutrition is associated with 50% of all deaths in children <5 years of age worldwide. The majority of these deaths are in combination with infection (namely bacterial pneumonia, diarrhoea, malaria, measles, and HIV disease). Malnutrition is also common in the elderly with a prevalence of 10–50% depending on the specific population studied. Nutritional status is worse in hospitalized or institutionalized older people. Although adequate data are not available, nutrition appears to have important effects on outcome in critical illness. Malnutrition can therefore be considered the most common cause of immunodeficiency worldwide.

There is a synergistic relationship between malnutrition and infection; malnutrition predisposes to susceptibility, severity, and persistence of infection and infection predisposes to malnutrition and vitamin deficiency illness. Nutritional energy demands are significantly elevated in acute infection, exacerbating deficiencies. The result is a vicious cycle of declining immunity, progressive weakening of physiological reserve, and breakdown of skin and mucosal barriers with increasing invasion by pathogenic organisms. This, in turn, leads to malabsorption, poor wound healing, increasing proportion of energy budget devoted to immunity, and accelerating catabolism. The deleterious effects of this process manifest to the greatest extent in individuals at the extremes of age, in pregnant mothers, and in individuals with chronic illness.

The immunological effects of malnutrition are complex and confounded by concomitant illness and micronutrient deficiency. Impaired cellular immunity, acute-phase protein function, and mucosal immunity are particularly important.

Vitamin and micronutrient deficiency

In addition to the classical clinical features, several vitamin and micronutrient deficiency illnesses have important effects on the immune system.

Vitamin A (retinol)

Deficiency causes xerophthalmia and keratomalacia. Important in maintaining the integrity of the epithelium, particularly in the respiratory and GI tracts. In children, there is a close and bi-directional synergy between vitamin A deficiency and measles infection. Vitamin A deficiency increases risk and severity of measles while measles depletes body stores of vitamin A. The combination kills an estimated 2 million children a year. In addition, vitamin A deficiency increases risk and severity of *Plasmodium falciparum* malaria and diarrhoeal illness.

Vitamin C (ascorbic acid)

Deficiency causes scurvy; essential for collagen synthesis in connective tissue and bone. Deficiency leads to a breakdown of mucosal surfaces and fractures. Interruption of epithelial integrity predisposes to infection. There is currently no firm evidence to support the use of vitamin C in preventing or treating the common cold.

Vitamin D (cholecalciferol)
Deficiency illness results in rickets and osteomalacia. In addition to its role in calcium homeostasis, vitamin D appears to have an important and wide-ranging role in modulating the innate and adaptive immune responses. This includes regulating the function of macrophages and the cellular immune response to *Mycobacterium tuberculosis*. There is an association between vitamin D deficiency and TB. This interaction is still not fully understood and there are still insufficient data to support the use of vitamin D supplementation in the treatment or prevention of TB.

Zinc
Trace mineral essential for enzyme function, protein synthesis, and metabolism. Important in the maintenance of epithelial integrity, and particularly important in immunity to diarrhoeal illness. Deficiency has broad effects on humoral and cellular immune function. Zinc supplementation reduces the duration and intensity of diarrhoeal illness and pneumonia.

Iron
The most common trace mineral deficiency. The relationship between iron deficiency and infection is complex; there is evidence of impairment in cell-mediated immunity but supplementation can favour infection with siderophilic bacteria and *Plasmodium* spp. (malaria).

Alcoholism and substance misuse

Alcoholism

Chronic alcohol use has direct deleterious effects on the immune system. The mechanisms are multiple and indistinct; there is suppression of the protective acute-phase response to initial infection, alongside defective phagocytic, APC, and T-lymphocyte function. Alcohol leads to decreased saliva production and impairment of the antimicrobial function of saliva and the oral mucosa. This appears to be a strong contributor to susceptibility to respiratory infection. Complications of chronic alcohol abuse such as chronic liver disease (→ see 'Chronic liver disease' p.190), bone marrow suppression, and impaired splenic function contribute to an increasingly profound state of immunosuppression. Behavioural risk factors that form part of the syndrome of alcoholism increase exposure to infection. These include frequent episodes of depressed conscious level with inadequate airway protective reflexes increasing the rate of micro-aspiration, alongside a strong association with smoking, malnutrition, repeated trauma, and poor self-care.

Bacterial pneumonia

Alcohol abuse is associated with increased incidence and severity of community-acquired pneumonia. Contributory factors include increased aspiration of upper airway secretions, salivary and oral mucosal immunity dysfunction, and impaired acute-phase and cellular immune response at the level of the alveolus. In addition, there is a strong association with smoking, COPD and functional hyposplenism (→ see 'Splenectomy and hyposplenism' p.199). *Streptococcus pneumoniae* remains the most common causative organism. *Klebsiella pneumoniae* forms part of the normal flora of the human mouth and bowel, and pulmonary infection is particularly associated with alcoholism. Alcohol-induced alterations in the volume and nature of saliva production, increased gastro-oesophageal reflux, and accelerated periodontal disease are putative mechanisms favouring growth of *K. pneumoniae* in the upper airways and subsequent contamination of the lower airways.

CNS infection

The incidence of bacterial meningitis in chronic alcoholism is higher than the background population, chiefly due to *S. pneumoniae*. Alcoholism is a significant risk factor for CNS *Listeria monocytogenes* infection. *L. monocytogenes*, an environmental organism, usually enters the body by oral ingestion. Translocation from the bowel may be aided by alcohol-induced liver damage. It is a facultative intracellular parasite and immunity relies mainly on macrophage function, which is depressed in alcoholism.

Tuberculosis

The correlation between alcohol use and risk of TB is well known. Although there are multiple factors that may contribute to this association (social circumstances, malnutrition, chronic lung disease, etc.), significant alcohol abuse does appear to independently elevate TB risk, potentially due to the effects of alcohol on cellular immunity.

Tropical infection

Melioidosis (*Burkholderia pseudomallei*) is caused by a Gram-negative organism found in soil and water and is a major public health problem in Southeast Asia and Northern Australia. Acute infection most commonly involves severe pneumonia and/or septicaemia but can involve many anatomical sites and can cause chronic infection. *Streptococcus suis* is a zoonosis resulting from exposure to pigs and is emerging as an important cause of meningitis in Asia. Alcoholism and liver disease appears to be a particular risk factor and there is evidence that these conditions facilitate gut translocation of *S. suis*. (➔ See '*Burkholderia pseudomallei*', p.354)

Substance misuse

Substance misuse is practically universal throughout human societies; major drugs of abuse worldwide include opiates, cocaine, cannabis, amphetamine-type stimulants, and other psychoactive substances. Many drugs of abuse appear to have direct or indirect negative effects on the immune system while the lifestyle and behaviour associated with the syndrome of addiction significantly increases exposure to infection. Opiates have direct immune depressing effects including impairment of neutrophil and macrophage phagocytosis and chemotaxis, altered cytokine production, and impaired lymphocytic function. Specific effects of cocaine and other stimulants on the immune system are yet to be elucidated; *in vitro* studies show that cocaine increases HIV replication in peripheral monocytes. Along the trafficking and distribution process, many narcotics are combined ('cut') with multiple substances in order to bulk out the volume. Some of these substances can have significant medical consequences. There are several documented occurrences of agranulocytosis in drug users, likely due to the inclusion of levamisole (an antiparasitic agent) into the drug supply.

Pulmonary infection

Pneumonia is common in substance misusers (~10 times increased risk). Smoking of heroin and crack (a free-base form of cocaine) results in severe thermal and chemical pulmonary damage. Marijuana and tobacco have well-documented damaging effects on the lungs. These result in structural lung damage (e.g. bullous lung disease, interstitial lung disease, and foreign body granulomatosis), impaired local lung defences, and ineffective mucociliary clearance. Frequent episodes of depressed conscious level increase the rate aspiration. Major organisms include *S. pneumoniae, S. aureus, H. influenzae, K. pneumoniae,* and *Escherichia coli*. IV drug use is a strong risk factor for pulmonary abscess, either as a complication of pneumonia or following haematogenous spread (e.g. from right-sided endocarditis). Infection is often polymicrobial and can include mouth organisms (e.g. *Peptostreptococcus* spp., *S. milleri* group, *Bacteroides* spp., *Prevotella* spp., and *Fusobacterium* spp.) as well as *S. aureus* and *K. pneumoniae*. The prevalence of TB (both active and latent disease) is considerably higher in the IV drug-using population. Poor compliance increases the risk of treatment failure and drug resistance.

Complications of intravenous injecting

Blood-borne viruses

Sharing of IV injecting paraphernalia is a major mechanism of transmission of blood-borne viruses such as HCV, HBV, and HIV. Injecting paraphernalia (e.g. needles, syringes, cotton filters, and 'cooking' equipment) are all sources of contamination and transmission.

Skin and soft tissue

Repeated injecting (intravenously, subcutaneously 'skin popping', or intramuscularly 'muscle popping') introduces multiple organisms into the skin and soft tissue leading to abscesses, cellulitis, and potentially necrotizing fasciitis. Failed attempts to inject into the vein and extravasation into surrounding tissues commonly initiates abscess formation, particularly as in addition to microbes, injected solutions are highly irritant and often induce tissue necrosis. Major organisms include *S. aureus* (including MRSA), *S. pyogenes* (group A streptococci), and other streptococci (e.g. *S. dysgalactiae* group C/G). Street drugs, particularly heroin, are often contaminated with clostridial spores including *Clostridium perfringens* (causing gas gangrene), *C. tetani* (causing tetanus; spasmodic paralysis), and *C. botulium* (causing wound botulism; flaccid paralysis). Contamination of street drugs with anthrax (*Bacillus anthracis*) also periodically occurs and causes large black, necrotic, painless ulcer-like skin lesions (cutaneous anthrax).

Cardiovascular infection

Repeated bacteraemia resulting from injecting commonly leads to bacterial endocarditis (both right and left sided) and infected venous thrombus. *S. aureus* accounts for >50% of endocarditis in IV drug users while viridans streptococci and enterococci are the next most common. Other mouth organisms (besides viridans streptococci) occur often as a result of licking needles (to 'clean' and to 'lubricate' the needle); these include *Haemophilus parainfluenzae, Aggregatibacter actinomycetemcomitans, Cardiobacterium hominis, Eikenella corrodens,* and *Kingella kingae* (the 'HACEK' organisms). Contaminated tap water (used to 'cook up' heroin) has caused *Pseudomonas aeruginosa* infection while lemon juice (used to dissolve heroin) is known to have caused *Candida albicans* infection. Transmission of malaria (*Plasmodium vivax*), relapsing fever (*Borrelia recurrentis*), and Chagas disease (*Trypanosoma cruzi*) have all been described through needle sharing.

Behaviour and lifestyle

Risk-taking behaviour is common among drug users; multiple sexual partners (including transactional sex) predispose to STDs including HIV, syphilis, gonorrhoea, and chlamydia.

Other conditions associated with immunosuppression

The number of chronic medical conditions predisposing to specific infections or generally increasing the risk and severity of infection continues to grow. The list in Table 9.3 is by no means exhaustive:

Table 9.3 Other conditions associated with immunosuppression

Condition	Immune defect or associated infection
Gastrointestinal conditions	
Coeliac disease	Active disease invariably causes functional hyposplenism (unclear mechanism); pneumococcal, Hib, and meningococcal vaccination should be considered.
Inflammatory bowel disease	Elevated risk of bacterial translocation and bacteraemia due to mucosal disease and therapeutic immunosuppression. Intraluminal disease also occurs at increased frequency due to the disruption in the gut mucosal immunity; infectious gastroenteritis and *Clostridium difficile* are important complications
Colonic malignancy	Disrupted colonic mucosa favours extraluminal spread of colonic bacteria; *Streptococcus gallolyticus* (formerly *S. bovis*) is well documented as a cause of endocarditis in association with colonic malignancy (~50% of bacteraemias have concomitant colorectal tumours)
Rheumatological conditions	
Rheumatoid arthritis, autoimmune connective tissue diseases, vasculitides	The hallmark of rheumatologic disease is abnormal and inappropriate immune functioning. Although this can be thought of as an overzealous immune response to host or innocuous antigens, this abnormal immune functioning also means that appropriate immune responses are dysfunctional. Thus, in the absence of therapeutic immunosuppression, active rheumatological disease is an immune compromised state. Ironically, appropriate therapeutic immunosuppression may lead to an improvement in immune defence against infection
Neurological conditions	
Degenerative conditions, e.g. multiple sclerosis, motor neuron disease, myasthenia gravis, spinal injury, stroke	Increased susceptibility to infection in neurological conditions is mainly caused by indirect effects of disease complications. Progressive degenerative neurological conditions such as multiple sclerosis and motor neuron disease predisposed to recurrent and persistent infection due to factors such as deteriorating respiratory function, immobility, and abnormal bladder and bowel function. Many neurological conditions have an autoimmune basis leading to impaired appropriate immune function and complications from therapeutic immunosuppression. Patients with spinal injuries are at risk of the complications of immobility, colonization with resistant organisms, and abnormal autonomic response to severe infection

Condition	Immune defect or associated infection
Genetic conditions	
Down syndrome	Defects of the immune system are well recognized as part of the complications of Down syndrome. These include a reduction in the number and function of T and B cells, impaired specific antibody responses, and defects of neutrophil chemotaxis. Abnormal structural complications involved increased gastro-oesophageal reflux and abnormal ear canal anatomy. Respiratory tract infections are particularly common. Vaccination is important in these patients
Myotonic dystrophy	Associated with hypogammaglobulinaemia due to reduced antibody survival
Radiation and environmental	
Ionizing radiation(medical, industrial, or use as a weapon)	Directly damages DNA causing impaired cell division and apoptosis. Within hours following significant ionizing radiation, there is a decline in the number of immune cells, particularly lymphocytes. Rapidly dividing tissues are particularly affected, interrupting mucosal barriers in the gut and leading to translocation of gut flora
Ultraviolet radiation(sun exposure)	Chronic sun exposure alters and disrupts immune function in the skin. This contributes to diminished immune surveillance of abnormal cells and the development of skin cancer
Chemicals and toxins	
Numerous environmental and industrial chemicals have deleterious effects on the immune system	
Aflatoxins	A series of toxins produced by fungi (*Aspergillus* spp.) that contaminate staple crops, particularly in tropical regions of the world. Chronic exposure leads to DNA damage and immunosuppression alongside hepatic damage
Heavy metals (arsenic, cadmium, copper, gold, iron, lead, zinc)	Directly suppress bone marrow and lymphocytic function
Pesticides (organophosphates, organochlorines)	Directly suppress bone marrow and lymphocytic function
Aromatic amines (e.g. benzidine)	Impairment of cellular immunity
Aromatic hydrocarbons (e.g. benzene)	Impairment of cellular immunity

Travel in the immunocompromised

Introduction

With increasing globalization, travel, and therefore novel exposure, is growing in the immunocompromised. An evaluation of the degree of immune compromise should be made. (Box 10.1).

Box 10.1 Degrees of immune compromise

Not significantly immunocompromised
- Steroid therapy limited to short (5–7 days) oral course, inhaled, topical, intra-articular preparations or >1 month after completing withdrawal from long-term steroids.
- HIV with CD4 count >500/μL.
- Malignancy with last chemotherapy >3 months ago and in remission.
- HSCT >2 years with no ongoing immunosuppressive treatment and no GvHD.
- Autoimmune conditions (e.g. SLE, inflammatory bowel disease, rheumatoid arthritis, or multiple sclerosis) not on immunosuppressant drugs and not experiencing an exacerbation of disease.

Mild to moderate immunocompromise
- Asymptomatic HIV with CD4 count of 200–500/μL.
- Chronic medical conditions (e.g. diabetes mellitus, chronic liver disease, chronic renal disease, splenectomy/functional hyposplenism).

Severe immunocompromise
- Long term (>2 weeks), high-dose (>20 mg/day prednisolone) corticosteroid use.
- Solid organ transplant recipient on immunosuppressant medication (e.g. ciclosporin, tacrolimus, sirolimus, azathioprine, or mycophenolate).
- HSCT recipients (<2 years of transplantation or still on immunosuppressive drugs).
- Current chemotherapy (within 3 months) for cancer (excluding tamoxifen).
- Immunosuppressive drugs for the treatment of other conditions (e.g. cyclophosphamide, azathioprine, etc.).
- Biological agents that are immunosuppressive or immunomodulatory (e.g. TNF blockers such as etanercept and infliximab and other monoclonal antibodies such as rituximab and alemtuzumab).
- Active haematological malignancy or metastatic solid organ malignancy.

Source: data from Kotton, C.N. et al. Advising Travelers With Specific Needs: Immunocompromised Traveler. In *CDC Health Information for International Travel*. Atlanta, USA: Oxford University Press & Centers for Disease Control and Prevention. Copyright © 2014 Centers for Disease Control and Prevention/OUP.

Pre-travel advice

Appropriate pre-travel advice includes an assessment of the degree of compromise, intended destination and activities, vaccination, prophylaxis, access to medication, and appropriate medical care. Standard travel advice applies. General travel considerations are listed in Box 10.2.

Box 10.2 Travel considerations

- Accident prevention: road traffic accidents, swimming/drowning.

- Sunlight hazards: sun screen and skin care.

- Insect bite and sting prevention.

- Animals: rabies prevention.

- Drinking water: safe drinking water practices.

- Women's health and feminine hygiene.

- Access to essential medication while travelling.

- Travel insurance.

- Malaria prevention (see 'Malaria prophylaxis' p.223).

- Air transport: including deep vein thrombosis prevention.

- Sexual health and contraception: including prevention of HIV.

- Heat and cold illness prevention.

- Altitude illness prevention.

- Food hygiene: prevention of intestinal infection and diarrhoea.

- Risks associated with specific activities, e.g. diving, winter sports.

- Travelling with drugs including import controls etc.

- Emergency treatment access and evacuation planning.

- Immunization (see 'Immunizations' p.222).

Immunizations

Where indicated, immunization is vital to reducing the risk of disease in immunocompromised travellers. Inactivated or subunit vaccines are considered safe in all forms of immunocompromise. Additional booster vaccinations may be necessary with defective immune response. While the efficacy of the vaccine may be reduced (in terms of provoked immune response), they may be more effective as immunocompromised patients are more likely to suffer severe disease from infection. Live attenuated vaccines (e.g. BCG, MMR, oral polio vaccine, and yellow fever) have the potential to cause vaccine-associated disease and are therefore contraindicated in severe immunocompromise. All travellers should be up to date with routine vaccinations (unless contraindicated) in line with the latest national guidance.

Routine vaccinations

UK guidance can be found at ℘ https://www.gov.uk/government/publications/the-complete-routine-immunisation-schedule.

This currently includes vaccination against diphtheria, tetanus, pertussis, polio, *Haemophilus influenzae* type b, hepatitis B, pneumococcus, rotavirus, meningitis B and ACWY (all inactivated or subunit), in addition to MMR (live attenuated).

Additional vaccinations

Recommended in specific patient groups include annual influenza vaccination for children 2–8 years old, those >65 years old and chronic medical conditions (e.g. chronic renal failure, chronic liver failure, and diabetes), shingles vaccination in those >70 years old.

Travel-associated vaccinations

Up-to-date recommendations for travel vaccination can be found at:
- NICE Guidance: ℘ https://cks.nice.org.uk/
  immunizations-travel#!topicsummary.
- National Travel Health Network and Centre: ℘ http://www.
  travelhealthpro.org.uk/.
- Public Health England 'The Green Book' (2013) guidelines on
  immunization: ℘ https://www.gov.uk/government/publications/
  immunisation-against-infectious-disease-the-green-book-front-cover-
  and-contents-page.

Vaccinations considered safe in the immunocompromised

Diphtheria, tetanus, pertussis, *H. influenzae* type b, pneumococcus, hepatitis A, hepatitis B, meningococcal, rabies, inactivated typhoid vaccine, Japanese encephalitis, inactivated influenza, and inactivated polio.

Vaccinations contraindicated in the immunocompromised

The following vaccinations are contraindicated in severe immunocompromise and a consideration of the risks and benefits needs to be made in mild-to-moderate immunocompromise: BCG vaccine, oral live polio, MMR, herpes zoster, live oral typhoid vaccine, yellow fever, and live attenuated influenza vaccine.

Malaria prophylaxis

Malaria prophylaxis is recommended for all immunocompromised patients travelling to areas where it is indicated. Up-to-date recommendations and risk assessments for specific geographic regions can be found at the National Travel Health Network and Centre website (🖰 http://www.travelhealthpro.org.uk/).

The options are the same as for the non-immunocompromised: mefloquine, atovaquone/proguanil, doxycycline, and chloroquine and/or proguanil (in specific regions with little or no resistance). Interactions with concurrent medications should be checked. Bite avoidance and early presentation if unwell should be emphasized.

Infections associated with specific geographic regions

Travellers, both immunocompromised and not, remain susceptible to the usual infectious agents that cause respiratory, urinary, skin, GI infections etc. in human populations across the world.

Several organisms that are commonly associated with infection in the immunocompromised have a fairly ubiquitous global distribution (e.g. *Pneumocystis* pneumonia, CMV, *Toxoplasma gondii*, *Cryptosporidium* spp., *Candida* spp., *Aspergillus* spp., and *Cryptococcus neoformans*).

The following summary of geographical associations with specific infections omits pathogens that could be considered universal in all human populations, both immunocompromised and not. It is by no means exhaustive. Rather, it is designed to provide a broad idea of infections that may be relevant to immunocompromised travellers. In an age of modern air travel, it is becoming increasingly difficult to confidently determine firm geographical distributions for many infections.

Prophylaxis for specific infections beyond routine prophylaxis (e.g. malaria chemoprophylaxis) and specific recommendations for particular immunocompromised conditions (e.g. *Pneumocystis* pneumonia prophylaxis etc.) must be made on a case-by-case basis depending on the degree of immunocompromise, destination, and intended activities (e.g. antibiotic prophylaxis for traveller's diarrhoea).

North Africa and the Middle East

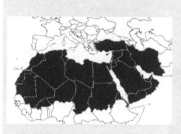

Major infections

Malaria Present along the southern border of the Sahara but almost absent from African countries north of the Sahara. Malaria transmission does occur on the Arabian peninsula, principally in Yemen. Malaria is also present in Iran, South East Turkey, and the border with Syria (*Plasmodium vivax*).

TB Present across North Africa and the Middle East. Incidence in the region ~50–100/100,000.

HIV Prevalence low in the Arabian peninsula and Middle East. Much higher prevalence in Western North Africa (e.g. Algeria, Mali, and Mauritania).

Meningococcal meningitis Neisseria meningitidis is especially prevalent across the Sahara ('meningitis belt') and outbreaks are particularly associated with the Hajj pilgrimage to Mecca.

Hepatitis B and C Highly endemic throughout North Africa.

Other significant infections

In addition to more cosmopolitan or usual pathogens consider:
Bacteria, enteric fever (*Salmonella typhi* and *paratyphi*), leptospirosis (*Leptospira* spp.), brucellosis (*Brucella* spp.), cholera (*Vibrio cholerae*). *Rickettsia*: Mediterranean spotted fever (*R. conorii*), epidemic typhus (*R. prowazekii*), murine typhus (*R. typhi*), *R. felis*, Anthrax (*B. anthracis*); especially in Turkey.

Viruses Hepatitis B and C—highly endemic throughout North Africa. Hepatitis A and E. Rabies. Middle East respiratory syndrome coronavirus (MERS-CoV)- associated with dromedary camels in the Middle East. Measles. Chikungunya, Dengue, Rift Valley Fever, Toscana, Sindbis, Sandfly, Crimean Congo Haemorrhagic fever and West Nile Viruses have all been reported in the region. Yellow fever (only Sudan).

Parasites Cutaneous and visceral leishmaniasis occurs across North Africa. Schistosomiasis: common particularly in Egypt and Northern Sudan. *Echinococcus granulosis* is hyperendemic and present throughout the region. *Trichinella* spp. (uncooked meat), *Giardia intestinalis, Cryptosporidium, Wuchereria bancrofti* still present in Yemen. Geohelminth infections (*hookworms, Strongyloides* and *Ascaris*). *Entamoeba histolytica*.

Fungi Globally distributed species (e.g. *Candida* spp., *Aspergillus* spp., *C. neoformans*).

Sub-Saharan Africa

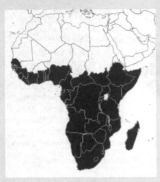

Major infections

Malaria Hyperendemic throughout most of the region with stable year-round transmission. Absent from the lower parts of South Africa. Chloroquine resistant *P. falciparum* is almost universal.

TB Highly prevalent, in conjunction with the HIV epidemic. Significant MDR and XDR, particularly in South Africa/Swaziland. Majority of the region has incidences of >250/100,000.

HIV Very high prevalence throughout the region. Prevalences >4% over large areas and as high as 18% in parts of South Africa and East Africa.

Meningococcal meningitis (*Neisseria meningitidis*) is common.

Other significant infections

In addition to more cosmopolitan or usual pathogens consider:
Bacteria Enteric fever (*S. typhi* and *paratyphi*), leptospirosis (*Leptospira* spp.), brucellosis (*Brucella* spp.), cholera (*V. cholerae*), bubonic plague (*Yersinia pestis*) (especially Madagascar), Relapsing fever (*Borrelia recurrentis*), Leprosy (*Mycobacterium leprae*), Rickettsia; epidemic typhus (*R. prowazekii*), murine typhus (*R. typhi*), tick typhus (*R. conorii, R. africae*), anthrax (*Bacillus anthracis*).

Viruses Measles, yellow fever, dengue, Chikungunya virus, Zika virus, hepatitis A, B, C, E, viral haemorrhagic fevers (e.g. Ebola, Marburg haemorrhagic fever, Lassa fever, Crimean–Congo haemorrhagic fever, Rift Valley fever), rabies virus, HTLV-1.

Parasites Trematodes; Schistosomiasis (*Schistosoma mansoni, S. haematobium*), liver flukes (*F. hepatica*), Lung fluke (*Paragonimus* spp.). Nematodes; Geohelminth infections (hookworms, *Strongyloides* and *Ascaris*), Trichinella spp. Protozoa; African trypanosomiasis (*Trypanosoma brucei gambiense* and *Trypanosoma brucei rhodesiense*), *G. intestinalis*, Cutaneous and visceral leishmaniasis (*Leishmania* spp.). Cestodes; echinococcosis (*E. granulosis*), *T. saginata, T. solium*. Filarial nematodes; lymphatic filariasis (*Wuchereria bancrofti*), Onchocerciasis (*Onchocerca volvulus*), *Loa loa, Mansonella streptocerca,* Others; *Entamoeba histolytica, Cryptosporidium* spp.

Fungi *Histoplasma capsulatum* var. *duboisii* is localized to western and central Africa and to Madagascar.

Indian subcontinent

Major infections

Malaria Present across most of the region, including India, Afghanistan, Pakistan, and Nepal. Risk is highest in north-eastern states of India.

TB Moderate to high incidence, ~50–250/ 100,000 across the region.

HIV Prevalence is low (<0.3% in India), rising prevalence in urban centres.

Dengue fever, enteric fever (S. typhi and paratyphi), and scrub typhus Common causes of febrile illness.

Other significant infections

In addition to more cosmopolitan or usual pathogens consider:
Bacteria Widespread antibiotic resistance in India, enteric fever (*S. typhi* and *paratyphi*), melioidosis (*Burkholderia pseudomallei*), leprosy (*Mycobacterium leprae*). Rickettsial infection, mainly scrub typhus (*Orientia tsutsugamushi*) (*Leptospira* spp.), brucellosis (*Brucella* spp.), cholera (*V. cholerae*).

Viruses Dengue fever, Japanese encephalitis, rabies is endemic, Chikungunya fever, hepatitis A, B, C, E, yellow fever, Nipah, Zika, Hantaviruses, Crimean Congo haemorrhagic virus, West Nile Virus, Kyasanur forest virus.

Parasites Entamoeba histolytica, Giardia intestinalis, Cyclospora cayetanensis, Cryptosporidium spp., Dientamoeba fragilis, Taenia saginata, T. solium, E. granulosus, S. stercoralis and other geohelminths, Fasciola hepatica and other liver flukes. Trichinella spp. (uncooked meat). Cutaneous and visceral leishmaniasis (*Leishmania* spp.), Filarial nematodes (*Wuchereria bancrofti, Brugia malayi*), Schistosomiasis (*S. haematobium* and *S. mansoni*)

Fungi Penicillium marneffei, newly endemic in several states of India, particularly Manipur, particularly in HIV (CD4 count <100 cells/μL), aspergillosis, histoplasmosis, cryptococcosis.

Southeast Asia (including Indonesia and the Philippines)

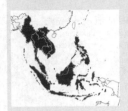

Major infections

Malaria Present throughout the region, including Indonesia and the Philippines, transmission in most parts is unstable and seasonal. *P. knowlesi* malaria is present on the island of Borneo. The proportion of *P. falciparum* is declining in favour of *P. vivax*. Chloroquine and mefloquine resistance is widespread in SE Asia and resistance to artemisinins is beginning to develop (Thai–Burma and Thai–Cambodia borders).

TB Incidence is high with incidence up to 750/100,000 in parts of SE Asia. One-third of the world's MDR TB in the region.

HIV Prevalence is high in parts of SE Asia (>1% in Thailand), lower in Indonesia (0.4%) and the Philippines (<0.1%).

Dengue fever and Scrub typhus Common causes of fever.

Streptococcus suis and melioidosis (B. pseudomallei) Important causes of severe bacterial infection in the region.

Chronic hepatitis B carriage is common.

Other significant infections

In addition to more cosmopolitan or usual pathogens consider:
Bacteria S. suis, B. pseudomallei, rickettsial infection including scrub typhus (*O. tsutsugamushi*), murine typhus (*R. typhi*), leptospirosis (*Leptospira* spp.), enteric fever (*S. typhi* and paratyphi), Brucella, cholera.

Viruses Japanese encephalitis virus (JEV), dengue, Nipah (Borneo), rabies, Chikungunya fever, hepatitis A, B, C, E, yellow fever. Influenza (H1N1)/avian influenza (H5N1) particularly associated with Southeast Asia.

Parasites Schistosomiasis (*S. mekongi, S. japonicum*), E. histolytica, G. intestinalis, C. cayetanensis, Cryptosporidium spp., D. fragilis, T. saginata, T. solium, E. granulosus, S. stercoralis and other geohelminths, F. hepatica and other liver flukes (*Clonorchis/ Opisthorchis* spp.), *Gnathostoma* spp. (raw seafood), *Paragonimus westermani*, (raw seafood), eosinophilic meningitis (*Angiostrongylus cantonensis*), lymphatic filariasis (*Wuchereria bancrofti, Brugia malayi*, and *B. timori*), *Trichinella* spp. (uncooked meat).

Fungi P. marneffei, endemic in Southeast Asia (especially Northern Thailand and Vietnam) and southern China. H. capsulatum.

China and the Far East

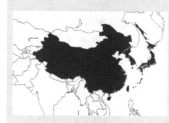

Major infections

Malaria Low prevalence but present in south and central China. *P. falciparum* is restricted to southern China (Yunnan and Hainan), also present in Korea (North and South). Absent from Japan, Taiwan, and Hong Kong.

TB Incidence is moderate, ~100/100,000.

HIV Prevalence low (0.1% in China and Japan).

Other significant infections

In addition to more cosmopolitan or usual pathogens consider:

Bacteria Rickettsial infection including scrub typhus (*O. tsutsugamushi*), murine typhus (*R. typhi*), Japanese spotted fever (*Rickettsia japonica*). Leptospirosis (*Leptospira* spp.), enteric fever (*S. typhi* and paratyphi), brucellosis (*Brucella* spp.), cholera (*V. cholerae*), bubonic plague (*Yersinia pestis*), anthrax (*Bacillus anthracis*), tularaemia (*Francisella tularensis*).

Viruses JEV, dengue, rabies, HTLV-1 (Japan), hepatitis A, B, C, E, SARS coronavirus.

Parasites Schistosomiasis (*S. mekongi, S. japonicum*), *E. histolytica, G. intestinalis, C. cayetanensis, Cryptosporidium* spp., *D. fragilis, T. saginata, T. solium, E. granulosus, S. stercoralis* and other geohelminths, *F. hepatica* and other liver flukes (*Clonorchis/Opisthorchis* spp.), *Gnathostoma* spp., *Trichinella* spp. (uncooked meat), eosinophilic meningitis (*A. cantonensis*).

Fungi *P. marneffei*, endemic in Southeast Asia (especially Northern Thailand and Vietnam) and southern China.

Australasia and Oceania

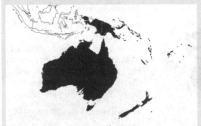

Common and major infections

Malaria
Hyperendemic (*P. falciparum* and *P. vivax*) in lowland areas of the island of New Guinea, Solomon Islands, and Vanuatu. Absent from Australia, New Zealand, and Polynesia.

TB Highly endemic on the island of New Guinea and Melanesia, incidences ~250–750/100,000. Low prevalence in Australia and New Zealand.

HIV Rising prevalence in populated parts of the island of New Guinea (>0.7% in Papua New Guinea). Low prevalence in Australia and New Zealand.

Dengue Tropical Australia and New Guinea.

Other significant infections

In addition to more cosmopolitan or usual pathogens consider:

Bacteria B. *pseudomallei* (tropical Australia and New Guinea), leptospirosis (*Leptospira* spp.), brucellosis (*Brucella* spp.), cholera (*V. cholerae*), Rickettsial infection: scrub typhus (*O. tsutsugamushi*), Murine typhus (*Rickettsia typhi*), Queensland tick typhus (*Rickettsia australis*), Flinder's Island spotted fever (*Rickettsia honei*).

Viruses Chikungunya, Ross River virus, Murray Valley encephalitis, Zika virus, Nipah, hepatitis A, B, C, E, Barmah Forest virus, Hendra virus, lyssavirus, HTLV-1.

Parasites Lymphatic filariasis (*W. bancrofti* or *B. malayi*) endemic in Papua New Guinea, Melanesia, and Polynesia. *E. histolytica, G. intestinalis*, eosinophilic meningitis (*A. cantonensis*). *Trichinella* spp. (uncooked meat), Strongyloidiasis (*S. stercoralis*), *A. lumbricoides, T. trichiuria*, hookworm species and other geohelminths, liver flukes (*F. hepatica*).

Fungi Globally distributed species (e.g. *Candida* spp., *Aspergillus* spp., *C. neoformans*).

Western and Northern Europe

Major infections

Malaria Not endemic.

TB Incidence low <75/ 100,000, higher in immigrant communities.

HIV Prevalence is low (~0.3%).

Other significant infections

In addition to more cosmopolitan or usual pathogens consider:
Bacteria Widespread use of antimicrobials means that resistant organisms are common. *Clostridium difficile*. Important but less common infections include *Borrelia* spp., tularaemia (*Francisella tularensis*), leptospirosis, *Listeria monocytogenes*, and *Legionella pneumophila*.

Viruses Influenza, hepatitis B and C—common in IV drug users. Tick-borne encephalitis (Scandinavia), Puumala virus (Scandinavia), HTLV-2.

Parasites *Leishmania infantum* causes visceral leishmaniasis in the Mediterranean region. *G. intestinalis, Blastocystis, D. fragilis*.

Fungi Globally distributed species (e.g. *Candida* spp., *Aspergillus* spp., *C. neoformans*).

Eastern and Southern Europe

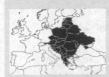

Major infections

Malaria Not endemic.

TB Incidence up to 250/100,000 in parts (e.g. Romania, Estonia, Latvia, Ukraine), rates of MDR and XDR are high.

HIV Prevalences >1% in parts (e.g. Estonia, Latvia, Ukraine).

Other significant infections

In addition to more cosmopolitan or usual pathogens consider:
Bacteria Drug-resistant bacteria including MRSA common. Important but less common infections include *Borrelia* spp., leptospirosis, *L. monocytogenes*, *L. pneumophila*, *Brucella melitensis*, *Yersinia* spp., tularaemia (*F. tularensis*).

Viruses Hepatitis B and C—common in IV drug users. Hepatitis A outbreaks are common, tick-borne encephalitis, Crimean–Congo haemorrhagic fever, HTLV-2.

Parasites *L. infantum* causing visceral leishmaniasis is present in the Mediterranean region, *G. intestinalis*, *E. granulosus*, *E. histolytica*, *Cystoisospora belli*, *Microsporidia*.

Fungi Globally distributed species (e.g. *Candida* spp., *Aspergillus* spp., *C. neoformans*).

Russian Federation and Central Asia

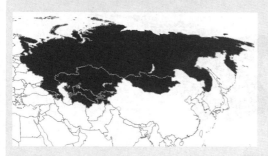

Major infections

Malaria (*P. vivax*) is present at low prevalence and transmission is unstable in focal areas of Russia bordering Central Asia and in wetlands close to Moscow.

TB Incidence up to 250/100,000 in parts of Russia and Central Asia (e.g. Kazakhstan), rates of MDR and XDR are high.

HIV Prevalence >1% in Russia, lower in Central Asia.

Other significant infections

In addition to more cosmopolitan or usual pathogens consider:

Bacteria Drug-resistant bacteria including MRSA common. Important but less common infections include Lyme disease (*Borrelia* spp.), leptospirosis (*Leptospira* spp.), *L. monocytogenes*, *L. pneumophila*, brucellosis (*B. melitensis*), bubonic plague (*Yersinia pestis*), anthrax (*B. anthracis*).

Viruses Hepatitis B and C—common in IV drug users. Hepatitis A outbreaks common. Hepatitis E, tick-borne encephalitis, Crimean–Congo haemorrhagic fever.

Parasites *G. intestinalis*, *E. granulosus*, *E. histolytica*, *C. belli*, *Microsporidia*.

Fungi globally distributed species (e.g. *Candida* spp., *Aspergillus* spp., *C. neoformans*).

North America

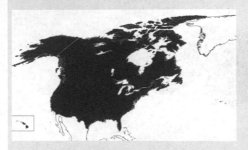

Major infections

Malaria not endemic.

TB Incidence low (<5/100,000).

HIV Prevalence is low (0.6%).

Other significant infections

In addition to more cosmopolitan or usual pathogens consider:
Bacteria Widespread antibiotic resistance including community-acquired MRSA, ESBL/AmpC, and CPE, *C. difficile*, *L. pneumophila* (air conditioning units etc.), *L. monocytogenes*. Tick-borne infection (mainly from Northeast and upper Midwest): *Borrelia* spp., Rocky Mountain spotted fever (*Rickettsia rickettsii*), *Ehrlichia, Anaplasma*. Southern tick-associated rash illness (STARI), tularaemia (*F. tularensis*), Leptospirosis (*Leptospira* spp.).

Viruses Saint Louis encephalitis, eastern equine encephalitis, western equine encephalitis, West Nile fever (introduced from Africa and spread throughout the United States and southern Canada), Dengue—occasional outbreaks in Florida, Texas, and Hawaii. HTLV-2. Rabies remains present.

Parasites *Trichinella* spp., and *T. gondii* are common in Arctic regions due to consumption of wild animals. *G. intestinalis, Cryptosporidium* spp., *Ascaris lumbricoides, Cyclospora cayetanensis* (especially Midwest).

Fungi Dimorphic fungi acquired via spore inhalation: histoplasmosis—*H. capsulatum* is endemic in the Mississippi and Ohio River valleys. *Coccidioides immitis*—SW United States and parts of South America, *Blastomyces dermatitidis*.

Central America and the Caribbean

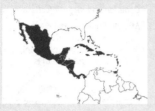

Common and major infections

Malaria Present in most lowland regions of Central America as well as Haiti and the Dominican Republic in the Caribbean. Mainly due to *P. vivax*.

TB Incidence ~25/100,000 in Central America while ~80/100,000 in the Caribbean.

HIV Low prevalence in Central America but high prevalence in parts of the Caribbean (e.g. Jamaica 1.6%).

Other significant infections

In addition to more cosmopolitan or usual pathogens consider:

Bacteria Enteric fever (*S. typhi* and *paratyphi*), leptospirosis (*Leptospira* spp.), *L. monocytogenes*, Rickettsial infections including Rocky Mountain spotted fever (*Rickettsia rickettsii*), cholera (*V. cholerae*) (especially Haiti and Dominican Republic).

Viruses Dengue, Zika, Chikungunya, Hantavirus, West Nile virus (Mexico), HTLV-1 (Caribbean), rabies, measles.

Parasites *T. saginata*, *T. solium*, *Trichinella* spp., Chagas disease (*Trypanosoma cruzi*), *Leishmania* (cutaneous, mucosal, and visceral), *S. mansoni* present but now rare on several Caribbean islands. *A. lumbricoides*, *T. trichiuria*, hookworm species and other geohelminths filariasis (*W. bancrofti*) (Haiti), *C. belli*, *G. intestinalis*, *Cryptosporidium* spp., *Cyclospora cayetanensis* (especially Mexico), *Entamoeba histolytica*.

Fungi Dimorphic fungi acquired via spore inhalation: histoplasmosis—*H. capsulatum* (Central America and many of the Caribbean islands). Pulmonary coccidioidomycosis (*Coccidiodes* spp.) (especially Mexico).

South America

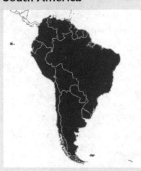

Common and major infections

Malaria Endemic, mainly in tropical Brazil and Northern parts of the continent. Mainly *P. vivax* but *P. falciparum* is present.

TB Incidence 40–60/100,000, highest in Andean regions (e.g. Peru and Bolivia).

HIV Overall prevalence ~0.5%. Higher in urban centres.

Other significant infections

In addition to more cosmopolitan or usual pathogens consider:

Bacteria enteric fever (*S. typhi* and *paratyphi*), brucellosis (*Brucella* spp.), *L. monocytogenes, Bartonella* spp., rickettsial infection (including *R. rickettsii*). leptospirosis (*Leptospira* spp.), anthrax (*Bacillus anthracis*).

Viruses Dengue, Zika, measles, yellow fever (jungle), HTLV-1, *Hantavirus*, hepatitis A, B, C, E, Saint Louis encephalitis, eastern equine encephalitis, Venezuelan equine encephalitis, oropouche virus.

Parasites Chagas disease (*T. cruzi*), Leishmania (cutaneous, mucosal, and visceral; *Leishmania* spp.), Schistosomiasis (*S. mansoni*), Cestodes; *Taenia solium, T. saginata*, hookworms, *Lagochilascaris minor, A. lumbricoides, S. stercoralis, Toxocara canis, Angiostrongylus* spp., Filarial nematodes; lymphatic filariasis (*Wuchereria bancrofti*), Onchocerciasis (*Onchocerca volvulus*), *Entamoeba histolytica*.

Fungi Dimorphic fungi acquired via spore inhalation: *Paracoccidioides brasiliensis. C. immitis, Sporothrix schenckii* (especially Peru).

The unwell returning traveller

Key features of the history

- *Degree of immune suppression*: assess degree of compromise.
- *Destination*: exactly where has the patient been?
- *Timing*: incubation periods, duration of exposure, and season.
- *Exposures*: sexual exposure; activities (e.g. freshwater swimming, jungle trekking, etc.); insect bites, bed net use, etc.; sources of food, drinking water, etc.; healthcare contact abroad; animal bites; and air conditioning.
- *Prophylaxis*: malaria chemoprophylaxis, and vaccinations (consider efficacy in severe immunosuppression).
- *Clinical syndrome*: CNS, pulmonary, GI, fever with eosinophilia, rash, jaundice, fever and bleeding, etc.

Incubation periods

The usual incubation periods for particular infections may be altered in the immunosuppressed patient. Box 10.3 shows incubation periods for common and important travel-related infections.

Box 10.3 Incubation periods for travel-related infections

- *Malaria*:
  - *Plasmodium falciparum* usually 7–14 days (~max. 90 days).
  - *P. vivax*/*P. ovale* usually 12–18 days (~max. 1 year).
  - *P. malariae* 18–40 days (~max. 1 year).
- *Dengue*: 4–8 days (~max. 3–14 days).
- *Acute HIV*: 10–28 days (~max. 6 weeks).
- *Acute schistosomiasis*: ~4–8 weeks.
- *Viral haemorrhagic fevers*: (e.g. Ebola, Marburg, etc.) 2–21 days (max. <21 days).
- *Rabies*: 1–3 months (~max. 1 week to 1 year).
- *Enteric fever*: (Salmonella spp.) 7–18 days (~max. 3–90 days).
- *Amoebic liver abscess*: several weeks to months.
- *Hepatitis A*: 14–50 days (max. < 9 weeks).
- *Hepatitis E*: 25–45 days (max. < 9 weeks).
- *Hepatitis B*: 90 days (60–150 days).
- *Chikungunya*: 2–4 days (~max. 1–14 days).
- *Leptospirosis*: 7–12 days (~max. 2–26 days).
- *Legionella*: 5–6 days (~max. 2–10 days).
- *Rickettsial infections*: 3–28 days.
- *Measles*: 7–18 days.
- *Arboviral encephalitis*: (JEV, West Nile virus, etc.) 3–14 days (~max. 1–20 days).
- *Campylobacter* spp.: 1–10 days.
- *Shigella* spp.: 12 hours–4 days.
- Enterotoxigenic *Escherichia coli*: 1–4 days.
- *Leishmania*: visceral: 10 days to years.

Clinical syndromes

Malaria and HIV must be excluded in all unwell travellers returning from endemic areas. Consider the following conditions in addition to more usual causes:

Undifferentiated fever

Malaria, dengue, other arboviruses (e.g. chikungunya, zika), leptospirosis, typhoid and paratyphoid, rickettsial infection, tuberculosis, acute HIV infection, African and American trypanosomiasis, viral haemorrhagic fevers (Lassa, Ebola, Marburg), brucellosis, visceral leishmaniasis.

Fever with CNS signs

Malaria, bacterial meningitis (*Neisseria meningitidis, Streptococcus pneumoniae, Haemophilus influenzae*), viral encephalitis (HSV, JEV, West Nile virus, enterovirus), leptospirosis, listeriosis, rickettsial infection, African trypanosomiasis, rabies and TB.

Fever with respiratory symptoms

Influenza, legionella, Middle East respiratory syndrome (MERS), SARS, melioidosis, TB, Q fever (*Coxiella burnetii*), pertussis, rickettsial infection, ascariasis (Loeffler's syndrome), Katayama fever (acute schistosomiasis), meliodosis, histoplasmosis, and coccidioidomycosis.

Fever with gastrointestinal symptoms

E. coli (enterotoxigenic *E. coli*), *Campylobacter* spp., *Salmonella* spp., *Shigella* spp., amoebic dysentery (*E. histolytica*), hepatitis A virus, Cholera, *Vibrio parahaemolyticus*, *Yersinia* spp.

Fever with rash (often accompanied by thrombocytopenia)

Dengue, rickettsial infection, measles, Chikungunya, Zika, meningococcal infection and rubella.

Fever with jaundice

Viral hepatitis (HAV, HEV, acute HBV), leptospirosis, malaria, amoebic liver abscess and yellow fever.

Fever with eosinophilia

Alongside allergic reactions, classically associated with parasitic infections; nematodes (e.g. *Strongyloides stercoralis*), trematodes (schistosomiasis, flukes), filarial nematodes (e.g. lymphatic filariasis, onchocerciasis), cestodes (e.g. *Taenia* spp.). Myiasis (e.g. C. *anthropophaga*), scabies.

Further reading

1. Kotton CN, Freedman DO. Advising travelers with specific needs: immunocompromised travelers. In: CDC Health Information for International Travel ('The Yellow Book'). Centers for Disease Control and Prevention; 2014. ℘ https://wwwnc.cdc.gov/travel/yellowbook/2018/advising-travelers-with-specific-needs/immunocompromised-travelers
2. Public Health England. 'The Green Book' (2013) guidelines on immunization: ℘ https://www.gov.uk/government/publications/immunisation-against-infectious-disease-the-green-book-front-cover-and-contents-page

Section 3

Microbiology

Viruses

Introduction

Viral infections are particularly important in the immunocompromised and are a leading cause of death in SOT and HSCT. They represent a particular challenge to the clinician as they can present non-specifically, disease can progress rapidly, and treatment options have variable efficacy.

Two further important features of viral infection contribute to their significance. The first is the ability of some viruses (particularly the human herpesviruses) to establish latency and reactivate in circumstances of reduced immune suppression. This makes viruses such as CMV, EBV, HSV, and VZV key pathogens in the immunocompromised. The second feature is the association between certain viruses and the development of malignancy (e.g. EBV, HPV). The oncogenic potential of these infections and the failure of immune surveillance is exacerbated in the immunocompromised.

Fortunately, developments in molecular diagnostic techniques, particularly PCR, have made a significant contribution to the rapid diagnosis of these infections allowing for earlier and more effective treatment.

Human herpesviruses

The eight human herpesviruses are divided into alpha, beta, and gamma sub-families on the basis of their genomic and biological properties (Table 11.1).

Herpesviruses have a linear, double-stranded DNA genome inside an icosahedral capsid; this is surrounded by a protein tegument and enclosed within an outer lipid envelope containing glycoprotein spikes. They all share the capacity to produce latent infection in their natural host, during which the viral genome persists in cells, usually as a closed circle (episome), expressing only a limited subset of genes.

The diseases they cause may result from primary infection or reactivation of latent virus and tend to be more severe in immunosuppressed patients. The gamma herpesviruses (γ) can induce cell transformation, and are associated with specific tumours.

Table 11.1 Herpesviruses

Name/designation (subfamily)	Site of latency
Herpes simplex virus 1/HHV-1 (α)	Sensory ganglia
Herpes simplex virus 2/HHV-2 (α)	Sensory ganglia
Varicella zoster virus/HHV-3 (α)	Sensory ganglia
Epstein–Barr virus/HHV-4 (γ)	B lymphocytes (oropharyngeal epithelium)
Human Cytomegalovirus/HHV-5 (β)	Monocytes ($\pm$ epithelial cells)
HHV-6 (β)	Monocytes, T lymphocytes
HHV-7 (β)	—
Kaposi's sarcoma-associated virus/HHV-8 (γ)	Uncertain

Cytomegalovirus (CMV/HHV-5)

With a diameter of 150–200 nm, CMV is one of the largest viruses known to cause human disease. Its genome encodes >200 proteins, including some that downregulate the immune system and contribute to its immunosuppressive properties. Two proteins, US2 and US11, are known to target major histocompatibility complex class 1 molecules for degradation. This impairs viral antigen presentation on infected cells, thus interfering with T-cell recognition and is a possible mechanism for viral latency.

Epidemiology

CMV is most commonly acquired during childhood and early adulthood. It can be transmitted transplacentally, through the birth canal and via breastmilk. In childhood, transmission is mostly through saliva and later in life via sexual contact. Transmission can also occur via blood transfusions and transplantation. CMV infection is globally ubiquitous with a seroprevalence reaching ~70% in some urban US adult populations and 100% in some developing countries.

After primary infection, the virus establishes latency in leucocytes, endothelial cells, renal epithelial cells, and salivary glands and persists lifelong. These sites of latency act as both viral reservoirs for onward transmission and foci of reactivation during periods of immunocompromise.

Clinical features

In the immunocompetent, primary infection may be asymptomatic, a nonspecific febrile illness, or an infectious mononucleosis-like syndrome characterized by fever, lymphocytosis, and lymphadenopathy.

Those at greatest risk of severe CMV disease are patients with advanced HIV infection, transplant recipients, and the fetus. Common presentations in these groups include the following:

HIV infection

(➔ See also Chapter 5.)

- *Ocular*: unilateral blurred central vision, 'floaters', or photopsia (flashing lights) are the commonest manifestations of CMV retinitis in HIV (usually when CD4+ T-cell count <50 cells/μL). If left untreated it results in subacute progressive retinal destruction leading to irreversible blindness.
- *CNS*: polyradiculopathy (weakness and diminished reflexes in lower extremities, urinary retention) or ventriculoencephalopathy (delirium, confusion, and/or focal neurological abnormalities).
- *Respiratory*: pneumonitis (dyspnoea, fever, and cough).
- *GI tract*: oesophagitis, gastritis, ileitis, colitis, pancreatitis, or hepatitis.

SOT recipients

Reactivation may be triggered by a combination of allostimulation, allograft rejection, and/or pharmacological immunosuppression. The highest risk group for primary disease is CMV-seronegative patients who receive an allograft from a CMV-seropositive donor. The GI tract is the most common site of disease in CMV-negative SOT recipients.

The transplanted organ is also at higher risk for organ-specific invasive CMV disease. CMV pneumonitis following lung transplant is the most rapidly life-threatening and requires prompt empiric initiation of antiviral treatment.

HSCT recipients

CMV disease in HSCT recipients presents as either CMV syndrome (fever, myalgia, and myelosuppression) or tissue-invasive disease (pneumonitis being the most common and severe). Allogeneic HSCT recipients require more immunosuppression than autologous recipients and are therefore at higher risk of CMV disease.

Neonates

Most cases of intrauterine infection and congenital CMV arise from primary maternal CMV infection in pregnancy. The risk is highest if infection occurs in the first half of pregnancy. Congenital CMV infection, known as cytomegalic inclusion disease, usually manifests as jaundice, petechiae, hepatosplenomegaly, microcephaly, chorioretinitis, and cerebral calcification and is often rapidly fatal.

Other at-risk groups

Biological therapy

Patients receiving the anti-CD52 monoclonal antibody alemtuzumab (for treatment of lymphoma) are at particular risk of CMV disease (either CMV syndrome or tissue-invasive disease).

Therapeutic immunosuppression or malignancy

Other immunosuppressive treatments and malignancies (especially haematological) also increase the risk of CMV disease.

Immunocompetent

Primary disease can occur in any CMV-seronegative patient.

Diagnosis

Molecular techniques

Quantitative PCR (qPCR)

The most widely used method and generates huge numbers of copies of a CMV target gene sequence. As well as allowing rapid quantification of viral load it can detect non-viable virus and early disease prior to seroconversion.

Real-time qPCR

Within a closed system, the target gene sequence is simultaneously amplified and detected. This reduces the risk of contamination and enables quick turnaround time. The assay can be performed on stored specimens containing degraded virus.

Both the absolute level of CMV viral load and the rate of increase are useful in predicting those at risk of clinical disease. The main drawbacks with current molecular methods are the potential for contamination and the lack of standardization between assays (e.g. different target gene sequences and different sample types).

Non-molecular assays

Serology

Although unreliable in the diagnosis of CMV disease in the immunocompromised, CMV serology still has a role in risk stratification (as a marker of prior exposure) in those awaiting transplant, HIV-infected patients, and in pregnancy.

Antigen detection

Antigen detection of the CMV matrix protein pp65 within neutrophils has been shown to be both sensitive and specific but its reliance on adequate neutrophil numbers makes it less reliable than PCR in the immunocompromised.

Histopathology

Demonstrating the presence of virus in biopsy samples is still essential for the diagnosis of tissue-invasive disease. The presence of the virus in tissue (most commonly lung, GI, and liver samples) can be demonstrated by staining and microscopy to show viral inclusion disease or using *in situ* hybridization techniques to detect viral DNA.

When to use these diagnostic techniques?

Screening, surveillance, and prevention

CMV serology is used to determine the risk of primary infection in pregnancy, reactivation in HIV infection, and to assess the prior exposure of both recipient and donor in transplantation. If a seronegative individual receives an organ from a seropositive donor, they are at high risk for primary disease and benefit from antiviral prophylaxis. For 8–12 weeks post transplantation, it is now routine to collect weekly blood samples for CMV qPCR assays. If the viral load exceeds a certain threshold (assay dependent), pre-emptive antiviral therapy is started. Trends in viral load for an individual patient (assuming the same assay is used) are more useful for predicting CMV disease than absolute viral load number.

Primary diagnosis

Definitive diagnosis requires the demonstration of CMV in the relevant clinical specimen in the context of suggestive clinical signs and symptoms. Quantitative real-time PCR is now the main modality for diagnosing CMV disease in the immunocompromised. Whole blood is considered the most sensitive and convenient specimen for CMV PCR assays but they can be performed on a wide range of samples including CSF (in suspected CMV encephalitis or polyradiculopathy), BAL samples (in suspected CMV pneumonitis), aqueous humour (in suspected retinitis), tissue biopsies (in suspected organ invasive disease), and heel-prick blood samples (Guthrie test) or urine in the neonate.

Monitoring response to treatment

Serial qPCR (or pp65 antigen) can be used to guide duration of treatment and predict risk of relapse. A rising viral load while on treatment suggests drug-resistant CMV.

Interpretation of test results

HIV infection
(See Chapter 5.)

Retinitis
Anti-CMV therapy is usually initiated on finding the characteristic funduscopic appearances, but if confirmation is needed, the virus can be demonstrated by PCR of the aqueous humour. The presence and titre of CMV DNA can usefully distinguish active from inactive CMV retinitis and aqueous humour viral load can be used to monitor response to therapy.

Polyradiculopathy and ventriculoencephalitis
The sensitivity of CSF PCR is >90% for the diagnosis of neurological CMV disease and serial CSF viral loads may be used to monitor response to therapy.

GI disease
The GI tract is the most common extra-ocular site of CMV disease in HIV infection and any part of the tract may be affected. Diagnosis requires *endoscopic* visualization of the characteristic lesions and biopsy for confirmation of the pathognomonic inclusion bodies. The biopsied tissue can also be tested for CMV by culture, PCR or *in situ* hybridization.

Pneumonitis
The diagnosis of CMV pneumonitis can be difficult as isolating CMV does not usually differentiate asymptomatic infection from active pneumonitis. Approximately half of HIV-infected patients have CMV isolated from pulmonary secretions sampled during bronchoscopic examination. Very high levels of CMV DNA (or antigen) in secretions or demonstration of virus in tissue samples support the diagnosis of true invasive disease.

HSCT patients
(See Chapter 8.)
CMV viral load in whole blood, measured by qPCR, is generally a good marker of disease severity but in suspected pneumonitis, viral load in bronchial secretions is more predictive.

Frequent viral load monitoring (once or twice weekly) in the post-transplant period is recommended to detect rising viraemia and guide initiation of pre-emptive treatment. Monitoring the decline in viral load once on treatment is useful to guide duration of treatment, predict risk of relapse, and monitor for drug resistance.

SOT patients
(See Chapter 7.)
In GI disease, a characteristic pattern of mucosal ulceration is seen on endoscopy and CMV can be detected in biopsies of these lesions by *in situ* hybridization or PCR.

While definitive confirmation of the diagnosis requires demonstration of CMV in biopsies of the affected tissue, more rapid tests such as PCR on more accessible samples such as whole blood, may point to the likely diagnosis. CMV hepatitis in liver transplant recipients may be difficult to distinguish from GvHD and liver biopsy is the only reliable option as the distinction is essential. GvHD requires an increase in immunosuppression whereas CMV hepatitis requires reducing immunosuppression and initiating antiviral treatment. Initiation of pre-emptive treatment on detection of viral DNA in the peripheral blood has been shown to greatly reduce the incidence of CMV disease in the post-transplant period.

An example of a CMV viral load monitoring protocol is found in Table 11.2.

Once on antiviral treatment, serial measurement of CMV DNA can be used to monitor response. The half-life of decline in CMV viral load when on treatment is ~3 days and patients with slower declines are at higher risk for subsequent relapse. In most centres at least two negative PCR results a week apart are required prior to cessation of antiviral therapy.

Congenital CMV infection

Diagnosis is confirmed by testing the neonate's urine for CMV DNA using qPCR. More recently it has been shown that CMV PCR on the dried blood sample from the Guthrie test is also very effective (100% sensitive and 99% specific in one study). The CMV viral load (in blood or urine) of these infants has been shown to correlate to the severity of their clinical symptoms.

Treatment

Oral valganciclovir or IV ganciclovir are recommended as first-line treatment. Valganciclovir is preferred, except in cases of life-threatening disease or where oral intake is not appropriate or gut absorption is impaired (e.g. severe CMV colitis). The main side effects are myelosuppression and renal toxicity. Antiviral dose should always be adjusted for creatinine clearance.

Treatment should be continued for a minimum of 2 weeks following viraemia eradication. Secondary prophylaxis is not routinely recommended.

Dose reduction of immunosuppressive therapy should be considered in severe CMV disease, non-responding patients, patients with high viral loads, and leucopenia. IV immunoglobulin may be considered for severe forms of CMV disease.

Table 11.2 CMV viral load monitoring protocol

CMV load copy no (plasma)Log copies/mL	CMV load copy no (whole blood)	Interpretation/action
CMV *not* detected	CMV *not* detected	No evidence for systemic CMV infection, continue monitoring
CMV detected but <300	CMV detected but <500	CMV present but below quantifiable level. Send repeat sample in 24–48 hours
300–1000	500–3000	Active CMV infection. Send repeat sample and consider treatment if clinically indicated or rising viral load
>1000 (preferably in 2 consecutive samples)	>3000	Active CMV infection. Send repeat sample and commence pre-emptive treatment (do not wait for second result before starting treatment)

Resistance may occur due to UL97 phosphotransferase and UL54 DNA polymerase mutations. The risk of resistance developing is increased if the antiviral dose is reduced during therapy (e.g. if adverse events occur), so this should be avoided. In cases of severe leucopenia, consider adjunctive granulocyte-colony stimulating factor before stopping antiviral therapy. CMV PCR monitoring should be performed weekly during treatment to monitor response. Ganciclovir resistance should be suspected if there is persistence or an increase in viral load or clinical progression of CMV disease despite adequate exposure to the drug for 3 weeks.

Foscarnet is the empirical alternative antiviral treatment in the presence of serious CMV disease and suspected ganciclovir resistance where no genotypic study is available.

Refer to

British Transplantation Society (BTS) guidelines ℅ https://bts.org.uk/guidelines-standards/ for guidelines related to infection in SOT.

British Committee for Standards in Haematology, British Society of Blood and Marrow Transplantation and the UK Clinical Virology Network joint guidelines ℅ http://www.clinicalvirology.org/guidelines/ for guidelines related to infection in HSCT.

British HIV Association (BHIVA) and British Infection Association (BIA) ℅ http://www.bhiva.org/Guidelines.aspx for guidelines related to infections in HIV.

Epstein–Barr virus (EBV/HHV-4)

Discovered in 1964, EBV, or HHV-4, is a member of the Gammaherpesvirinae subfamily. It has an important association with cancer in the immunocompromised. The virus establishes latency in the B lymphocytes following primary infection and as these cells proliferate, the number of cells available to carry the virus increases. In an immunocompetent individual, specific cytotoxic T lymphocytes control the amount of B-cell proliferation. In an immunocompromised patient lacking functioning T cells, latent EBV infection may reactivate to cause lymphoproliferative disease, which may ultimately progress to malignancy.

Epidemiology

Primary infection usually occurs in infancy and EBV antibodies are found in nearly 90% of all adult populations. Primary infection is usually either asymptomatic or causes mild fever and lymphadenopathy. If primary infection occurs in adolescence, ~50% of cases develop the combination of pharyngitis, lymphadenopathy, and high fever termed infectious mononucleosis. Splenomegaly and hepatomegaly may also occur but CNS or cardiac involvement is rare and in the immunocompetent host, EBV is almost never fatal.

There are three groups of the immunocompromised in which EBV has more severe effects:

Congenital immunodeficiency

(➲ See Chapter 8.)

In children with conditions such as congenital T-cell deficiency or X-linked lymphoproliferative syndrome, where T-cell function is absent or severely impaired, EBV infection leads to severe hepatic necrosis and bone marrow failure and is usually rapidly fatal. Other congenital conditions such as chronic active EBV (CAEBV), where T-cell function is impaired, present with an infectious mononucleosis-like illness that fails to resolve and has a high morbidity and mortality.

HIV infection

(➲ See Chapter 5.)

With increasingly suppressed T-cell immunity, virus-induced B-cell proliferation causes EBV-associated lymphoproliferative disorders. Patients infected with HIV may develop non-malignant lymphoproliferative diseases, such as follicular hypoplasia, primary lymphoid hyperplasia, and oral hairy leucoplakia, as well as lymphoid, muscular, and epithelial cell malignancies.

Post-transplant lymphoproliferative disorders (PTLD)

(➲ See Chapter 8.)

PTLD is one of the most common post-transplant malignancies and a well-recognized complication of both SOT and allogeneic HSCT. Most cases of PTLD are associated with EBV infection, either as a consequence of reactivation post transplantation or primary infection. In cases of primary infection, EBV may be acquired from the donor graft or, less commonly, from environmental exposure. PTLD has an overall incidence of

1–2% and the risk depends on pre-existing EBV serostatus, the immuno-suppressive regimen used, and the type of organ transplanted. Transplant patients who are EBV seronegative at the time of transplant are at highest risk. Primary EBV infection while being treated with immunosuppressive drugs significantly increases the risk of developing PTLD. This is particularly common in the paediatric transplant population.

Additional risk factors in the HSCT population include the intensity and duration of immunosuppressive therapy, an unrelated donor, T-cell-depleted allografts, and use of ATG and immunosuppression to prevent GvHD. PTLD can manifest variously, ranging from benign polyclonal hyper-plasia to malignant lymphoma (➲ see Chapter 8).

Clinical features

Most cases of PTLD occur within 1 year post transplant, with onset and severity correlating to the intensity of the immunosuppression used. A rising blood level of plasma EBV viral load by qPCR measurement should raise concern for PTLD. Lymph nodes, liver, lung, kidney, bone marrow, spleen, CNS, tonsils, and salivary glands are common sites of involvement. Patients may present with non-specific symptoms or signs such as fever, weight loss, and lymphadenopathy. Other features may include hepatosplenomegaly, GI symptoms (including obstruction), pul-monary symptoms, and CNS symptoms. Involvement of the allografted tissue can cause declining organ function and failure of the transplant may be the presenting feature.

Diagnosis

Serological assays

Detect three EBV antigens; early antigen (EA), viral capsid antigen (VCA), and Epstein–Barr nuclear antigen (EBNA). These are used to determine pre-transplant serostatus and assess risk, but serology is of limited use in diagnosing acute infection in the immunocompromised.

Molecular testing

qPCR is the most accurate option for detecting and monitoring the overall EBV burden. It allows early detection of EBV replication with the goal of restoring adequate immune function to control viral replication. Although both peripheral blood mononuclear cells and plasma may be used, a higher positive predictive value is achieved with plasma.

Histopathology

The definitive diagnosis of PTLD is made by finding histopathological evi-dence of lymphoproliferation, commonly with the presence of EBV DNA, RNA, or protein detected in tissue.

Treatment

There is no specific treatment for EBV infection. Reduction in immunosup-pression is the first step in managing PTLD. Aciclovir has some activity and is often trialled, along with corticosteroids, but without an evidence base. Rituximab is used for later disease.

Refer to

British Transplantation Society (BTS) guidelines ✍ https://bts.org.uk/guidelines-standards/ for guidelines related to infection and PTLD in SOT.

British Committee for Standards in Haematology, British Society of Blood and Marrow Transplantation and the UK Clinical Virology Network joint guidelines ✍ http://www.clinicalvirology.org/guidelines/ for guidelines related to infection and PTLD in HSCT.

British HIV Association (BHIVA) and British Infection Association (BIA) ✍ http://www.bhiva.org/Guidelines.aspx for guidelines related to infection in HIV.

HHV-8

A gammaherpesvirus which, like EBV, has the capacity to cause cancer in the immunocompromised. In its latent state only a small subset of its genes are expressed and there is no viral replication. It is the causative agent of Kaposi's sarcoma (KS), primary effusion lymphoma, and some forms of multicentric Castleman disease.

Epidemiology

Seropositivity data vary widely by region, with reported rates of 5–10% in the general US population and >40% in some African populations. Rates of seropositivity also vary widely between different patient groups; it is rare in children, ~3.5% in blood donors, ~20% in transplant patients, and >40% in men who have sex with men. The mode of transmission is still not entirely clear but it is thought to be transmitted sexually as well as through saliva, blood transfusion, and organ transplantation.

Clinical features

In immunocompetent hosts, HHV-8 infection is usually asymptomatic, though it may cause a flu-like syndrome ± maculopapular rash. In the immunocompromised, severe disease with fever, splenomegaly, and pancytopenia can result. HIV-associated KS is the commonest cancer seen in HIV-infected men who have sex with men and an iatrogenic form of KS is seen in SOT patients. HHV-8 is not known to cause cancer in the immunocompetent, except in African endemic KS. Post-transplant KS is most frequently encountered in kidney transplant recipients but can arise following transplantation of any organ. Post-transplant KS normally affects the skin with only a small proportion having visceral involvement.

Diagnosis

As primary HHV-8 infection is usually asymptomatic, a clinical diagnosis of primary infection is rarely made. A presumptive diagnosis of KS is usually made on the basis of the characteristic skin lesions, but should be confirmed by biopsy.

Histology

KS and Castleman disease are usually diagnosed histologically with antibodies to the virus's latency-associated nuclear antigen used to demonstrate the presence of HHV-8 in the tissue sample. Viral DNA can also be detected by PCR of the tissue

Serology

~85% of people with KS, in whom HHV-8 DNA has been detected in lesions, will have antibodies to HHV-8 detectable by IFA. As the highest-risk transplant is from a seropositive donor to a seronegative recipient, determination of HHV-8 serostatus may be performed prior to transplant.

NAAT

Clinical applications of PCR for HHV-8 disease are limited.

Treatment

There is little evidence base for the antiviral treatment of HHV-8; ganciclovir has *in vitro* activity but no good clinical evidence. KS, primary effusion lymphoma, and Castleman disease are treated in a variety of ways with chemotherapy; however, ARVs and immune reconstitution are often sufficient treatment for limited KS.

HHV-6

HHV-6 is genetically and biologically similar to CMV and is a known cause of severe disease in the immunocompromised, most notably encephalitis among HSCT recipients.

Epidemiology

Seroprevalence among adults in industrialized nations is in the range of ~70–95% and the most common route of transmission appears to be via saliva from mother to infant. It infects various cells but has a tropism for astrocytes, oligodendroglia, and microglia in the brain.

Clinical features

Acute HHV-6 causes roseola infantum (Sixth disease) and usually presents with fever, fussiness, and rhinorrhoea in young children. The characteristic rash of roseola is only described in ~25% of cases. As childhood infection is near universal, almost all immunocompromised patients are at risk of reactivation. HHV-6 reactivation occurs in up to 50% of allogeneic HSCT recipients. Viremia is usually detected 14–21 days post transplant.

HHV-6 encephalitis

Usually presents with a combination of confusion, coma, seizures, speech disturbance, and headaches. Most cases have been reported in allogeneic HSCT recipients, but it has also been reported rarely in SOT recipients and in immunocompetent individuals. In HSCT recipients, reactivation may present with a rash.

HHV-6 pneumonitis

Occurs in HSCT recipients, though the association is less clear than with encephalitis due to the frequent presence of other pathogens in the diagnostic respiratory samples (e.g. PCP, adenovirus, and CMV).

Diagnosis

HSCT recipients developing signs of encephalitis should, after brain MRI, have their CSF sampled and sent for HHV-6 qPCR. A peripheral blood should also be sent. HHV-6 encephalitis can be diagnosed in allogeneic HSCT recipients with characteristic clinical findings in whom HHV-6 DNA is detected in the CSF without other causes identified.

Treatment

Ganciclovir is often used, though with little evidence base.

Herpes simplex virus (HSV-1 and HSV-2)

HSV-1 and HSV-2 are morphologically similar alphaherpesviruses. Their genomes share only ~50% sequence homology, so they are easily distinguished by molecular diagnostics. HSV-1 typically establishes latency in the trigeminal ganglia and HSV-2 in the sacral nerve root ganglia. Reactivation, presenting with lesion formation at the peripheral site, can be triggered by various stimuli including stress, fever, ultraviolet light, and immunosuppression.

Intact cellular immunity is required for the initial containment of primary infection and prevention of reactivation; the immunocompromised are thus at risk of severe, recurrent, and disseminated infection.

Epidemiology

HSV is present worldwide and humans are the only known reservoir. HSV-1 is transmitted by saliva, usually during childhood, whereas HSV-2 is transmitted through sexual contact in almost all cases. In the US, seroprevalence in the general population is ~60% for HSV-1 and ~20% for HSV-2. Worldwide, >90% of people are seropositive for HSV-1 by the fourth decade of life.

Clinical features

In the immunocompetent, infection is often subclinical, but HSV-1 may cause gingivostomatitis and ulceration ('cold sores') and HSV-2 recurrent painful vesicular genital lesions. Both HSV-1 and HSV-2 can cause severe disease in the immunocompetent, most notably encephalitis and neonatal infections.

Risk factors for increased severity of HSV infection include HIV infection, malignancy, organ transplantation, malnutrition, pregnancy, and advanced age.

Transplant recipients (SOT and HSCT)

Most cases of reactivation occur at the time of maximal immunosuppression, usually about 3 weeks post transplant. Reactivation has been reported in ~60% of SOT patients not receiving prophylaxis, with about 50% of these developing symptomatic lesions. Primary infection, which can be acquired through transplantation of an infected organ, tends to be more severe than reactivation, with higher risk of dissemination to the lungs, GI tract, liver, and skin. HSV pneumonia is associated with significant mortality (~75%) for SOT patients. Encephalitis is rare after SOT. Among HSCT recipients, reactivation of HSV occurs in up to 70% of those who are seropositive prior to transplantation. Most oncologists routinely use prophylaxis in this group as HSV infection is difficult to distinguish clinically from chemotherapy-induced mucositis.

HIV infection

Associated with more severe and chronic HSV lesions and increased rates of asymptomatic shedding of genital HSV-2.

Diagnosis

Molecular

Detection of viral DNA in CSF by PCR is now the gold standard for the diagnosis of HSV encephalitis. It is fast and has a sensitivity and specificity in the region of 98% and 94% respectively. PCR testing is positive within the first 24 hours of onset of symptoms and remains positive during the first 7 days of antiviral treatment. 0.5–1 mL of CSF is required for most HSV PCR assays and specimens should be stored refrigerated or frozen until testing. PCR on blood may be performed if disseminated disease is suspected.

Viral culture

Characteristic cytopathic effect can be seen within 48 hours of inoculation, but culture is now rarely used due to its longer turnaround time and lower sensitivity compared to molecular methods.

Direct antigen detection

Cells scraped from the base of lesions can be stained with fluorescent antibody. This can be performed in 2–3 hours.

Serology

Of limited diagnostic value in the immunocompromised as most have recurrent infections.

Treatment

Aciclovir and the prodrug valaciclovir are the treatments of choice. Prophylactic or early presumptive treatment is most effective. Encephalitis is treated with IV aciclovir (infused slowly to reduce the risk of crystalluria) for at least 14 days. Encephalitis may itself be a side effect of aciclovir, especially in renal failure. Ganciclovir or foscarnet may be used if aciclovir is unavailable.

Refer to

British HIV Association (BHIVA) and British Infection Association (BIA) http://www.bhiva.org/Guidelines.aspx for guidelines related to infection in HIV.

Association of British Neurologists and British Infection Association (BIA) National Guidelines https://www.britishinfection.org/guidelines-resources/published-guidelines/ for guidelines related to HSV encephalitis.

Varicella zoster virus (VZV/HHV-3)

VZV has the smallest genome (~71 known genes) of all the human herpes-viruses. It causes two distinct clinical entities: varicella and herpes zoster. Varicella, or chicken pox, is characterized by fever, malaise, and vesicular rash and is usually a benign infection of childhood in the unvaccinated population. On resolution of the varicella, the virus becomes latent in the dorsal and trigeminal ganglia where it remains for the lifetime of the host.

Reactivation of the virus from latently infected neuronal cells results in herpes zoster ('shingles') and presents as a painful vesicular rash, usually in the dermatomal distribution of the sensory nerve ganglion in which the virus was latent. Pain after resolution of the vesicular rash, post-herpetic neuralgia, is the most common complication of zoster.

Immunocompromised patients, particularly those with impaired cellular immunity, are at risk of severe disease from VZV. Primary infection with VZV during pregnancy has major implications for both maternal and fetal health.

Epidemiology

VZV had a worldwide distribution and transmission is solely from human to human. Seropositivity rates among adults in the US and Europe are >95% (lower in the tropics).

VZV is acquired via inhalation of aerosolized particles and first infects the mucous membranes of the respiratory tract before spreading to regional lymph nodes. The incubation period is 10–21 days.

It is highly contagious and both varicella and disseminated zoster require airborne isolation precautions due to their transmissibility via the respiratory route. There is a risk of rapid and extensive transmission in susceptible populations and therefore prompt diagnosis of infected patients and health care workers is critical.

Though usually benign, complications may be severe and include pneumonia (more common in adults) and CNS involvement ranging from benign cerebellar ataxia to meningoencephalitis.

Varicella pneumonia following primary infection in pregnancy complicates ~10–20% of maternal infections. If the mother acquires VZV during the early gestational period (up to week 20), the fetus is at risk of congenital varicella syndrome (limb hypoplasia, eye damage, and skin lesions). The live attenuated VZV vaccine can result in disease in the severely immunocompromised and is contraindicated in these groups. (➔ See Chapter 8.)

Clinical features

In the immunocompromised, the primary infection rash can persist for weeks accompanied by high fever and the risk of dissemination. Zoster is also more severe and prolonged in the immunocompromised with skin lesions extending beyond the primary dermatome and across the midline. Systemic involvement such as pneumonia, hepatitis, and encephalitis may occur.

In the immunocompromised, severe disease is not always preceded by the typical vesicular rash, so rapid diagnostic testing is needed to initiate appropriate antiviral therapy. Cutaneous dissemination is often accompanied by visceral involvement and in immunosuppressed transplant patients this is a life-threatening emergency. Disseminated VZV has been documented in both SOT recipients and in patients with haematological malignancies undergoing chemotherapy.

VZV reactivation occurs in up to ~35 % of allogeneic HSCT recipients within 1 year of transplant and up to half of these patients will develop disseminated VZV (pneumonitis/hepatitis/pancreatitis/meningoencephalitis). HIV-infected patients with low CD4 counts are at increased risk of the neurological and ophthalmological complications of zoster.

Diagnosis

The diagnosis can usually be made clinically based on the typical lesions. In the immunocompromised, however, it may present atypically, and sometimes with no preceding rash.

Molecular

PCR has become the most widely used diagnostic assay. VZV DNA can be detected in crusted lesions, CSF, ocular fluid, lungs, liver, brain, whole blood, plasma, and peripheral blood mononuclear cells. VZV DNA levels in the blood appear to rise simultaneously with the onset of clinical disease and therefore, unlike CMV or EBV, there is no benefit in monitoring levels to guide pre-emptive therapy.

Serology

Used to determine the patient's immune status prior to transplant, but is less useful in diagnosing active infection. Pre-transplant seropositivity means increased risk of post-transplant reactivation whereas those who are VZV seronegative prior to transplant are at increased risk for primary infection.

Congenital varicella syndrome

Following acute maternal infection, PCR testing of fetal blood or amniotic fluid for VZV DNA between weeks 17–21 of gestation may be undertaken, along with detailed ultrasound imaging, to assess risk of fetal damage. Normal imaging and negative PCR suggest a low risk of congenital varicella syndrome.

Treatment

Immunocompromised hosts with primary varicella should be treated with IV aciclovir for at least 7–10 days followed by oral therapy once all lesions have healed, the patient is afebrile, and there is no evidence of visceral involvement. Duration of oral therapy will depend on individual circumstances.

Treatment of zoster should be with IV aciclovir for at least 7 days or until all lesions have dried and crusted.

Refer to

British HIV Association (BHIVA) and British Infection Association (BIA) ℘ http://www.bhiva.org/Guidelines.aspx for guidelines related to infection in HIV.

British Infection Society (BIS) guidelines on the treatment of chickenpox: ℘ https://www.britishinfection.org/guidelines-resources/published-guidelines/.

Association of British Neurologists and British Infection Association (BIA) National Guidelines ℘ https://www.britishinfection.org/guidelines-resources/published-guidelines/ for guidelines related to VZV encephalitis.

Public Health England (PHE) guidelines on the use of immuno-globulin: ℘ https://www.gov.uk/government/publications/immunoglobulin-when-to-use.

Royal College of Obstetricians and Gynaecologists guidelines on chickenpox in pregnancy: ℘ https://www.rcog.org.uk/en/guidelines-research-services/guidelines/.

HHV-7

First isolated in 1990, this betaherpesvirus shares genomic homology with CMV and HHV-6. It infects CD4+ T lymphocytes and establishes latency following primary infection.

Infection usually occurs early in life and may be associated with a febrile illness and symptoms similar to exanthema subitum. HHV-7 is known to reactivate following immunosuppression but the spectrum of disease associated with it remains unclear.

Epidemiology

The prevalence of HHV-7 in transplant patients has been up to ~50% in some surveys.

Clinical features

No clinical syndrome has yet been clearly associated with HHV-7 infection and immunosuppression. One study reported an association of HHV-7 reactivation with the occurrence of GvHD, vomiting, fatigue, and fever in children following bone marrow transplant.

Diagnosis

Usually made using paired sera in the immunocompetent and antigenaemia and/or PCR in the immunosuppressed. Without a defined disease state, interpretation of laboratory results is not clear.

Treatment

None known, nor does it appear to be indicated.

Hepatitis viruses

These are a group of five unrelated viruses that particularly affect the liver and are designated hepatitis A, B, C, D, and E. The collection of these viruses into a single group is historical and several other viruses also cause hepatitis (Table 11.3).

Table 11.3 Summary of the five hepatitis viruses

	Hepatitis A	Hepatitis B	Hepatitis C	Hepatitis D	Hepatitis E
Genome	ssRNA (+)	dsDNA	ssRNA (+)	ssRNA (−)	ssRNA (+)
Transmission	Faeco-oral	Blood, body fluids	Blood	Blood, body fluids	Faeco-oral
Incubation	15–50 days	45–160 days	14–180 days	(= HBV 45–160 days)	15–60 days
Clinical disease	Acute hepatitis (rarely fulminant)	Spectrum of acute (including fulminant) and chronic hepatitis	Usually chronic hepatitis (rarely acute)	Only viable in presence of HBV. Exacerbates HBV disease.	Acute hepatitis (including fulminant)
Initial screening test	HAV IgM HAV IgG	HBsAg HBcAb	HCV IgG	HDV IgG	HEV IgM & IgG
Confirmatory	HAV IgM	PCR (blood)	PCR (blood)	PCR (blood)	PCR (blood)

Hepatitis A

A single-stranded, positive-sense, non-enveloped, RNA virus (picornavirus).

Epidemiology

Distributed worldwide and associated with poor sanitation and overcrowding; endemic throughout much of the developing world. Can also occur as sporadic epidemics. Humans are the only known reservoir. Transmitted by the faeco-oral route (either direct contact or by ingestion of contaminated food or water). Viral shedding in the stool is highest during the prodromal phase prior to symptoms.

Clinical features

Incubation 15–50 days (average 28 days). Infection may be subclinical, and this is more common in children. Causes an acute self-limiting hepatitis and does not establish chronicity. Clinical features include anorexia, nausea, vomiting, abdominal pain, fatigue, malaise, and fever. These may be followed by myalgia, arthralgia, jaundice, and right upper quadrant pain. LFTs are elevated alanine aminotransferase/aspartate transaminase > alkaline phosphatase. Rarely can cause fulminant hepatitis (<1%), relapsing disease, prolonged cholestasis, and triggering of autoimmune hepatitis. Acute HAV can be considerably more severe in the immunosuppressed and there is an increased risk of fulminant hepatic failure. Pre-existing liver disease (including chronic hepatitis B and C) is a particular risk factor for complicated disease.

Diagnosis

Serology

Acute infection is determined by the detection of anti-HAV IgM antibodies in serum, these are present by the onset of symptoms. Past infection is determined by the detection of anti-HAV IgG antibodies; this usually confers lifelong immunity. Sensitivity of serological testing may be impaired in immunosuppressed states.

Molecular

HAV RNA can be detected in blood and stool earlier than antibodies and prior to the onset of clinical disease but may then become undetectable. Clinical utility is limited but may be helpful in specific scenarios.

Treatment

Usually treated symptomatically with advice to avoid paracetamol and alcohol. Fulminant disease may require transplantation.

Prevention can be achieved by passive immunization (pooled immunoglobulin), or active immunization HAV vaccine. Consideration of prophylaxis is important in travellers who are immunosuppressed. The immunocompromised generally have good serological responses to vaccination, but may have a poorer response and the development of immunity may take longer.

Refer to
Public Health England (PHE) guidelines on the use of immuno-globulin: https://www.gov.uk/government/publications/immunoglobulin-when-to-use.

Public Health England (PHE) 'The Green Book' (2013) guidelines on immunization: https://www.gov.uk/government/publications/immunisation-against-infectious-disease-the-green-book-front-cover-and-contents-page.

Hepatitis B

A double-stranded DNA virus with a very small genome consisting of 3200 base pairs and four open reading frames.

Epidemiology

Distributed globally and represents a major public health challenge. Results in >850 million deaths per year globally as a result of cirrhosis and hepatocellular carcinoma. Endemic to much of Africa and Asia/Western Pacific. Transmission occurs via contact with infected blood (and body secretions such as semen). In hyperendemic regions this occurs commonly by vertical transmission perinatally, or horizontally by direct contact in early childhood. In economically developed regions, transmission usually occurs due to the exchange of blood as a result of IV drug-using practices or by sexual transmission. Other modes of transmission include the transfusion of contaminated blood or blood products and needle-stick injury.

Clinical features

Incubation is 45–160 days. Infection acquired early in life is much more likely to result in chronic disease (80–90% of infants infected during the first year of life). Of infections acquired in adulthood, only 5–10% develop chronic disease. ~30% of chronic infections lead to cirrhosis and/or hepatocellular carcinoma. HBV can cause acute hepatitis (more commonly if acquired in adulthood) and rarely fulminant hepatic failure (<1%). Acute HBV presents with malaise, nausea, abdominal pain, and jaundice. Chronic infection can lead to cirrhosis, liver failure, and hepatocellular carcinoma. Extrahepatic manifestations include glomerulonephritis and arthropathy.

HBV in the immunosuppressed

HBV disease is exacerbated by immunosuppression as a result of enhanced viral replication. Acute infection is less likely to be cleared spontaneously, more likely to result in fulminant disease, and chronic infection (with its complications) is more common. Pre-existing liver disease (including HCV infection) worsen prognosis of HBV infection.

Reactivation

HBV reactivation can occur in patients with previously resolved or inactive infection. This occurs in patients following SOT or HSCT, patients infected with HIV, and patients on immunosuppressive medication (cytotoxic chemotherapy, long-term corticosteroids, immunomodulatory biological agents).

Diagnosis

Serology

Diagnosis is based on antibody and antigen detection.
- Screening for HBV infection: HBV surface antigen.
- Tests if HB replication: HBeAg, anti-HBe, (HBV DNA).
- Evidence of previous vaccination: HBV surface antibody (in the setting of negative HBV surface antigen and HBV core antibody).
- Evidence of resolved infection: HBV core antibody (in the setting of negative HBV surface antigen and HBV surface antibody) (NB can also represent inactive infection, resolving infection, or may be a false-positive result) (Table 11.4).

Table 11.4 Interpretation of serological tests in hepatitis B

	HB surface antigen	Anti-HB surface (total antibody)	Anti-HB core IgM	Anti-HB core (total antibody)
Vaccinated	Negative	Positive	Negative	Negative
Acute infection	Positive	Negative	Positive	Positive
Resolved infection	Negative	Positive	Negative	Positive
Chronic infection	Positive	Negative	Negative	Positive
Inconclusive[a]	Negative	Negative	Negative	Positive

[a] Possibilities are: 1. resolved infection (most likely); 2. false positive anti HBc; 3. low level chronic infection; 4. resolving acute infection.

Molecular

PCR for HBV DNA. Titres reflect disease activity.

Ultrasound and elastography (Fibroscan®)

Ultrasound assessment for structural damage (cirrhosis) and to examine for hepatocellular carcinoma. Elastography (Fibroscan®) where available, provides a non-invasive test of liver elasticity (fibrosis).

Histology

Liver biopsy determines the degree of liver damage/disease activity.

Treatment

Acute disease is treated symptomatically with advice to avoid paracetamol and alcohol. Fulminant disease may require transplantation. Chronic active disease treatment is based on peginterferon alfa and nucleoside/nucleotide analogues. Prophylactic treatment may be started prior to the initiation of immunosuppression in patients with inactive or resolved infection. Prevention is important including immunization and post-exposure prophylaxis.

Refer to

European Association for the Study of the Liver (EASL) treatment guidelines: ℜ https://www.easl.eu/research/our-contributions/clinical-practice-guidelines.

Public Health England (PHE) 'The Green Book' (2013) guidelines on immunization: ℜ https://www.gov.uk/government/publications/immunisation-against-infectious-disease-the-green-book-front-cover-and-contents-page.

Public Health England (PHE) guidelines on the use of immunoglobulin: ℜ https://www.gov.uk/government/publications/immunoglobulin-when-to-use.

Hepatitis C

A single-stranded, positive-sense RNA virus (flavivirus). There are multiple variants of the virus, divided into at least seven genotypes and subdivided further into subtypes. Most common genotypes in the UK, Europe, and US are 1, 2, and 3.

Epidemiology

Worldwide distribution, ~180 million infected globally. Transmission is via contact with infected blood and, most commonly as a result of unsafe IV drug-using practices or transfusion of contaminated blood products. Other mechanisms of transmission include healthcare-associated infection (e.g. re-use of needles for injection, needle-stick injuries, unsafe haemodialysis practice, etc.), unsafe folk remedies, tattoo, or acupuncture practice. Sexual transmission or vertical transmission is rare.

Clinical features

Incubation is ~14–180 days, with ~75% of acute infections asymptomatic or with a mild non-specific illness. Severe or fulminant hepatitis is rare, although may be more common in the Far East. ~85% of acute infections will result in chronic infection, with the remaining 15% spontaneously clearing the virus (usually clearance <6 months). Chronic HCV infection leads to liver cirrhosis in 15–30% within 20 years.

HCV in the immunosuppressed

Although a large amount of hepatocellular damage in HCV infection is related to the host immune response, progression of liver fibrosis is accelerated by immunosuppression (e.g. advanced HIV, post SOT). In addition, there is a lower rate of spontaneous recovery from acute infection. Viral load is significantly higher, particularly with impaired cellular immunity. Initiation of immunosuppression in chronic HCV can lead to a flare in hepatitis.

Diagnosis

Serology

Anti-HCV IgG antibodies in serum is the initial screening test. Detectable by 6–8 weeks following infection. A serological test does not exist to differentiate between acute and chronic infection and is reliant on previous negative antibody results. The sensitivity of HCV serology can be markedly reduced in immunosuppression (e.g. antibody responses may be delayed or absent in HIV).

Molecular

PCR for HCV RNA in serum allows determination of active disease.

Ultrasound and elastography (Fibroscan®)

Ultrasound assessment for structural damage (cirrhosis) and to examine for hepatocellular carcinoma. Elastography (Fibroscan®) where available, provides a non-invasive test of liver elasticity (= fibrosis).

Histology
Liver biopsy determines the degree of liver damage/disease activity.

Treatment

Treatment of HCV has become highly effective and is rapidly evolving. Therapy is based on direct-acting antiviral combinations depending on genotype. The aim is to achieve a sustained virological response defined as undetectable HCV RNA 12 weeks or 24 weeks after treatment completion. In general, immunosuppressed patients are treated with the same regimens as immunocompetent patients. However, there may be significant drug interactions (e.g. with ARV medications). There is no vaccine.

Refer to
European Association for the Study of the Liver (EASL) treatment guidelines: ℘ https://www.easl.eu/research/our-contributions/clinical-practice-guidelines.

Hepatitis D

Hepatitis delta virus is a defective RNA virus, only able to replicate in the presence of the hepatitis B virus. Consists of a single-stranded circular RNA and delta antigen core enclosed in hepatitis B surface antigen-containing envelope.

Epidemiology

Transmitted in the same manner as hepatitis B. Vertical transmission is rare. Complicates ~5% of HBV infections. Higher prevalence areas include the Mediterranean, Middle East, Asia, and parts of Africa.

Clinical features

Co-infection or superinfection of HBV with HDV increases the risk and severity of chronic disease.

Diagnosis

Serology
Anti-HDV IgM and IgG antibodies in serum.

Molecular
PCR for HDV RNA in serum.

Treatment

No effective specific antiviral treatment, pegylated interferon has been used with limited sustained virological response.

HDV infection is prevented by hepatitis B immunization (➔ see 'Hepatitis B' p.92).

Hepatitis E

A single-stranded positive-sense RNA virus.

Epidemiology

Global distribution, associated with economically less-developed regions of the world but is increasingly recognized in the economically developed world. There are four genotypes associated with human infection. Transmission is faecal–oral, usually through contaminated food and water. Transmission via blood products or vertical mother-to-child transmission is possible. Zoonotic transmission (from pigs) may also occur.

Clinical features

Incubation is 15–60 days. A majority of infections result in mild non-specific illness or are asymptomatic. Symptomatic disease presents with anorexia, nausea, vomiting, abdominal pain, fever, diarrhoea, and jaundice. LFTs are consistent with an acute hepatitis. Illnesses usually self-limiting by ~6 weeks. Chronic disease does not occur in immunocompetent hosts. Risk of severe disease is increased by pregnancy, pre-existing liver disease, and malnutrition.

HEV in immunosuppression and chronic disease

Chronic HEV infection can occur in the immunosuppressed. This has been described in patients with HIV infection, following SOT and HSCT, and in patients receiving rituximab. This can lead to cirrhosis. Reducing immunosuppression can result in HEV clearance.

HEV in pregnancy

Acute HEV infection during pregnancy is associated with a mortality rate of up to 25%. The highest risk may be acquisition of infection during third trimester.

Diagnosis

Serology

Anti-HEV IgM antibodies are usually present by the onset of clinical disease, and are suggestive of an acute infection. Anti-HEV IgG antibodies are also usually present. A rising IgG titre (>fivefold in ~2 weeks) is also suggestive of acute infection. There is a high rate of false negatives in moderate to severely immunocompromised hosts.

Molecular

Detection of HEV RNA in serum or stool. Although not usually employed, may be particularly helpful in the immunocompromised. HEV RNA is detectable in serum for longer than in the stool (~6 weeks post infection).

Treatment

Symptomatic, avoid paracetamol and alcohol. Fulminant disease may require transplantation.

Refer to

British Transplantation Society (BTS) guidelines ℛ https://bts.org.uk/guidelines-standards/ for guidelines related to hepatitis E infection in SOT.

Retroviruses

Human immunodeficiency virus (HIV)
➲ See Chapter 5.

Human T-lymphotropic virus (HTLV)
The human T-cell lymphotropic viruses are single-stranded RNA retroviruses. HTLV-1 is associated with two clinical disease entities in humans; adult T-cell leukaemia/lymphoma and HTLV-1-associated myelopathy/tropical spastic paraparesis. It is has been linked to other clinical conditions including uveitis, dermatitis, and other neurological conditions.

Epidemiology
Areas of high endemicity include sub-Saharan Africa, South America, the Caribbean, parts of the Middle East, Japan, and parts of the South Pacific. Transmission is via contact with infected blood including vertical transmission from mother to child (including via breast milk), sexual transmission, IV drug-using practices, and transfusion of contaminated blood products.

Clinical features
The vast majority of infections are asymptomatic, with clinical disease in ~5% of infections. Acute infection is non-specific or asymptomatic. HTLV-1 virus is trophic for lymphocytes and can exert an immunomodulatory effect. This has been associated with defective immunity to infection, in particular *Staphylococcus aureus* and *Strongyloides stercoralis* infection.

Adult T-cell leukaemia/lymphoma
Four clinical forms: acute, lymphomatous, chronic, and smouldering. May present with skin lesions, lytic bone lesions, hypercalcaemia, lymphadenopathy, and pulmonary infiltrates.

HTLV-1-associated myelopathy/tropical spastic paraparesis
A progressive, degenerative myelopathy resulting in motor and sensory abnormalities in the lower extremities. Features include spasticity, hyperreflexia, ankle clonus, extensor plantar responses, and lumbar pain.

Diagnosis
Serology
Anti-HTLV-1 IgM and IgG antibodies in serum.

Molecular
PCR for HTLV-1 proviral DNA in serum and CSF samples.

Treatment
Asymptomatic HTLV-1 infection is not treated. There is no proven specific treatment for HTLV-1-associated myelopathy/tropical spastic paraparesis. Corticosteroids may slow progression/improve symptoms. Treatment for adult T-cell leukaemia/lymphoma is similar to regimens for advanced NHL.

Respiratory viruses

There is increasing awareness that RNA respiratory viruses such as influenza, respiratory syncytial virus (RSV), parainfluenza, human metapneumovirus, human rhinovirus and coronavirus cause significant morbidity, graft failure, and even death in transplant recipients.

The clinical presentation of respiratory infections, particularly in lung transplant recipients, is often atypical and manifestations may be as subtle as a change in pulmonary function testing. The RNA respiratory viruses do not generally cause a specific syndrome but are associated with a spectrum of clinical presentations including coryzal and flu-like illnesses, laryngitis, bronchitis, and croup. In the immunocompromised, these infections more frequently progress to pneumonia with an increased risk of co-infection and death. They are also associated with an increased risk of acute and chronic graft rejection. Prolonged viral shedding increases the risk of the emergence of antiviral resistance.

While often clinically indistinguishable, the availability of antiviral therapy, particularly for influenza, and the need for infection control mean that diagnosing the correct virus is clinically important.

In general, it is best to cast the net wide and perform a screen for the common respiratory viruses at first evaluation of the patient.

All these viruses are highly contagious and have caused outbreaks in transplant wards. Patients should be moved to a private room and appropriate infection control methods put in place once a respiratory viral infection is suspected.

Influenza

Influenza viruses are enveloped, single-stranded RNA viruses whose segmented genomes allow for re-assortment and antigenic variation. They are divided into types A, B, and C; types A and B are classically associated with 'influenza-like' illness while type C usually leads to a milder cold-like illness. Influenza A viruses are further classified by specific surface glycoprotein spikes possessing either neuraminidase (N) or haemagglutinin (H) activity.

Epidemiology

Influenza causes worldwide outbreaks and epidemics of acute respiratory illness. Transmission is through aerosolized droplets and in the immunocompetent the average duration of shedding is 5 days. This may be significantly prolonged in the immunocompromised.

Clinical features

The major complication in the immunocompromised is pneumonia, which often includes bacterial co-infection, most commonly with *Streptococcus pneumoniae*, *Staphylococcus aureus*, or *Haemophilus influenzae*. Other less common complications include CNS disease (encephalitis, aseptic meningitis), myocarditis, pericarditis, myositis, and toxic shock syndrome. Risk factors for severe disease include lymphopenia, infection soon after transplant, paediatric age group, and allogenic HSCT recipients. Acute and, particularly in lung transplant patients, chronic rejection can occur following influenza. Mortality is historically high but appears to be lower with the use of antiviral therapy.

Diagnosis

During an outbreak, diagnosis in an immunocompetent patient can be made clinically. However, in an immunocompromised patient with sudden-onset severe pulmonary disease, it is important to unequivocally identify the causative pathogen.

Specimens

The optimal specimens are nasopharyngeal aspirates, washings, and swabs (washings are more sensitive than swabs). Specimens from more than one respiratory site and taken on more than one day will increase sensitivity.

Point-of-care testing

Rapid antigen and immunofluorescence tests can be useful screening tools but are less sensitive (~60%) than molecular tests. A negative rapid test should usually be followed up by a more sensitive test such as PCR. A positive result should be considered diagnostic of influenza and antiviral therapy commenced for all immunosuppressed patients.

Definitive laboratory testing

Reverse transcriptase PCR testing is the most sensitive and specific test for influenza and nasopharyngeal washes are the preferred initial specimen. If there are lower respiratory tract signs, a bronchoscopy should be considered early in the illness and the bronchoalveolar fluid sent to the lab. PCR can also be used to monitor response to therapy, although a positive signal may persist for several weeks after replication has ceased.

Treatment

As immunocompromised patients are considered at high risk of death, treatment with IV oseltamivir is indicated. If oseltamivir resistance is suspected, then zanamivir is suggested.

Refer to

Public Health England (PHE) ℘ https://www.gov.uk/government/publications/influenza-treatment-and-prophylaxis-using-anti-viral-agents for guidelines on seasonal influenza treatment.

Public Health England (PHE) ℘ https://www.gov.uk/government/publications/avian-influenza-guidance-and-algorithms-for-managing-human-cases for guidelines on avian influenza.

European Conference on Infections in Leukaemia (ECIL) guidelines on influenza infection in leukaemia and HSCT: ℘ https://www.ebmt.org/Contents/Resources/Library/ECIL/Pages/ECIL.aspx.

Public Health England (PHE) 'The Green Book' (2013) guidelines on immunization: ℘ https://www.gov.uk/government/publications/immunisation-against-infectious-disease-the-green-book-front-cover-and-contents-page.

Respiratory syncytial virus (RSV)

These are enveloped, single-stranded, negative-sense RNA viruses belonging to the family Paramyxoviridae and the genus *Pneumovirus*. Subtypes A and B are simultaneously present in most outbreaks, with A subtypes causing more severe disease.

Epidemiology

RSV disease is seasonal and often overlaps in mid-winter with the influenza season. It is globally dispersed and is the most common cause of lower respiratory tract infection in children <1 year old.

Clinical features

In the general population, RSV commonly causes infection of the upper respiratory tract resulting in rhinitis, cough, and sometimes fever. In young children, however, it is a very significant pathogen, causing up to ~90% of hospitalizations for bronchiolitis, ~40% for pneumonia, and ~30% for tracheobronchitis. In the immunocompromised, there are increased complication rates and a higher rate of mortality. Risk factors for progression to lower respiratory tract disease include a history of prior lung disease, lymphopenia, and onset of upper respiratory tract infection prior to HSCT. Most centres defer stem cell transplant until RSV has been cleared.

Diagnosis

Point-of-care testing

A nasopharyngeal sample sent for rapid antigen testing is the usual first line, but these rapid tests have variable sensitivity and may be particularly insensitive in the immunosuppressed. Endotracheal or BAL samples have been shown to improve sensitivity.

Definitive laboratory testing

If rapid antigen testing is negative, a sample should be sent for testing with a more specific assay such as PCR, direct fluorescent antibody, or culture.

A positive result with any of these assays in an immunocompromised host mean that therapy should be considered and continued until viral replication has ceased.

Treatment

Ribavirin is commonly used in immunocompromised patients. The main side effect is myelosuppression and haemolytic anaemia. There is no good evidence for the use of immunotherapy including palivizumab.

Refer to

Haemato-oncology subgroup of the British Committee for Standards in Haematology (BCSH), the British Society for Bone Marrow Transplantation (BSBMT) and the UK Clinical Virology Network guidelines on respiratory viral infections in haematological malignancy and HSCT: ℬ http://www.b-s-h.org.uk/guidelines/.

Parainfluenza viruses

These viruses are enveloped, single-stranded RNA viruses and belong to the Paramyxoviridae family, which also includes measles, mumps, RSV, and human metapneumovirus. Of the four recognized serotypes affecting humans, parainfluenza 3 is most prevalent among transplant patients.

Epidemiology

These viruses are found throughout the world and infections occur year round. They are acquired via droplet inhalation. By adulthood, >90% of individuals have antibodies to parainfluenza viruses, though these are only partially protective against subsequent infection.

Clinical features

Parainfluenza viruses cause a disease spectrum from the common cold, croup, and bronchiolitis to pneumonia. Progression to pneumonia is more likely in HSCT recipients, patients with leukaemia, and SOT recipients (particularly lung transplants). Parainfluenza has been associated with acute rejection in lung transplant recipients. Other risk factors for progressive lower tract disease in transplant recipients include anti-lymphocyte therapy, GvHD, young age, and steroid use.

Diagnosis

PCR of nasopharyngeal aspirates or BAL samples. There are no rapid antigen tests for parainfluenza. Viral culture and antigen tests are slower and less sensitive respectively.

Treatment

No specific treatment.

Refer to

Haemato-oncology subgroup of the British Committee for Standards in Haematology (BCSH), the British Society for Bone Marrow Transplantation (BSBMT) and the UK Clinical Virology Network guidelines on respiratory viral infections in haematological malignancy and HSCT: ℑ http://www.b-s-h.org.uk/guidelines/.

Human metapneumovirus

Human metapneumovirus is a recently described (2001) single-stranded, negative-sense, non-segmented RNA virus with a similar clinical and epidemiological profile to RSV.

Epidemiology

Distributed worldwide and thought to be transmitted by direct contact with secretions rather than small particle aerosols. Most common in late winter/ early spring in Europe and symptomatic infections tend to be in young children and older adults.

Clinical features

Should be considered as a potential cause of respiratory illness in all immunocompromised patients. One study showed that up to 25% of lung transplant patients had infections due to human metapneumovirus.

Diagnosis

PCR on respiratory samples is the test of choice. Human metapneumovirus is increasingly included in multiplex PCR respiratory virus panels. If PCR is not available, direct fluorescent antibody testing or culture are alternatives.

Treatment

No specific treatment. Co-infection with bacteria, fungi, and other viruses is common and should be sought in all cases.

Refer to

Haemato-oncology subgroup of the British Committee for Standards in Haematology (BCSH), the British Society for Bone Marrow Transplantation (BSBMT) and the UK Clinical Virology Network guidelines on respiratory viral infections in haematological malignancy and HSCT: ℛ http://www.b-s-h.org.uk/guidelines/.

Human rhinoviruses

Human rhinoviruses are single-stranded RNA viruses and members of the picornavirus family. There are >100 serotypes of human rhinoviruses.

Epidemiology

Human rhinoviruses are among the most common causes of colds in children and adults and have seasonal peaks in late autumn and early spring. They are also thought to be important triggers of asthma exacerbations. Transmission occurs when virus is deposited on the nasal mucosa, although some aerosol transmission may occur. Symptoms typically occur within 12 hours of inoculation.

Clinical features

Available data suggest that human rhinoviruses are likely to be the commonest cause of respiratory viral infections in the immunocompromised and cause disease ranging from mild coryzal illness to life-threatening pneumonia.

Diagnosis

Nasopharyngeal samples for respiratory viral PCR (or direct fluorescent antibody).

Treatment

No specific treatment. Careful screening for co-infection or complicating pathogens should be performed.

Refer to

Haemato-oncology subgroup of the British Committee for Standards in Haematology (BCSH), the British Society for Bone Marrow Transplantation (BSBMT) and the UK Clinical Virology Network guidelines on respiratory viral infections in haematological malignancy and HSCT: ℛ http://www.b-s-h.org.uk/guidelines/.

Coronaviruses

These enveloped, membrane bound RNA viruses typically cause mild coryzal illnesses. They are named after their crown-like appearance on electron microscopy. There are five known clinically significant human coronaviruses and these include severe acute respiratory syndrome coronavirus (SARS-CoV), which caused a short-lived epidemic in 2003, and Middle East respiratory syndrome coronavirus (MERS-CoV). MERS and SARS are both zoonoses (Box 11.1).

Epidemiology

They are found throughout the world and associated respiratory infections peak in winter. They probably account for up to 10% of all acute upper respiratory tract infections in adults. Transmission is via direct contact with infected secretions or large aerosol droplets. MERS-CoV is associated with dromedary camels and both MERS-CoV and SARS-CoV are readily transmitted in healthcare settings.

Box 11.1 Multipathogen testing for respiratory viral infections

It is often impossible to distinguish viral respiratory infections clinically, particularly in the context of a lung transplant patient. An initial broad screen for likely viral pathogens is therefore a prudent approach.

Several antigen detection kits are available which use pools of monoclonal antibodies to detect multiple viral pathogens. These can be applied directly to the patient specimen. Commercial assays are available which screen for influenza A and B, parainfluenza 1–3, RSV, and adenoviruses and these have been widely tested in both immunocompetent and immunosuppressed populations. Similarly, there are several multiplex PCR kits, which screen for gene targets of the common respiratory viruses. These nucleic acid amplification techniques usually provide the highest yield and are becoming more widely used.

Clinical features

Severe pneumonia has been described in coronavirus infections in the immunocompromised, including patients with HIV. There is also an association between coronavirus infections, acute rejection, and bronchiolitis obliterans in lung transplant recipients.

Diagnosis

Respiratory samples for viral PCR or immunofluorescence antigen detection.

Treatment

No specific treatment.

Refer to

Public Health England (PHE) guidelines on Middle East Respiratory Syndrome Coronavirus (MERS-CoV).
https://www.gov.uk/government/collections/middle-east-respiratory-syndrome-coronavirus-mers-cov-clinical-management-and-guidance.

Other viruses of particular relevance in the immunocompromised

Adenoviruses

Adenoviruses are non-enveloped, double-stranded DNA viruses that cause a wide range of clinical disease in humans. >50 serotypes have been described and while they generally cause mild, self-limiting illness in the immunocompetent, they may lead to severe disease in certain immunocompromised groups. The best described association is with haemorrhagic cystitis in HSCT recipients.

Epidemiology

Adenoviruses have a worldwide distribution, with seropositivity rates approaching 100% by 10 years of age. They are a major cause of febrile illnesses in young children and typically cause self-limiting GI, conjunctival disease, or respiratory disease. Transmission can be faecal–oral, via exposure to infected tissue/blood, direct conjunctival inoculation, or inhalation of aerosolized droplets. Incubation periods range from 2 to 14 days depending on the mechanism of transmission and the viral serotype.

In the immunocompromised, adenovirus infection may disseminate leading to end-organ damage and a higher mortality. The most severe adenovirus disease occurs in HSCT transplant patients, among whom mortality from disseminated disease can be as high as 75%.

Clinical features

HSCT patients

The onset of adenoviral disease usually occurs during the first 100 days post transplant. Incidence ranges from 5% to 50% and it is more common in allogenic transplants, acute GvHD, T-cell depleted grafts, and children. Disease usually presents with respiratory, GI or genitourinary symptoms; these range from mild coryzal symptoms to severe pneumonia or mild diarrhoea to haemorrhagic colitis and severe hepatitis. While genitourinary disease can cause an interstitial nephritis, it is more commonly associated with haemorrhagic cystitis. Outcomes can be poor (untreated mortality ~25% in all symptomatic patients) and may be associated with graft failure or delay in engraftment. Co-infection, with pathogens such as CMV and *Aspergillus* spp. is common and contributes to the poor outcome.

SOT recipients

Invasive adenoviral disease occurs in up to 10% of SOT recipients and the transplanted organ is the most common site of infection (with the exception of renal transplant patients in whom haemorrhagic cystitis is the most common form of disease). Additional risk factors for adenoviral disease among SOT recipients include renal or hepatic transplant, serological donor–recipient mismatch, T-cell depletion, and paediatric age group.

Diagnosis

Screening and treatment response

PCR of whole blood is used as a screening method and has a proven impact in the paediatric HSCT population. Adenoviral DNA in the blood predicts the onset of disease and sequential quantitative monitoring of viral load when on treatment may indicate the likelihood of therapeutic response. Most who respond to therapy do so within the first two doses of antiviral agent.

Other specimens and techniques

PCR, viral culture, or direct antigen assays of upper nasopharyngeal, throat, urine, and stool or rectal samples will detect viral shedding. Additional testing of blood and specimens from affected sites (e.g. BAL in patients with pneumonia; urine in patients with haemorrhagic cystitis; CSF in patients with CNS involvement; and tissue biopsies in patients with colitis, nephritis, or hepatitis) may be needed to diagnose adenovirus infection.

Treatment

Although there is no randomized controlled trial evidence, cidofovir is often used as treatment in immunocompromised hosts. Renal toxicity is a limiting factor.

Refer to

European Conference on Infections in Leukaemia (ECIL) guidelines on adenovirus infections in leukaemia and HSCT: ℅ https://www.ebmt.org/Contents/Resources/Library/ECIL/Pages/ECIL.aspx.

Enteroviruses

Enteroviruses are small (~30 nm diameter), non-enveloped viruses with single-stranded RNA genomes encoding ~11 known gene products. There are >100 distinct serotypes currently described in the *Enterovirus* genus, which forms part of the Picornaviridae family. Clinically, enteroviruses are usually grouped into polioviruses, non-polio enteroviruses (group A and B coxsackieviruses, echoviruses), and parechoviruses.

Epidemiology

Enterovirus infections are globally distributed, with markedly higher rates in summer and autumn in temperate climates and year-round transmission in tropical regions. In the US, 10–15 million symptomatic non-polio enterovirus cases occur annually.

Antibodies to the more commonly circulating serotypes are seen in up to 80% of adults. Highest rates of infection and disease are among infants and children and males have a much higher risk of disease than females.

Human enterovirus infections require direct contact with the virus shed in faeces or from the upper respiratory tract and only small inoculums of infectious virus are needed to establish infection. The incubation period is generally 7–14 days. Virus can be shed in the faeces for months. Protective immunity to enterovirus infection is serotype specific and antibody response is the most important factor in limiting disease and eliminating the virus.

Clinical features

Most enterovirus infections are asymptomatic in the immunocompetent. If symptomatic, an acute non-focal febrile illness in infants <1 year is the most usual manifestation. Herpangina (painful vesicles on the palate, uvula, and tonsils) is most often seen in children aged 1–7 years. Hand, foot, and mouth disease, most commonly associated with Coxsackievirus A-16 and enterovirus-71, is characterized by cutaneous lesions on the distal extremities and vesicular stomatitis. Enterovirus-71-associated hand, foot, and mouth disease has been associated with severe CNS disease, including brainstem encephalitis and acute motor neurone disease.

Among the immunocompromised, severe manifestations, including encephalitis and myocarditis, are well documented in children with acute leukaemia and outbreaks have occurred on oncology wards. Children with X-linked agammaglobulinaemia or adults with common variable immunodeficiency are at particular risk of severe enteroviral disease. These patients, with defective B lymphocytes, may suffer a variety of CNS disorders, such as headache, lethargy, ataxia, tremor, seizures, and weakness, as well as a dermatomyositis-like syndrome and chronic hepatitis.

Diagnosis
Depending on the clinical syndrome, enterovirus infection can be detected in multiple specimen types, including blood, CSF, urine, stool, and tissue.

Molecular methods
PCR of CSF, serum, plasma, stool, urine, respiratory, and tissue specimens. Detecting the virus may represent asymptomatic colonization or prolonged shedding and does not always imply causality for the illness under investigation.

Other techniques
Culture is an option for CSF, stool, and respiratory specimens but PCR is preferable due to its greater sensitivity and faster turnaround time. Immunohistochemistry and *in situ* hybridization are appropriate for tissue specimens.

Treatment
No specific antiviral treatment is available. Normal human IV immunoglobulin has been used in B-cell deficient patients.

Refer to
Association of British Neurologists and British Infection Association (BIA) National Guidelines: ◈ https://www.britishinfection.org/guidelines-resources/published-guidelines/ for guidelines related to enterovirus encephalitis.

European Academy of Neurology (EAN) guidelines on meningoencephalitis: ◈ https://www.ean.org/Reference-Center.2699.0.html.

Parvovirus B19

Parvovirus B-19, of the genus *Erythrovirus*, is the predominant parvovirus pathogen in humans. Of the three described genotypes, genotype 1 is most prevalent in the US and Europe. Since its discovery in 1975, parvovirus B19 has been linked to fifth disease (or erythema infectiosum), polyarthralgia/polyarthritis, fetal hydrops, transient aplastic crises, and chronic red cell aplasias.

The only known host for parvovirus B19 is humans and it infects erythroid precursor cells. Transmission normally occurs by the respiratory route. Destruction of erythroid precursor cells and consequent drop in circulating reticulocytes usually follows about a week later.

It is a highly stable virion and persists despite the standard heat treatment of blood products. It can therefore be transmitted in products such as albumin, immunoglobulin, and pooled factor VIII and IX concentrates.

Epidemiology
Parvovirus B19 infections occur worldwide, either sporadically or in clusters. Acquisition begins in childhood and by early adulthood ~50% of people are seropositive. All immunocompromised groups are at risk, but those with an impaired antibody response are most susceptible, as it is the production of neutralizing antibodies that leads to the elimination the virus.

Clinical features
Immunocompetent
In children, ~50% of infections are symptomatic and may cause the classic 'slapped cheek' facial rash. In adults, symmetrical polyarthralgias predominate, most often wrists, knees, and hands, and can last for months. In healthy individuals, with a normal red cell lifespan of ~120 days, the drop in haematocrit is moderate and not clinically significant.

Immunocompromised
Most immunocompromised patients with pre-existing immunity will be able to mount a sufficient antibody response to infection but in some, neutralizing antibodies are not produced and viraemia persists. This persistent active infection may lead to chronic pure red cell aplasia. Neutropenia, agranulocytosis, pancytopenia, and thrombocytopenia may also develop due to bone marrow involvement. Immune-mediated symptoms such as rash and arthralgia are not observed unless antibody develops or IV immunoglobulin is administered. Parvovirus B19 infection should be considered in patients with haematological malignancies on chemotherapy who have an unexplained severe anaemia with reticulocytopenia.

The use of rituximab, which inhibits B cells, has been linked to persistent parvovirus B19 infection in lymphoma patients.

Numerous cases of pure red cell aplasia due to parvovirus B19 infection have been documented in SOT recipients, particularly renal transplant patients, and may occur weeks to years after transplantation.

Infection may result from primary infection (via the respiratory route or blood products) or from endogenous reactivation. Exposure to the prolonged shedding from other immunocompromised hosts has been implicated in outbreaks in transplant and oncology wards.

Fetal infection
Results from transplacental transmission of the virus, leading to interruption of fetal erythropoiesis and subsequent anaemia. In a minority of such cases, parvovirus-associated myocarditis and severe anaemia lead to heart failure, fetal hydrops, and fetal demise.

Diagnosis
Whole-blood qPCR for parvovirus B19 DNA is of greatest value in establishing a diagnosis and monitoring. Recurrence of pure red cell aplasia, suggested by a falling haematocrit, should prompt serial measurement of viral load. Trends in viral load are useful as no data are currently available to correlate specific viral loads with disease. Levels of DNA fall as antibodies develop or are administered, but low levels can be detected in blood and tissue samples for years after symptoms have resolved.

Treatment
No specific antiviral treatment available.

Refer to
Public Health England (PHE) guidelines, including guidelines on management of infection in pregnancy: ℰ https://www.gov.uk/guidance/parvovirus-b19.

Lymphocytic choriomeningitis virus (LCMV)

A negative-sense single-stranded RNA virus. Member of the family Arenaviridae.

Epidemiology
Worldwide, wherever there are rodent populations. Zoonosis particularly associated with rodents including mice, rats, and hamsters. These can be chronically infected and the virus is mainly excreted in the urine and faeces. Humans acquire infection following contact with these secretions or by inhalation of contaminated particles. Vertical transmission from mother to child occurs. Seroprevalence ~5% in some populations.

Clinical features
Flu-like illness, headache, meningism. Rarely orchitis, parotitis, myopericarditis, or arthritis. CSF typically lymphocytic like other viral meningitis. Disease may be severe or fatal in the immunosuppressed.

Transplant-associated disease
There are several described cases of transmission from transplant donor to recipient leading to fatal disease due to multisystem organ failure.

Congenital infection
Congenital infection can result in birth defects, including hydrocephalus and chorioretinitis.

Diagnosis
Serology
Anti-LCMV IgM and IgG antibodies in serum.

Molecular
PCR for LCMV RNA in serum and CSF samples.

Treatment
Supportive, no specific treatment of proven benefit although ribavirin has been used in severe disease in the immunocompromised.

Refer to
US Centers for Disease Control and Prevention (CDC) ℰ https://www.cdc.gov/vhf/lcm/index.html for more information.

Human papilloma viruses (HPV)

Small, circular, double-stranded DNA viruses. They infect epithelial cells of the skin and mucosal surfaces and are oncogenic, causing a variety of pre-malignant or overtly malignant conditions. There are in excess of 200 types.

Epidemiology

HPV infections transmitted from skin surface to skin surface and are the most common STD in the world. Vertical transmission from mother to child also occurs. Seroprevalence varies between type and population; anogenital HPV infection has particularly high prevalence in individuals with multiple sexual contacts. The most common types worldwide are types 16 and 18.

Clinical features

HPV infects epithelial cells, most infections are asymptomatic and resolve spontaneously or present as skin lesions (e.g. warts). Infection typically resolves within 12 months; however, infection may persist in latent form. This may lead to squamous metaplasia or neoplasia.

Disease associations include cervical cancer, anal cancer, other genital cancers (vulva, vagina, penis), and oropharyngeal cancer. Impaired cell-mediated and humoral immunity removes immunological control of the virus. This can result in widespread, persistent, and recurrent warts and increased prevalence of HPV-associated malignancy. This is best described in SOT recipients and HIV infection.

Diagnosis

Viral warts are usually diagnosed clinically. Specific virological testing is possible (serology or PCR for HPV DNA) but rarely used.

Screening for HPV-associated cancers is, however, widely used, particularly for cervical dysplasia and neoplasia.

Treatment

No specific treatment. Skin lesions can be removed by a variety of methods (e.g. cryotherapy, liquid nitrogen, trichloroacetic acid, and surgical removal).

Vaccination against the most common types is available.

Refer to

British Association for Sexual Health and HIV (BASHH) ✍ https://www.bashh.org/guidelines for guidelines on anogenital warts.

Public Health England (PHE) 'The Green Book' (2013): ✍ https://www.gov.uk/government/publications/immunisation-against-infectious-disease-the-green-book-front-cover-and-contents-page.

British HIV Association (BHIVA) and British Infection Association (BIA) ✍ http://www.bhiva.org/Guidelines.aspx for guidelines related to vaccination in HIV infected patients.

Polyomaviruses: BK virus (polyomavirus hominis 1)

BK virus is a small, non-enveloped, double-stranded DNA virus, associated with renal and genitourinary tract disease. It is named with the initials of the patient in whom it was first identified in 1971 and is a member of the Papovaviridae family. It can withstand heating to 50°C for 30 minutes with minimal effect on its infectivity. It is thought to remain latent in renal tubular epithelial cells after primary infection and is a cause of haemorrhagic cystitis and nephropathy in transplant recipients.

Epidemiology
Serological studies have indicated a wide prevalence range, from 30% to 90%, in the US and Europe. Route of transmission has not yet been proven but oral and/or respiratory are considered the most likely.

Clinical features
Haemorrhagic cystitis
The most prevalent BK virus-associated complication and occurs in 10–25% of bone marrow transplant recipients. Diagnosis is considered when post-engraftment BMT patients present with haematuria, dysuria, urgency, frequency, or suprapubic pain. Complications include severe bleeding, clot formation, urinary tract obstruction, and renal failure.

BK virus-induced nephropathy
Occurs in up to 10% of kidney transplant recipients and, on average, the diagnosis is made at ~44 weeks after transplantation. There is a trend towards an increasing prevalence of BK virus-induced nephropathy in renal transplant patients treated with potent immunosuppressive medications such as tacrolimus and mycophenolate.

BK virus-induced ureteral stenosis
Occurs in ~3% of renal transplant patients. Because the transplanted kidney is not innervated, renal transplant patients with ureteral stenosis do not usually present with pain or discomfort but rather with urinary obstruction and laboratory findings of elevated serum creatinine levels.

Diagnosis
Urinary PCR
Detection of BK viruria and renal insufficiency in the appropriate clinical setting is diagnostic of BK virus-induced nephropathy. Although detection of BK virus DNA with PCR in the urine of patients with haemorrhagic cystitis is sensitive, it is non-specific because asymptomatic BK viruria is common. However, an increased BK viral load in the urine along with haematuria points to the diagnosis.

Serum PCR
BK virus DNA can be detected in the blood of kidney transplant recipients. PCR detection of BK virus DNA in the blood has a negative predictive value of 100% and a positive predictive value of 50% and is therefore of most clinical utility in ruling out BK virus nephropathy rather than confirming it. BK virus is usually not detected in the blood of patients with haemorrhagic cystitis or ureteral stenosis.

Histopathology
Renal biopsy is often used in the diagnosis of nephropathy but is associated with a false-negative rate of up to 30% due to the focal nature of the disease.

Treatment
There is no specific antiviral treatment, but reduction of immunosuppression, IV immunoglobulin, and leflunomide have been tried.

Refer to

European Conference on Infections in Leukaemia (ECIL) guidelines on BK virus infections in leukaemia and HSCT: ℘ https://www.ebmt.org/Contents/Resources/Library/ECIL/Pages/ECIL.aspx.

Polyomaviruses: JC virus (polyomavirus hominis 2)

JC virus shares ~75% nucleotide homology with the BK virus and also bears the initials of the patient from whom it was first isolated in 1971. It is associated with progressive multifocal leucoencephalopathy (PML). Detection of JC virus in urine of healthy adults indicates that the virus is present in a state of latency in the kidney and immunohistochemical staining shows viral proteins in the kidney tubular epithelial cells. In immunosuppressed patients, asymptomatic urinary shedding occurs in up to 50% of patients.

Epidemiology

JC virus is thought to have only one major serotype and virus-specific antibodies tend to be detected around the age of 10 years and then steadily increase during adulthood to 50–70% prevalence. Routes of transmission have not been definitively proven but oral and respiratory routes are likely.

   Primary infection with JC virus is asymptomatic, after which the virus becomes clinically latent. In PML, JC virus infects oligodendrocytes and astrocytes in the brain causing a lytic infection resulting in the destruction of the myelin sheath. Pathological examinations of PML lesions show extensive demyelination of the affected areas.

Clinical features

PML usually begins insidiously with changes in intellect, affect, motor function, or sensory loss. It then progresses rapidly, giving rise to multifocal neurological signs and death, usually within a year. Prior to effective ARV therapy, PML developed in 2–4% of patients with HIV.

   ~80% of cases of PML are seen in patients with HIV, ~13% in patients with haematological malignant diseases, ~5% in transplant recipients, and ~2% in those with chronic inflammatory diseases. A relatively new group of patients with PML has emerged among those treated with immunomodulatory medications for malignant diseases or autoimmune diseases. Examples include patients treated with natalizumab for multiple sclerosis or Crohn's disease, rituximab for lymphoma or lupus, and efalizumab for psoriasis.

Diagnosis

Brain biopsy

This is the gold standard for the diagnosis of PML with sensitivity in the range of 65–95% and a specificity of 100%. Histology shows demyelinated areas with reactive gliosis, enlarged and bizarre astrocytes, and macrophages containing phagocytosed myelin and cellular debris. These lesions are located in both cortical and subcortical regions of the brain. The presence of JC virus in these lesions can be demonstrated by fluorescent antibody staining.

CSF examination

Usually non-specific, with a mild pleocytosis, slightly elevated protein, and a normal glucose. PCR detection of JC virus in CSF had a sensitivity of ~70–90% and a specificity of ~90–100% before the widespread use of HAART, but the sensitivity has decreased to ~60% in patients with HIV presenting with PML while on HAART.

Treatment

There is no specific antiviral treatment. Reduction in immunosuppression, discontinuation of immunosuppressant medication or ARV drug initiation in HIV are recommended.

Refer to

British HIV Association (BHIVA) and British Infection Association (BIA) http://www.bhiva.org/Guidelines.aspx for guidelines related to infection in HIV.

Acknowledgement

This chapter was kindly reviewed by Dr Ian Bowler, Consultant in Infectious Diseases and Microbiology, Oxford University Hospitals NHS Trust.

Parasites

Introduction

While all human parasitic infections can cause disease in the immunocompromised, those described in this chapter are of particular concern due to their prevalence and/or severity.

With the exception of *Strongyloides stercoralis* and *Sarcoptes scabiei*, all are protozoan. Protozoa (meaning 'first life') are unicellular eukaryotes that have been recently reclassified, along with certain algal and fungal groups, into the kingdom Protista. Protozoa are the motile protists and are further grouped, based on their method of locomotion, into amoebae, flagellates, ciliates, and sporozoans.

Given the fragility of the immunocompromised state and potential for rapid deterioration, presumptive treatment covering the most likely pathogens is often started prior to confirmation of microbiological diagnosis.

Toxoplasma gondii

T. gondii is an obligate intracellular protist, whose definitive host (where sexual reproduction occurs) is the cat family. The two life-cycle stages of the parasite found in humans are the trophozoites/tachyzoites and the bradyzoites/cyst stages. The trophozoites are crescentic actively proliferating intracellular stages. They parasitize many tissues, including the CNS, lungs, heart, and lymphoid organs. The cysts contain the more quiescent, slowly developing bradyzoites and are found mostly in the brain, skeletal and cardiac muscle, and the eye. Following ingestion of *T. gondii* oocysts, sporozoites enter the intestinal epithelial cells and, following rapid intracellular proliferation, rupture the cell and invade adjacent cells. Dissemination occurs via the blood and lymphatics to distant tissues. Once the tissue cysts form, the pathogen becomes quiescent and these cysts are the latent reservoir of disease.

In the immunocompetent, infection rarely causes disease and lifelong asymptomatic latent infection ensues. In the immunodeficient, disease can result from primary infection but more commonly results from reactivation and uncontrolled proliferation of latent tissue cysts.

Epidemiology

T. gondii has a worldwide distribution, seropositivity rates are highly variable (~10% among US adults but up to ~80% in some parts of Brazil). Human infection occurs through ingestion of the infective oocyst stage, most commonly in raw or undercooked meat, but also through ingestion of anything contaminated by cat faeces. Transplacental transmission may occur causing congenital toxoplasmosis and transmission is also possible through transplant of infected organs, blood transfusion, and needle-stick injury.

Patients with HIV, who are *T. gondii* seropositive and not on antimicrobial prophylaxis, have a high chance of reactivation and disease if their CD4 count drops to <100 cells/μL.

Clinical features

In all immunocompromised patients, blurred vision, eye pain, red eye, and floaters should prompt consideration of toxoplasma chorioretinitis.

HIV infection

CNS infection usually presents with headache, confusion, fever, focal neurological deficit, or seizures. Pulmonary toxoplasmosis presents with cough, fever, and dyspnoea and may be clinically indistinguishable from tuberculosis, cryptococcosis, PCP, or histoplasmosis. Chorioretinitis presents as visual impairment and/or eye pain. In some patients infected with HIV, gastric toxoplasmosis has been noted as the first manifestation of disease.

Transplant recipients

HSCT recipients are at particular risk for severe disseminated toxoplasmosis due to reactivation of latent disease. In SOT recipients, *T. gondii* may be transmitted by and cause disease in the transplanted organ (e.g. myocarditis in cardiac transplant). Disseminated toxoplasmosis should be considered in culture-negative sepsis, especially if there are neurological signs, respiratory signs, or unexplained skin lesions.

Neonates

Congenital toxoplasmosis occurs when parasites cross the placenta during primary maternal infection. In ~90% of infections, the pregnant woman will be asymptomatic. Congenital infections are particularly severe if the infection occurs during the first or second trimester of pregnancy. Initial symptoms in the neonate may include retinochoroiditis, cerebral calcification, and occasionally microcephaly or hydrocephalus, but signs and symptoms of congenital CNS involvement may not manifest for several years.

Diagnosis

Serology

Assays to detect antibody in blood or CSF are first line, but given the impaired/delayed antibody response in the immunocompromised and the very high general seropositivity, results must be interpreted with caution. Definitive diagnosis is demonstrated by a rising antibody titre, an IgM immunofluorescence assay (IFA) titre ≥1:64 or an IgM enzyme-linked immunosorbent assay (ELISA) titre >1:256. The absence of specific IgG antibodies weighs heavily against the diagnosis of reactivation toxoplasmosis in immunocompromised patients.

In patients with advanced HIV, a suggestive clinical history, a positive specific IgG test, and typical radiographic findings (multiple ring-enhancing brain lesions) are usually given a trial of anti-*Toxoplasma* chemotherapy. Treatment of patients with toxoplasmosis usually leads to clinical and radiographic improvement within 7–10 days. A diagnostic brain biopsy is indicated if there is failure to improve within this time frame.

Molecular techniques

PCR can be performed on CSF, serum, BAL fluid, and ocular tissue. However, the absence of *Toxoplasma* DNA does not exclude toxoplasmosis. The sensitivity of PCR depends on context; it is higher when used on amniotic fluid to confirm congenital toxoplasmosis than when used to detect reactivation in, for example, patients with HIV. PCR amplification of *Toxoplasma* DNA in CSF has a high predictive value, but relatively low sensitivity. In patients who can safely undergo lumbar puncture, analysis of CSF should be performed to look for evidence of *T. gondii*, as well as other infectious and non-infectious causes of CNS disease.

Histology

A stained (Giemsa/haematoxylin and eosin/immunoperoxidase) brain or bronchoalveolar biopsy sample showing tachyzoites confirms the diagnosis of toxoplasmosis.

Treatment

The preferred initial regimen is sulfadiazine and pyrimethamine plus folinic acid for 6 weeks followed by maintenance therapy. In sulpha allergic patients, pyrimethamine plus clindamycin is recommended. Atovaquone and TMP–SMX have also been used but experience is limited. Corticosteroids should not be used routinely in the absence of signs of raised intracranial pressure. Refer to

Refer to
British HIV Association (BHIVA) and British Infection Association (BIA) ♒
http://www.bhiva.org/Guidelines.aspx and Infectious Diseases Society of
America (IDSA) ♒ http://www.idsociety.org/PracticeGuidelines/ for up-
to-date guidelines.

Cryptosporidium species

Intracellular protist parasites of the class Apicomplexa and associated with GI and biliary disease in vertebrates. Of the 20 or so species identified, two cause most human disease: *C. parvum*, which can also cause disease in other vertebrates and *C. hominis*, which infects primarily humans.

Oocysts are ingested by mouth and excyst in the small bowel to release four banana-shaped motile sporozoites which attach to the epithelial cell wall. The sporozoites mature asexually into meronts, which release merozoites intraluminally. These can reinvade host cells, resulting in autoinfection, or can undergo sexual maturation to form new oocysts which can either excyst within the host GI tract or pass out into the environment. Oocysts are infectious and can remain viable for many months at a wide range of temperatures. They are also chlorine resistant, so drinking water must be boiled.

Epidemiology

Cryptosporidium spp. are a major cause of diarrhoea worldwide, with seropositivity rates of up to ~35% in North America and Europe. Transmission is via ingestion (± inhalation) of oocysts and spread can be person to person, water/foodborne, or animal to person. *C. hominis* infections are often foreign travel or day-care associated, whereas *C. parvum* is usually associated with farm animal contact.

The organisms reside in gut epithelial cells and cause secretory diarrhoea that may lead to malabsorption. They are associated with sporadic water-related outbreaks of self-limiting diarrhoea among immunocompetent hosts and chronic severe diarrhoea among the immunocompromised.

Clinical features

Immunocompetent

Following an incubation period of 7–10 days, infection classically causes a frothy, watery diarrhoea, abdominal cramps, anorexia, and low-grade fever. It can occasionally be more persistent and requires IV fluid replacement. Chronic cryptosporidiosis in infants has been linked to failure to thrive.

Immunocompromised

Particularly in HIV infection, cryptosporidiosis can cause severe and life-threatening disease. If the CD4 count is <200 cells/μL, infection may be chronic, severe, and also involve the lungs, gall bladder, liver, and pancreas. Patients with SCID and haematological malignancies are also at risk of disseminated cryptosporidiosis. Its auto-infective oocyst stage may explain why a small inoculum can lead to overwhelming infection in the immunosuppressed.

Diagnosis

Several specimens of stool (or sputum samples if respiratory symptoms) may be needed.

Antigen immunoassays

IFA or ELISA to detect *Cryptosporidium* antigen in stool are sensitive and specific first-line diagnostic tests.

Microscopy
Modified acid-alcohol fast staining is used to look for the oocysts (4–6 μm diameter). Stool concentration techniques increase sensitivity.

PCR
Increasingly used in reference laboratories and allows speciation, which can be useful in outbreak investigation. If available, PCR is the diagnostic method of choice as it is more sensitive than microscopy.

Treatment
Treatment is mainly supportive. In HIV, initiation of HAART offers the best outcome. Nitazoxanide is approved for use in the immunocompetent but there is little evidence of efficacy in the immunocompromised. Paromomycin and azithromycin have also been used, although evidence of benefit is very limited.

Refer to
British HIV Association (BHIVA) and British Infection Association (BIA) ♒ http://www.bhiva.org/Guidelines.aspx and Infectious Diseases Society of America (IDSA) ♒ http://www.idsociety.org/PracticeGuidelines/ for up-to-date guidelines.

Cyclospora cayetanensis

C. cayetanensis is an intracellular coccidian parasite causing diarrhoeal illness. Humans are thought to be the only natural hosts.

Epidemiology

C. cayetanensis has emerged as a worldwide cause of severe and prolonged diarrhoeal illness in the immunocompromised. It is most commonly reported in Latin America, India, and SE Asia. Unlike *Cryptosporidium*, the oocysts passed in fresh stool are not infective, therefore direct faeco-oral transmission and auto-infective cycles do not occur. The oocysts take days to weeks to sporulate (become infective) after being passed in the stool. As with *Cryptosporidium*, the oocysts are not killed by chlorination, so boiling water is recommended.

Clinical features

Suspect in unexplained, prolonged diarrhoea in returning travellers from tropics and sub-tropics. Median incubation is 7 days from ingestion and the presentation is often with anorexia, nausea, flatulence, fatigue, abdominal cramping, watery diarrhoea (may contain blood or mucus), low-grade fever, and weight loss. In the immunocompetent, 3–4 days of diarrhoea are usual with relapses lasting up to 7 weeks. In the immunocompromised, symptoms may persist for up to 12 weeks and may include biliary disease. Like *Cryptosporidium*, it may also infect the lungs and cause respiratory symptoms.

Diagnosis

Collect three stool samples at 2- or 3-day intervals for microscopy ('OCP' (ova, cysts and parasites)). Send stool as fresh as possible. The samples are centrifuge concentrated and then stained with a modified acid-fast or safranin stain to allow visualization of the oocysts. The oocysts are bigger (8–10 μm diameter) than those of *Cryptosporidium* (4–6 μm). Ultraviolet autofluorescence microscopy is a fast and sensitive, though non-specific, method of visualizing oocysts in stool.

Treatment

TMP–SMX is the recommended treatment. Nitazoxanide or ciprofloxacin are alternatives.

Refer to

British HIV Association (BHIVA) and British Infection Association (BIA) ℅ http://www.bhiva.org/Guidelines.aspx and Infectious Diseases Society of America (IDSA) ℅ http://www.idsociety.org/PracticeGuidelines/ for up-to-date guidelines.

Cystoisospora belli (formerly *Isospora belli*)

C. belli is a diarrhoea-causing coccidian parasite, similar to *Cryptosporidium*, and another cause of chronic and severe diarrhoea in the immunocompromised. It is the only species of *Cystoisospora* known to infect humans. The parasite completes its life cycle within the human host and immature oocysts are excreted in stool. No other reservoir hosts are known.

Epidemiology

Globally distributed, though most prevalent in the tropics and sub-tropics, particularly South America and India. Transmission is through ingestion of water or food contaminated with mature, sporulated oocysts.

Clinical features

Consider in HIV-infected patients with a low CD4 count returning from the tropics and presenting with persistent, non-bloody diarrhoea, weight loss, and eosinophilia. *C. belli* infection is also associated with acalculous cholecystitis and reactive arthritis in HIV.

Diagnosis

Send fresh stool samples for microscopy. Microscopic techniques include wet mount of fresh stool to look for oocysts (thin walled, ellipsoid, and ~30 μm long), acid-fast and/or auramine-rhodamine stains of concentrated stool, and ultraviolet autofluorescence.

If oocysts are not detected in stool, microscopic examination of duodenal aspirates or intestinal tissue biopsy may be diagnostic.

Treatment

TMP–SMX is recommended. As relapse is common, secondary prophylaxis is important (TMP–SMX three times/week) following acute treatment. Ciprofloxacin is an alternative but response is slower and may be incomplete. Pyrimethamine has been used but efficacy is unclear.

Refer to

British HIV Association (BHIVA) and British Infection Association (BIA) ℘ http://www.bhiva.org/Guidelines.aspx and Infectious Diseases Society of America (IDSA) ℘ http://www.idsociety.org/PracticeGuidelines/ for up-to-date guidelines.

Entamoeba histolytica

E. histolytica is a pseudopod-forming, non-flagellated protozoan parasite causing both intestinal disease (amoebic dysentery) and extra-intestinal disease (most commonly liver abscess). Its life cycle consists of an infective cyst stage and an invasive trophozoite form. The cyst is resistant to gastric acid and desiccation, and can survive in a moist environment for several weeks. There are three species of intestinal amoebae with identical morphological characteristics: *E. histolytica*, *E. dispar*, and *E. moshkovskii*. Infection is acquired by ingestion of amoebic cysts usually in food or contaminated water but venereal transmission through faecal–oral contact also occurs. Ingestion of a single cyst is sufficient to cause disease. The trophozoites emerge from the cysts in the small intestine, invade the epithelium, and cause disease by destroying host tissues.

Epidemiology

E. histolytica infection (amoebiasis) occurs worldwide and is second only to malaria as a protozoan cause of death. An estimated 40–50 million cases of amoebic colitis and liver abscess occur annually, resulting in 40,000–110,000 deaths. Most amoebic infections occur in Central/South America, Africa, and Asia. In economically developed countries, amoebiasis is most often seen in migrants or travellers from endemic areas.

Clinical features

The majority of *Entamoeba* infections are asymptomatic; this includes 90% of *E. histolytica* infections. *E. dispar* is generally considered non-pathogenic and most symptomatic disease is caused by *E. histolytica*. Reports of *E. moshkovskii* infection causing diarrhoea are becoming more frequent, but its pathogenic potential remains unclear.

Colonization with *E. histolytica* carries a low but definite risk of development of invasive amoebiasis and impaired cell-mediated immunity increases the risk of invasive disease with liver involvement.

Colonization with the morphologically identical parasite *E. dispar* is much more common than infection with *E. histolytica*.

Dysentery or colitis

Amoebic colitis typically presents with a several-week history of gradual-onset abdominal pain and tenderness, diarrhoea, and bloody stools. The appearance of amoebic colitis on colonoscopy may resemble that of inflammatory bowel disease, with granular, friable, and diffusely ulcerated mucosa.

Liver abscess

May present acutely with fever, right upper abdominal tenderness, and pain, or sub-acutely with weight loss, fever, and abdominal pain. Patients with liver abscess usually present without concurrent colitis, although some will have a history of dysentery within the last year. Amoebic abscesses are usually single and in the right lobe of the liver (~80% of cases) and patients are most commonly adult males.

Extra-intestinal disease

Pleuro-pulmonary disease results from liver abscess rupture into the pleural space or, more rarely, from haematogenous spread.

Cardiac infection can follow rupture of a liver abscess into the pericardium while brain abscesses result from haematogenous spread. Cutaneous amoebiasis, resulting from direct inoculation of stool in nappy-wearing infants or from anal intercourse in adults, may present as painful ulceration in the perineal/perianal region.

Diagnosis

Stool microscopy

The traditional first-line test for suspected amoebiasis. It is not very sensitive, however, so at least three stool samples should be sent. A direct saline wet mount is examined to look for motile trophozoites alongside a concentration step and a stained smear. Microscopic examination cannot differentiate *E. histolytica* from the non-pathogenic *E. dispar* or *E. moshkovskii* (unless red blood cells are seen within the trophozoite cytoplasm which is diagnostic of *E. histolytica*). In general, if the patient is symptomatic, the amoebae are assumed to be *E. histolytica*.

Stool antigen tests

Using monoclonal antibodies are sensitive, specific, rapid, easy to perform, and can distinguish between species. They are also commonly used as first-line tests. Distinguishing between species is vital as *E. dispar* colonization is much more common than *E. histolytica* infection.

Serology

May be useful, as infection with *E. histolytica* results in the development of antibodies whereas *E. dispar* infection does not. Antibodies are detectable within a week of acute infection and may persist for years. About 10–35% of uninfected individuals in endemic areas have anti-amoebic antibodies due to previous infection with *E. histolytica*. Negative serology is therefore helpful for exclusion of disease, but positive serology cannot distinguish between acute and previous infection. In amoebic liver abscess (or pleuropulmonary/cardiac/cerebral lesions), most patients do not have detectable parasites in stool and the presence of antibodies can be useful in diagnosis. Tests for antibodies to amoebae are ~90% sensitive for amoebic liver abscess and 70% sensitive for amoebic colitis.

Molecular methods

PCR of stool is much more sensitive than faecal antigen tests but is not yet widely available for diagnostic clinical testing.

Imaging

Ultrasound, CT, and MRI studies of the liver are equally sensitive at detecting amoebic abscesses but equally incapable of specifically differentiating amoebic from pyogenic abscesses.

Endoscopy

Colonoscopy may be helpful in the diagnosis of amoebic colitis if antigen detection tests are negative.

Treatment

Invasive disease is treated with metronidazole or tinidazole, followed by a luminal agent such as diloxanide furoate or paromomycin to eliminate intraluminal cysts.

Refer to

British HIV Association (BHIVA) and British Infection Association (BIA) ℰ http://www.bhiva.org/Guidelines.aspx and Infectious Diseases Society of America (IDSA) ℰ http://www.idsociety.org/PracticeGuidelines/ for up-to-date guidelines.

Free-living amoebae

These globally distributed environmental protozoa live freely without the need for a host and feed on bacteria and nutrients in moist soil, fresh water, and salt water. Four genera, Naegleria, Acanthamoeba, Balamuthia, and Sappinia cause human CNS disease and the immunocompromised are at increased risk.

There are two clinical entities caused by infection with these organisms: primary amoebic meningoencephalitis caused by Naegleria fowleri and granulomatous amoebic encephalitis caused by Acanthamoeba spp., *Balamuthia mandrillaris*, and *Sappinia pedata*.

Naegleria fowleri

N. fowleri is a free-living amoeba which inhabits most soil and freshwater habitats. The life cycle consists of trophozoite and cyst stages.

Epidemiology

There have been ~200 cases of primary amoebic meningoencephalitis documented worldwide (~50% in the US) since it was first reported in 1965. Most cases have been in healthy young people with a history of recent water-sport related activities. Amoebae enter through the nasal cavity and the organisms penetrate the nasal mucosa and migrate via the olfactory nerves to the brain. Haemorrhagic necrosis ensues and is concentrated in the olfactory bulbs and base of the brain.

Clinical features

Primary amoebic meningoencephalitis is an acute haemorrhagic meningoencephalitis characterized by a fulminant course with clinical and laboratory features that resemble acute bacterial meningitis. The period between contact with the amoebae and symptoms ranges from 2 to 15 days and, with very rare exceptions, the disease is rapidly fatal. In 1997, the first death was reported in a transplant recipient who received the organ from a donor who died of undiagnosed *N. fowleri* infection.

Diagnosis

CSF parameters are as for acute purulent bacterial meningitis but Gram stains and bacterial culture will be negative. Negative results for bacteria and common viruses in patients with acute meningoencephalitis should prompt the search for amoebae in the CSF. History of recent exposure (e.g. swimming in a lake) increases the likelihood of primary amoebic meningoencephalitis, but it is not always obtained.

Microscopy

CSF or sedimented CSF is placed under a cover slip and observed for motile trophozoites. Smears can be stained with Wright or Giemsa stains. It can be very difficult to distinguish amoebae from leucocytes and the motility of trophozoites is variable.

Brain biopsy

Brain tissue can be examined for trophozoites and sections stained with immunofluorescent anti-*N. fowleri* antibodies. *N. fowleri* can be cultured and isolated in non-nutrient agar coated with enteric bacteria.

Molecular methods
Multiplex PCR can rapidly identify the DNA of the major free-living amoebas in CSF, but is not yet widely available.

Imaging
In presumptive pyogenic meningitis with no bacteria detected in the CSF, basal arachnoiditis seen on contrast CT brain imaging should prompt consideration of primary amoebic meningoencephalitis.

Treatment
Unclear, however, there are anecdotal reports of successful treatment with careful intracranial pressure management and a variety of drugs including miltefosine, amphotericin B, and azithromycin.

Refer to
US Centers for Disease Control and Prevention (CDC) website: ℗ https://www.cdc.gov/parasites/naegleria/treatment-hcp.html for more information.

Acanthamoeba spp., *Balamuthia mandrillaris*, and *Sappinia pedata*

Acanthamoeba spp. are freshwater motile organisms and the commonest environmental amoebae. They exist in trophozoite and cyst stages. *Balamuthia mandrillaris* was first isolated in a baboon brain in the 1980s and ~200 human cases have been reported subsequently (mostly in the Americas). There has only been one reported human case of granulomatous amoebic encephalitis due to *Sappinia pedata*.

Epidemiology
Acanthamoeba spp. are globally ubiquitous and found in soil, air, and water. They may be transmitted via inhalation or direct skin contact. Although most cases are in patients with HIV and low CD4 counts, many other immunosuppressed states also predispose to infection. *Balamuthia mandrillaris* cases have been associated with activities such as dirt biking and gardening. Transmission via organ donation has been described in at least three clusters, including one asymptomatic donor. Animal faeces are likely to be a necessary component of the life cycle of *Sappinia pedata*.

Clinical features
Granulomatous amoebic encephalitis is a subacute or chronic meningo-encephalitis with focal granulomatous lesions in the brain; it should be considered in the differential diagnosis of CNS space-occupying lesions in all immunocompromised hosts. The presentation is over weeks to months and is usually a combination of headache, low-grade fever, confusion, drowsiness, lethargy, nausea/vomiting, stiff neck, and occasionally seizures and hemiparesis. Brain imaging shows single or multiple space-occupying lesions with ring enhancement, with the temporal and parietal lobes most commonly affected. *Acanthamoeba* spp. also cause skin infections. These are more common in patients with HIV (irrespective of CNS disease) and normally present as firm nodules which initially drain purulent material and progress to non-healing indurated ulcers.

Diagnosis

Brain biopsy

Haematoxylin and eosin staining demonstrates both trophozoites and cysts. If available, PCR applied to brain or other tissues provides a more rapid diagnosis.

Other samples

If skin or pulmonary lesions are present, biopsy of these may demonstrate trophozoites on microscopy. IFA and immunoperoxidase stains also help in identifying amoebae in biopsied tissue. Lumbar puncture is usually contraindicated due to risk of herniation, but if CSF is obtained, Giemsa staining of the sediment may reveal trophozoites. For eye and skin infections, swabs or tissue samples can be plated onto specialized growth media (non-nutrient agar with bacterial overlay) and the organisms cultured.

Treatment

Treatment of these conditions is unclear and usually consists of combination therapy. Drugs that have been used include flucytosine, pentamidine, fluconazole, sulfadiazine, azithromycin, and miltefosine. Amoebic keratitis has been treated with chlorhexidine, polyhexamethylene biguanide, and neomycin ± epithelial debridement. Evidence is lacking.

Refer to

US Centers for Disease Control and Prevention (CDC) ℘ https://www.cdc.gov/parasites/index.html for more information.

Microsporidia species

Microsporidia are primitive, eukaryotic, obligate intracellular organisms, closely related to fungi and capable of infecting a large number of invertebrate and vertebrate hosts. They became prominent in the medical literature during the mid 1980s due to their association with GI and systemic disease in patients with HIV infection. *Enterocytozoon bieneusi* is the most common species to infect humans and infection is mostly confined to the intestinal and biliary tract, although disseminated disease involving the kidneys, lungs, eyes, and other organs may occur.

Epidemiology

Microsporidia spores are environmentally widespread and normally enter the host via ingestion or inhalation. The incidence of intestinal microsporidiosis in HIV-infected patients has decreased in developed countries with the widespread use of HAART, but is increasingly reported in non-HIV immunocompromised patients such as transplant recipients.

Clinical features

The most common presentation is persistent, non-bloody, watery diarrhoea ± crampy abdominal pain in patients with HIV. Disseminated infections, mostly reported in SOT and HSCT recipients, can affect any organ system. Most cases of pulmonary microsporidiosis have been reported in patients with haematological malignancies or following bone marrow transplantation. Microsporidial brain abscess, sinusitis, endocarditis, myocarditis, osteomyelitis, cutaneous, and genitourinary infections have also been described.

Diagnosis

Microscopy

This may identify the spores in stool, body fluid samples, and biopsied tissue. Microsporidial spores stain pink using haematoxylin and eosin stain.

Culture

Culture has been successfully performed for many of the species that infect humans, using a number of different cell culture lines, including human diploid fibroblasts.

Molecular techniques

PCR, if available, can be used to detect *Microsporidia* and identify the species.

Treatment

Specific treatment is unclear. Restoration of immune function if possible is likely to resolve infection. Of the agents that have been used, albendazole is recommended initially. Nitazoxanide, albendazole, and itraconazole have also been used. For *E. bieneusi*, oral fumagillin has been used but is associated with significant toxicity.

Refer to

British HIV Association (BHIVA) and British Infection Association (BIA) ℘ http://www.bhiva.org/Guidelines.aspx and Infectious Diseases Society of America (IDSA) ℘ http://www.idsociety.org/PracticeGuidelines/ for up-to-date guidelines.

Trypanosoma cruzi

T. cruzi is a protozoan parasite and the causative agent of the zoonotic disease American trypanosomiasis (Chagas disease). In humans, *T. cruzi* is found in two forms; the extracellular trypomastigote stage in the blood and the intracellular amastigote stage in cells of mesenchymal origin such as reticuloendothelial, myocardial, adipose, and neuroglial cells. Reactivation of chronic *T. cruzi* infection may occur in patients with immunosuppression due to malignancy, chemotherapy, immunosuppressive transplant regimens, or HIV infection.

Epidemiology

Chagas disease is endemic in 21 Latin American countries and an estimated 8–10 million people are infected. Because of recent human migration patterns, the disease is now also becoming a public health concern in non-endemic areas. The vector, the triatomine beetle (reduviid/kissing bug), defecates during its blood meal and faecal material containing the parasite is inoculated through the bite wound or mucous membranes. Transmission may also occur congenitally, via transfusion of blood components, transplantation of infected organs, or via the consumption of contaminated food or drink.

Clinical features

In the immunocompetent host, acute infection occurs a week or two after inoculation and may include the characteristic 'Chagoma' skin lesion at the site of inoculation. About 20–30% of patients go on to develop the chronic disease, associated with cardiomyopathy, megacolon, and mega-oesophagus. Reactivation due to immunosuppression is characterized by a return to the high level parasite replication seen in acute disease.

Transplant recipients

T. cruzi infection may present with fever, signs of organ rejection, or skin lesions. Acute Chagas may rarely follow transplantation of infected tissue, but more commonly occurs as reactivation of latent disease due to transplant-related immunosuppression.

HIV infection

T. cruzi reactivation most commonly presents with CNS disease: meningo-encephalitis or brain abscesses. Acute myocarditis is the next most frequent manifestation of reactivation.

Diagnosis

Microscopy

Parasitaemia may be high in the acute phase or during reactivation and motile trypomastigotes may be visible on microscopy of fresh preparations of anticoagulated blood or in buffy coat preparations. Depending on presentation, other specimens such as CSF, bone marrow aspirate, and pericardial fluid may also be examined by wet preparation microscopy or Giemsa smear.

Serology
Two different assays should be used to detect IgG (usually ELISA and IFA) as individually they have poor sensitivity.

Molecular methods
The demonstration of rising parasite numbers by quantitative PCR in serial specimens is the most sensitive indicator of reactivation.

Xenodiagnosis and haemoculture
May also be attempted if the laboratory has capacity and other diagnostics are inconclusive.

Treatment

Benznidazole and nifurtimox are anti-trypanosomal drugs with proven efficacy. As benznidazole has the best safety and efficacy profile it is preferred.

Refer to
US Centers for Disease Control and Prevention (CDC) ℘ https://www.cdc.gov/parasites/chagas/health_professionals/tx.html for more information.

Leishmania species

The genus *Leishmania* comprises a heterogeneous group of vector-borne protozoa, with two stages to their life cycle; the amastigote, which resides in the macrophages of the mammalian host and the promastigote, found in the gut of the phlebotomine sandfly vector.

Human disease (leishmaniasis) is caused by nine different *Leishmania* species which tend to cause either visceral or cutaneous disease. The visceral form (also known as black fever, dumdum fever, and kala-azar) is predominantly caused by *L. donovani and L. infantum* (known as *L. chagasi* in Latin America) but can also occur with *L. mexicana and L. tropica*—species normally associated with cutaneous disease. Visceral leishmaniasis has been seen with increasing frequency in HIV-infected patients.

Epidemiology

The usual route of transmission is from the bite of an infected sandfly, but transmission may also occur via blood transfusion, needle sharing, sexual contact, and congenitally. Endemic areas include Africa, Asia, South and Central America, and the Mediterranean basin. The incubation period is normally between 2 and 6 months, but can range from less than a week to more than a year.

Clinical features

Once inoculated, the parasite is engulfed by tissue macrophages which travel in the bloodstream to the reticuloendothelial organs—liver, spleen, and bone marrow. Leishmania infection impairs cell-mediated immunity allowing proliferation and dissemination of the parasite. A granulomatous reaction occurs around infected cells and results in either sub-clinical disease and self-cure or the syndrome of visceral leishmaniasis. Classic clinical features include fever, malaise, weight loss, and splenomegaly. Laboratory tests may reveal hypergammaglobulinaemia, pancytopenia, immune complexes, and positive rheumatoid factor.

In endemic areas, patients often present with gradual-onset malaise, whereas in individuals from non-endemic regions, the onset can be acute with fever, diarrhoea, and anorexia and may be confused with typhoid or malaria. Untreated visceral leishmaniasis generally leads to death after weeks or years and secondary viral and bacterial infections are common. In patients infected with HIV, visceral leishmaniasis is a recurrent disease, the course of which is modified by the severity of immunosuppression. In patients with CD4 cell counts <50 cells/μL, infection of atypical sites may occur, including the GI tract, peritoneal space, lung, pleural space, and skin. The majority of patients with HIV present with classic visceral leishmaniasis but cutaneous lesions in visceral leishmaniasis with HIV infection are increasingly reported. These lesions are not always the typical ulcers and include subcutaneous nodules on the legs, hypo-pigmented lesions on the arms, or violaceous scaly plaques on the face.

Diagnosis

Though often made clinically, definitive diagnosis requires either demonstration of amastigotes in clinical samples, growth of promastigotes on culture, or detection of parasite DNA in patient samples. While acute disease may mimic many other diseases, the differential diagnosis of late-stage visceral leishmaniasis is confined to haematological and lymphatic malignancies.

Blood smears

Samples should be collected at night as the amastigote exhibits diurnal periodicity. Examination of buffy coat smears taken at night show a 66% recovery compared to only 46% on daytime samples.

Tissue aspirates

The highest yield tissue is the spleen (98% sensitive), although the risk of splenic laceration or bowel perforation associated with splenic aspiration means that bone marrow aspirates (80% sensitive) are more often used. Liver and lymph node biopsy are alternatives.

Culture

Buffy coat or splenic/bone marrow aspirates should be inoculated onto parasite growth medium and checked weekly (for 4 weeks) by microscopy to look for amastigotes. Sensitivity is generally 60–80 % and amastigotes are visible after 2 weeks.

Antigen detection

The K39 strip test, an immunochromatographic test for use on serum, has shown high sensitivity and specificity, but can remain positive for years after treatment, so cannot be used to diagnose relapse.

Molecular techniques

If available, PCR has higher sensitivity and specificity than smear or culture and is useful for assessment of treatment response as well as diagnosis and identification of the species. Sensitivity is higher when used on tissue samples (spleen/marrow) than on peripheral blood.

Treatment

Treatment of cutaneous leishmaniasis is highly individualized depending on *Leishmania* species, immunocompetence of the patient, and site of infection. Treatment options include topical therapy (e.g. with paromomycin), intralesional therapy (e.g. with sodium stibogluconate), and systemic therapy with miltefosine, amphotericin B, or pentavalent antimonials. The treatment of choice for visceral and mucosal leishmaniasis is liposomal amphotericin B. Miltefosine is a newer alternative.

Refer to

World Health Organization (WHO) management recommendations: ℘ http://www.who.int/leishmaniasis/resources/case_management/en/ and Infectious Diseases Society of America (IDSA) ℘ http://www.idsociety.org/PracticeGuidelines/ for up-to-date guidelines.

Strongyloides stercoralis

Strongyloidiasis is caused by infection with the soil-transmitted parasitic helminth *Strongyloides stercoralis* (and less commonly by *Strongyloides fuelleborni*). Infection occurs via skin contact with faecally contaminated soil. Larvae penetrate the skin, enter the circulatory system, are transported to the lungs, and penetrate the alveoli. After passing up the trachea, they are swallowed, moult twice in the small intestine, and mature into adult female worms. The adults live threaded in the duodenal epithelium producing eggs asexually which yield rhabditiform larvae. These non-infective rhabditiform larvae are either passed in the stool or transform into infective filaria and reinvade the gut mucosa or the perianal skin. *Strongyloides* is the only human helminth parasite of clinical importance that can complete its entire life cycle within human hosts (although sexual reproduction occurs during the free-living phase). This determines two important clinical features: the possibility of autoinfection and the development of persistent infections. The spectrum of disease ranges from chronic asymptomatic infection in the immunocompetent to dissemination and septic shock in the immunocompromised.

Epidemiology

More than 100 million people are infected worldwide and higher rates have been found among HIV-positive patients. In economically developed countries, *S. stercoralis* infection is very rare, but occasional clusters occur, often among farmers or miners. Humans are the principal host of *S. stercoralis*, but dogs, cats, and other mammals can also harbour the helminth and serve as reservoir hosts.

Clinical features

Immunocompetent

Chronic infections are usually asymptomatic or may lead to recurrent intestinal, respiratory (wheeze), cutaneous (larva currens), or systemic (weight loss) symptoms. Eosinophilia is usual.

Immunocompromised

The immunocompromised are at risk of hyperinfection syndrome (massive invasion of filariform larvae in the bowel ± the lungs) and disseminated strongyloidiasis (presence of larvae in the extra-intestinal/pulmonary sites such as the liver, heart, kidneys, CNS, and skin). If untreated, the mortality rate of hyperinfection and disseminated disease approaches 100%. Hyperinfection is most commonly associated with the administration of corticosteroids or cytotoxic drugs and it is therefore important to detect and eradicate *Strongyloides* infection prior to initiation of immunosuppressive therapy. Even short courses of corticosteroids have led to overwhelming hyperinfection and death. Severe strongyloidiasis can occur up to 65 years after the primary infection.

General symptoms of hyperinfection may include fever and chills, fatigue, weakness, and general body pain. This may be accompanied by abdominal symptoms (pain, diarrhoea, vomiting, and peritonitis), respiratory symptoms (wheeze, cough, haemoptysis, dyspnoea), cutaneous signs (petechiae, purpura, pruritic linear streaks on the buttocks/lower trunk), and CNS manifestations (meningitis).

Diagnosis

Microscopy

Allows visualization of rhabditoid larvae in stool specimens. Send either fresh, unpreserved stool or at least three preserved faecal samples collected on alternate days. Standard stool examination has low sensitivity (<50%) due to the low burden of larvae and their intermittent shedding. Specialized techniques, such as the agar plate method, increase sensitivity. In severe strongyloidiasis, eggs, larvae, and adult stages may also be detected in wet preparations of respiratory samples or in stained slides of lung tissue. If a rash is present, larvae may be visible in skin biopsies.

Endoscopy

Strongyloidiasis has a range of colonoscopic features, including oedema, serpiginous ulcerations, erosions, friable mucosa, and yellowish-white nodules. Biopsied material can be stained for histological examination.

Serology

Commercially available ELISA kits are available with sensitivities and specificities >90%, but may give false-negative results in the immunocompromised.

Molecular techniques

PCR assays for use on stool samples are in development.

Treatment

Ivermectin is the drug of choice with albendazole as an alternative. Caution is advised in patients who have travelled to west and central Africa, as treatment with ivermectin can lead to encephalopathy if there is concomitant infection with *Loa loa* (a filarial nematode). A blood film looking for *Loa loa* microfilaria before treatment with ivermectin is recommended. *Strongyloides* hyperinfection syndrome is also treated with ivermectin, although the addition of antibiotics to cover Gram-negative sepsis are recommended as this is a common accompanying complication. Ivermectin should continue until 2 weeks after the last positive stool sample to account for the autoinfection cycle.

Refer to

US Centers for Disease Control and Prevention (CDC) for up-to-date recommendations: https://www.cdc.gov/parasites/strongyloides/health_professionals/index.html.

Sarcoptes scabiei

S. scabiei is a microscopic arthropod that lives in cutaneous burrows and causes the pruritic dermatitis called scabies. A severe form known as Norwegian or crusted scabies, in which there are huge numbers of mites present, is associated with defects in cellular immunity, including AIDS and HTLV-1 infection.

Epidemiology

S. scabiei mites are transmitted by close skin-to-skin contact or via fomites (usually clothes and bedding). Outbreaks are common in hospitals and institutions such as prisons and nursing homes.

Clinical features

Severe itch is the predominant symptom and scratching often leads to excoriation and sometimes secondary infection. Scabies most commonly affects the hands (interdigital spaces), axillae, groin and buttocks. The classic sign of burrows may be absent in Norwegian scabies and instead there are hyperkeratotic, crusted, scaling, fissured plaques.

Diagnosis

Microscopy

Skin scrapings from infected area will show the mites, eggs, or faecal pellets. If skin scrapings are plated out for fungal culture on Saboraud's dextrose agar, serpiginous tracks will be seen. If the mites cannot be seen on mineral oil preparations of skin scrapings, encrusted scrapings can be left in a petri dish or small plastic box at room temperature for 12 hours. The mites will drop to the bottom of the container and can be seen with a magnifying glass or microscope.

Treatment

Clothing, bedding, etc. from infected patients and household/close contacts over the previous 4 days should be decontaminated by high-temperature washing and drying or dry cleaning. Recommended topical scabicides are permethrin or malathion. In severe cases, the addition of oral ivermectin is recommended.

Refer to

National Institute for Health and Care Excellence (NICE) ℘ https://cks.nice.org.uk/scabies for up-to-date guidelines.

Acknowledgement

This chapter was kindly reviewed by Dr Ian Bowler, Consultant in Infectious Diseases and Microbiology, Oxford University Hospitals NHS Trust.

Fungi

Introduction

Many fungal species considered of low inherent virulence or non-pathogenic in the immunocompetent have the potential to cause serious disease in the immunocompromised. The prevalence and importance of invasive fungal infections is probably greater now than ever before. The expansion of transplantation programmes, the increasingly widespread use of antibiotics, and the many new immunomodulatory drugs have coincided with the HIV epidemic resulting in increasing numbers of susceptible hosts. Patients with end-organ failure and malignancies now live much longer and many treatments and interventions breech protective barriers, disrupt immune function, and alter normal microbiota; all of which predispose to invasive fungal disease. Patient groups less obviously immunocompromised (e.g. patients with diabetes or those undergoing complex surgery) and patients with implanted medical devices or materials are also at increased risk (➔ see Chapter 1). Neutrophils and macrophages are the principal mediators of innate immunity against fungi, so neutropenic patients are highly susceptible to opportunistic fungal pathogens. The morbidity and mortality associated with invasive fungal infections in the immunocompromised is high; this is largely due to the fact that susceptible patients are usually very unwell to begin with. In addition, the emergence of drug-resistant strains and the lack of robust evidence on best treatment all contribute to poor outcomes.

The majority of fungal disease in the immunocompromised is still caused by the 'big two', *Aspergillus* spp. and *Candida* spp.; however, infection with less common hyaline and dematiaceous filamentous fungi are increasingly encountered. Fungi causing invasive disease in the immunocompromised are almost all saprophytic moulds that are widely distributed in nature and present globally. Only a few species such as *Histoplasma capsulatum* (North America) and *Penicillium* (*Talaromyces*) *marneffei* (SE Asia) are endemic to particular regions.

It is essential to correlate clinical, radiological, pathological, and laboratory findings in order to distinguish an invasive fungal species from a contaminant. The finding of a known pathogen, especially when in a significant amount, from a normally sterile site usually represents true infection.

Although there are clinical and radiological signs that point towards a fungal cause of infection, definitive diagnosis requires laboratory confirmation. This is in the form of one or more of the following:

• Positive culture.
• Microscopy with characteristic fungal elements seen in stained tissue/ body fluid.
• Elevated/rising titres of fungal antigens such as *Cryptococcus* or *Histoplasma* antigen, galactomannan for *Aspergillus*, or the more generic fungal antigen 1,3-beta-D-glucan (BD-glucan).
• Detecting the presence of fungal DNA.

Prophylactic antifungal therapy is used in many high-risk immunosuppressed patients as the diagnostic and monitoring tools are currently insufficient to accurately predict which patients will develop disease and require pre-emptive therapy.

Pathogenic fungi described in this chapter are categorized morphologically into filamentous fungi/moulds, yeasts, dimorphic fungi, and atypicals.

Filamentous fungi/moulds

These have branching hyphae, which can be either septate or non-septate and colourless (hyaline) or pigmented (e.g. dematiaceous moulds).

Aspergillus spp.

Aspergillus spp. are ubiquitous in nature; contact with and inhalation of the infectious conidia is a frequent event. Resulting disease, termed aspergillosis, includes allergy, respiratory tract invasion, skin infection, and extrapulmonary dissemination. Human disease is most commonly caused by four species: *A. fumigatus, A. flavus, A. niger*, and *A. terreus*.

Although *A. fumigatus* accounts for ~90% of invasive mould infections, there are regional differences and laboratories should be able to distinguish the four species, particularly as *A. terreus* is resistant to amphotericin B.

Epidemiology

Those at highest risk of invasive aspergillosis are HSCT and SOT (particularly heart, lung, and liver) recipients and those with prolonged severe neutropenia. Other high-risk groups include patients on prolonged courses of glucocorticoids, patients in ICU (particularly with underlying COPD), and those with impaired cellular immunity due to HIV or anti-autoimmune therapies. Hospital-acquired infection can occur and there are documented cases of patients having acquired aspergillosis in medical facilities with faulty ventilation systems or in healthcare clinics located near construction sites.

Clinical features

Focal infection

Invasive aspergillosis usually presents with lung involvement and in neutropenia, presentation is classically with pleuritic pain, fever, and haemoptysis. While chest X-rays may not reveal abnormalities (such as the 'halo' sign) in early disease, CT typically reveals focal lung lesions. Other presentations include tracheobronchitis (wheeze, cough, and dyspnoea), endophthalmitis (eye pain and visual changes), endocarditis (fever and embolic phenomena), skin lesions (red/violet plaques/papules, evolving into necrotic ulcers), and rhinosinusitis (nasal congestion, fever, and facial/orbital pain).

Disseminated infection

Invasion of the blood vessels can lead to dissemination to the brain, liver, kidneys, and skin. Dissemination is associated with poor outcome. CNS disease may present with seizures or focal neurological signs and mycotic aneurysms may rupture causing haemorrhagic stroke.

Diagnosis

Aspergillus conidia are constantly inhaled, so culture isolation of species from the airway may not indicate disease. The diagnosis of invasive aspergillosis in the lung is therefore based on the combination of a clinical picture consistent with the diagnosis and isolating the organism (or markers of the organism). Isolation of the organism from normally sterile sites is usually diagnostic, particularly if accompanied by evidence of tissue damage.

Microscopy

The most direct method is microscopy and culture of sputum and/or BAL specimens. A positive stain or culture should trigger treatment in those at risk of invasive aspergillosis. The BAL sample should also be sent for galactomannan antigen testing.

Biomarkers

- *Galactomannan* is a cell wall polysaccharide of *Aspergillus*, is relatively specific for invasive aspergillosis, and the assay can be used on serum or BAL fluid. Specificities and sensitivities of ~70% and 90% respectively for proven disease have been reported in meta-analyses of a galactomannan enzyme immunoassay. False positives have been reported for patients on IV piperacillin–tazobactam and in infections with other fungal species (*Fusarium*, *Histoplasma*, and *Penicillium*).
- *BD glucan* is a more general fungal cell wall component and can be detected in a wide variety of fungal infections including aspergillosis, candidiasis, and *Pneumocystis jirovecii*, but with the notable exception of *Cryptococcus*. Assessments of the BD-glucan assay are variable between studies but most report sensitivities and specificities in the range of 55–95% and 75–95% respectively.

Histopathology

If clinical and radiographic signs are suggestive, but fungal stain and culture of sputum and serum galactomannan are negative, bronchoscopy with BAL and/or biopsy should be considered in lung disease (and biopsy in extrapulmonary disease). Histopathological examination can usually distinguish *Aspergillus* spp., *Scedosporium* spp., and *Fusarium* spp. (septated hyaline hyphae with acute angle branching) from the Mucorales (broad, non-septate hyphae with right angle branching). This distinction is crucial as the Mucorales are not susceptible to the treatment of choice for *Aspergillus* which is voriconazole.

Treatment

Given the diagnostic difficulties, therapy is often commenced without definitive microbiological diagnosis. Initial therapy for severe invasive aspergillosis is with voriconazole. In severe or invasive disease, an echinocandin may be added to voriconazole. Alternative therapy with liposomal amphotericin B may be considered in patients at risk of liver toxicity with voriconazole, severe drug–drug interaction, or intolerance or allergy to azoles. Beware of the increased risk of nephrotoxicity with liposomal amphotericin B.

Clinical and radiological response to treatment should be carefully monitored. Cavitation of lesions indicating necrosis or a slight increase in lesion volume (especially in the context of recovery after absolute neutropenia) does not indicate an adverse outcome.

Therapeutic failure or refractory disease is not clearly defined but may include:

- dissemination of the clinical symptoms during treatment
- new or increased lesions in the CT scan performed 7–10 days after treatment onset (in the absence of recovery from absolute neutropenia), and/or
- no decrease in lesion size on CT performed at 15–21 days.

In these circumstances, switching to a different antifungal from that used during initial therapy is recommended.

Therapy should be maintained until radiological signs resolve, usually a minimum of 6–12 weeks. Prolonged oral voriconazole is sometimes given to treat possible residual microfoci of aspergillosis.

Surgery/debridement with wide margins is recommended in patients with the following:

- Endocarditis.
- Pericardium involvement.
- Foci close to large vessels.
- Chest wall invasion by lung injury (empyemas may also need surgical drainage and thoracotomy).
- Haemoptysis secondary to a pulmonary lesion.
- Skin and soft tissue involvement.
- Osteomyelitis.
- Sinusitis.
- CNS involvement.
- Endophthalmitis/panophthalmitis.

Refer to

European Society for Clinical Microbiology and Infectious Diseases (ESCMID) and European Respiratory Society (ERS) guidelines: ℜ https://www.escmid.org/.

Infectious Diseases Society of America (IDSA) ℜ http://www.idsociety.org/PracticeGuidelines/for up-to-date guidelines.

Mucormycosis (zygomycosis)

Moulds of the order Mucorales are found in soil. Inhalation of their spores is continuous, but disease only occurs in the context of impaired immunity. The genera found most frequently in human disease are *Rhizopus*, *Mucor*, and *Rhizomucor*. The disease entity caused by these organisms is known as mucormycosis (previously zygomycosis). On microscopy, the hyphae are broad and scarcely or non-septate, allowing easy distinction from *Aspergillus* spp.

Epidemiology

The most common risk factors are diabetes mellitus, particularly in keto-acidosis (*Rhizopus* spp. contain an enzyme, ketone reductase, which allows them to thrive in high-glucose, acidic conditions) and haematological malignancy. Other risk factors include transplant recipients (both SOT and HSCT), glucocorticoid treatment, iron overload (or treatment with deferoxamine), and contaminated traumatic injuries.

Clinical features

Mucormycosis can cause life-threatening rhino-orbital, pulmonary, and disseminated infection. It is the second most common mould infection in HSCT recipients, but is infrequent overall at most centres. Mucormycosis should be suspected in diabetic or acidotic patients presenting with sinusitis, altered mentation, and infarcted nasal or palatal tissue.

Rhino-orbital-cerebral infection
This is the most common presentation and starts with inhaled spores set-
tling in the paranasal sinuses of a susceptible host, most often a hyper-
glycaemic, acidotic diabetic. The usual presentation is with acute sinusitis
rapidly followed by erythema and cyanosis of the facial skin overlying the
sinuses. Black eschars may be visible in the palate or nasal mucosa.

Pulmonary mucormycosis
Usually presents with fever, haemoptysis, and dyspnoea. Pneumonia with
infarction and necrosis occurs and may spread to contiguous structures
such as the heart.

Diagnosis
The agents of mucormycosis do not contain either galactomannan or 1,2
beta-D-glucan in their cell walls so neither test is positive in mucormycosis.

Microscopy
Endoscopic biopsies from the sinuses should be sent for urgent microscopy
to look for the characteristic broad, non-septate hyphae. In pulmonary infection, staining and microscopy of sputum or BAL specimens may show
the characteristic hyphae but sensitivity is low.

Imaging
CT imaging or MRI can evaluate the degree of invasion. Imaging of the chest
may reveal the classic 'halo sign' of ground-glass attenuation surrounding a
nodule but this is common to all angio-invasive fungal infections.

Treatment
Acute infection is so aggressive and rapidly spreading that treatment is
often initiated before definitive tissue or microbiological diagnosis. Surgical
debridement in combination with liposomal amphotericin B is the treatment of choice. A second-line alternative is posaconazole. Prophylaxis with
posaconazole is recommended in an outbreak situation in patients with
neutropenia, GvHD, or previous mucormycosis.

Refer to
European Society of Clinical Microbiology and Infectious Diseases (ESCMID)
Fungal Infection Study Group (EFISG) and European Confederation of
Medical Mycology (ECMM) guidelines ✍ https://www.escmid.org/for fur-
ther information.

Fusarium spp.

Another environmental mould found in the soil and in association with
plants. Like *Aspergillus*, *Fusarium* spp. produce hyaline septate hyphae with
acute-angle branching in affected tissue but unlike *Aspergillus*, it may be recovered from blood cultures.

Epidemiology
Fusarium spp. cause keratitis and onychomycosis in the immunocompetent
but invasive and disseminated infections occur almost exclusively in severely
immunocompromised patients, particularly those with prolonged and profound neutropenia and/or severe T-cell immunodeficiency.

Clinical features
Refractory fever in a profoundly neutropenic patient with skin lesions ± a mould isolated from blood culture. Unlike aspergillosis, and most other invasive mould infections, fusarial infections in the immunocompromised yield a high frequency of positive blood cultures. Fusariosis may also present with sinusitis and pneumonia.

Diagnosis
Blood cultures
Blood cultures are positive in about 40% of cases of invasive fusariosis and usually become positive at 3 days of incubation in an aerobic bottle.

Microscopic and histopathological
Examination of sputum/BAL samples if available. Skin biopsies should be performed in all immunocompromised patients with suspicious skin lesions. Direct examination of a skin biopsy can demonstrate the organism within hours.

Biomarkers
Serum galactomannan antigen may be positive.

Treatment
Fusarium spp. are particularly resistant to antifungal agents; fluconazole, itraconazole, and echinocandins are often ineffective. Sensitivity to amphotericin B, voriconazole, and posaconazole is variable. Selecting the most active antifungal drug, restoring adequate immune response, and surgical debridement are the most important interventions in invasive fusariosis. Liposomal amphotericin is usually first choice with voriconazole as oral follow on. Variable susceptibility of *Fusarium* spp. to antifungal agents means that combinations are sometimes used.

Refer to
European Society of Clinical Microbiology and Infectious Diseases (ESCMID) Fungal Infection Study Group (EFISG) and European Confederation of Medical Mycology (ECMM) guidelines ⅋ https://www.escmid.org/for further information.

Scedosporium apiospermum (*Pseudoallescheria boydii*) and *Scedosporium prolificans*

There are two medically important species of the genus *Scedosporium*: *S. apiospermum* (this is the asexual form/anamorph and *P. boydii* is the sexual form/teleomorph) and *S. prolificans*. Both are ubiquitous in soil and water throughout the world and can cause invasive hyalohyphomycosis in the immunocompromised.

Epidemiology
Infection results from inhalation of spores or skin inoculation. Nosocomial outbreaks among immunocompromised patients have been linked to contaminated ambient air in hospitals. These fungi are the commonest filamentous moulds isolated from the airways of patients with cystic fibrosis. Disseminated disease occurs among patients with chronic glucocorticoid

use, chronic granulomatous disease, haematological malignancy, and transplant recipients.

Clinical features
Classically presents with fever, cough, sputum, pleuritic pain, malaise, etc. It may disseminate from the lungs to multiple organs and present with endophthalmitis, brain abscess (noted in near-drowning survivors), and skin lesions (purple with necrotic centre). Like *Aspergillus* it may produce fungal balls in bronchiectatic airways, sinuses, and old tuberculous lung cavities. It also causes white grain mycetoma.

Diagnosis
Blood cultures
Blood cultures are also useful for detection of *Scedosporium* in cases of disseminated disease. Special fungal media culture bottles are recommended when fungaemia is suspected.

Microscopy and histopathology
Specimens from potentially sterile sources such as BAL fluid, tissue biopsies, etc. can be examined microscopically and cultured.
    Because the various hyaline moulds have a similar appearance on microscopic examination, culture is essential for the speciation and drug-sensitivity testing needed for optimal treatment.

Treatment
Scedosporium spp. can be resistant to multiple antifungal agents. Voriconazole is generally the agent of choice but *S. prolificans* has a poor response and surgery is often required.

Refer to
European Society of Clinical Microbiology and Infectious Diseases (ESCMID) Fungal Infection Study Group (EFISG) and European Confederation of Medical Mycology (ECMM) guidelines ✍ https://www.escmid.org/ for further information.

Dematiaceous moulds/phaeohyphomycosis

These fungi (mostly moulds) contain melanin pigments in their cell walls and spores giving the hyphae a golden-brown appearance on microscopy. In the immunocompetent, they are most associated with dark-grained mycetoma, chromoblastomycosis, allergic disease, keratitis, and sinusitis. In the immunocompromised, they are more likely to cause the life-threatening syndromes of pneumonia, CNS infection, and disseminated fungal disease. The most commonly isolated species causing cerebral phaeohyphomycosis is *Cladophialophora bantiana*. Diagnosis is most often made by demonstration of pigmented fungal structures seen on biopsy sections and specimens are not cultured or speciated.

Epidemiology
The dematiaceous fungi are found throughout the world in soil and decaying vegetation but are more common in the tropics/subtropics. Exposure is thought to be from inhalation or minor trauma. Inhaled spores may settle in the sinuses and cerebral infections are thought to be due to extension from the adjacent paranasal sinuses. Most cases of pneumonia and disseminated disease and about half of the cases of cerebral phaeohyphomycosis occur in

immunocompromised patients. The majority of cases have been reported in SOT recipients, patients with malignancies, or HIV-infected IV drug users.

Clinical features

Consider in the differential diagnosis of brain abscess or pneumonia in the immunosuppressed, particularly in chemotherapy-induced neutropenia and post SOT. Also suspect in near drownings and traumatic injuries with significant environmental contamination.

Diagnosis

Diagnosis is by histopathological examination. Samples may include aspirated fluid or surgical resection of the brain abscess, BAL fluid in pneumonia, or skin biopsies. Microscopic examination of the fluid/tissue may reveal branching, septate hyphae which usually appear brown on haematoxylin and eosin staining or on KOH preparations.

Treatment

Requires both resection of the abscess and antifungal therapy with a combination of liposomal amphotericin and voriconazole.

Refer to

European Society of Clinical Microbiology and Infectious Diseases (ESCMID) Fungal Infection Study Group (EFISG) and European Confederation of Medical Mycology (ECMM) guidelines ℘ https://www.escmid.org/for further information.

Dermatophytes

Normally superficial infections of the skin, hair, and nails caused by fungi such as *Trichophyton, Microsporum*, or *Epidermophyton* groups. In the immunocompromised, these fungi may become invasive; the most common dermatophyte isolated in invasive disease is *Trichophyton rubrum*.

Epidemiology

Invasive dermatophytosis is rare even in the immunocompromised, but has been seen in transplant patients, patients with HIV infection, and those on chemotherapy or other immunosuppressive regimens.

Clinical features

Violaceous, erythematous, or bleeding nodules in an area of chronic dermatophyte infection such as the feet or buttocks. Invasive dermatophyte nodules can also appear on the face and trunk. Deeper cutaneous spread may present as an abscess. Annular erythematous plaques can appear anywhere on the body.

Diagnosis

Microscopy of skin scrapings or biopsy with KOH staining.

Treatment

Oral terbinafine may be necessary for deeper infection.

Refer to

British Association of Dermatologists guidelines http://www.bad.org.uk/healthcare-professionals/clinical-standards/clinical-guidelines for further information.

Other moulds

Moulds which in the past were considered contaminants, are increasingly recognized as pathogens in the immunocompromised.

Acremonium strictum

As well as being a known cause of peritonitis, pneumonia, bone infection, endocarditis, corneal infection and white grain mycetoma, A. *strictum* is now a recognized cause of disseminated disease in the immunocompromised. It is relatively resistant to common antifungal drugs.

Paecilomyces

Has been reported as a cause of disseminated infection, catheter-related infection, fungaemia, and pneumonia in the immunocompromised.

Scopulariopsis

Is capable of causing severe disseminated disease in the immunocompromised and has been recovered in cultures left to incubate at 30°C for >2 weeks.

Yeasts

Single-celled fungi that undergo asexual reproduction by budding or fission. Of the ~2000 described species, only a handful are known human pathogens and of these, *Candida* spp. are the most common. *Cryptococcus neoformans* is the yeast most able to cause invasive disease even in the absence of severe immunosuppression. Opportunistic yeast infections typically arise in patients with defects in mucosal barriers, cell-mediated immunity, or phagocyte numbers/function.

Candida spp.

C. albicans is a commensal yeast in the human oropharynx, gut, and vagina and can be detected as normal flora in up to 50% of people. Though classified as yeasts, some *Candida* spp., such as *C. albicans*, can develop hyphae. It is an opportunistic pathogen and causes disease in the context of defective mucocutaneous barriers or cell-mediated immunity. *Candida* spp. are the most common fungal pathogen to affect humans. There are >350 species of the genus *Candida* and while sharing similar phenotypic characteristics, they have significant differences, including susceptibility to antifungal drugs. About a dozen species are known to cause human disease and although *C. albicans* accounts for the majority of cases of invasive candidiasis, a growing proportion are due to the common non-albicans species such as *C. krusei*, *C. glabrata*, *C. tropicalis*, and *C. parapsilosis*.

C. albicans and *C. glabrata* together account for 70–80% of *Candida* spp. found in blood and deep tissue samples.

Epidemiology

Candida spp. are present globally and while mostly within/on their human or animal reservoirs, they can also be recovered from surfaces in the hospital environment. Risk factors for candidal infection include immunosuppression, particularly when cell-mediated immunity is damaged (e.g. HSCT and SOT recipients, advanced HIV infection, and diabetes), critical illness, indwelling devices, and the use of broad-spectrum antibiotics.

Clinical features

Candidal disease ranges from superficial dermatitis in the immunocompetent to deeply invasive and disseminated disease in the immunocompromised. In those with defective cell-mediated immunity, disease is usually mucocutaneous whereas in those with depressed neutrophil function, disease is more commonly invasive. Invasive candidiasis, defined by haematogenous spread to multiple viscera, can range in presentation from minimal fever to a severe sepsis syndrome and should be suspected in any patient with persistent neutropenia or other risk factors, who remains febrile despite broad-spectrum antibiotic therapy. Skin pustules/macules and eye signs (chorioretinitis) can be useful clues to haematogenous spread.

ICU patients account for the majority of episodes of candidaemia in most hospitals, followed by surgical units, particularly those with burns and trauma patients. Notable major risk factors in the ICU include central venous catheters, total parenteral nutrition, broad-spectrum antibiotic use, prior abdominal surgery, and extensive GI mucosal damage.

Non-albicans *Candida* species are increasingly commonly recovered from bloodstream infections:

- *C. glabrata*: though less virulent than *C. albicans*, is more resistant to azole drugs and tends to cause disease in patients with more severe underlying illness.
- *C. parapsilosis*: strongly associated with vascular catheters and prosthetics. Most isolates are fluconazole sensitive but have higher minimum inhibition concentrations to echinocandins
- *C. tropicalis*: associated with neutropenia, haematological malignancies, and HSCT recipients. Generally fluconazole sensitive.
- *C. krusei*: associated with neutropenia and haematological malignancies, intrinsically resistant to fluconazole.
- *C. auris*: some isolates have had elevated minimum inhibition concentrations for all three major classes of antifungal agents (azoles, polyenes, and echinocandins).

Other species reported include *C. keyfr*, *C. guilliermondi*, *C. lusitaniae*, *C. peeliculosa*, *C. haemulonii*, and *C. dubliniensis*.

Diagnosis

Blood culture

Blood culture remains the gold standard for candidaemia. *Candida* spp. in a blood culture should never be dismissed as a contaminant; it should always prompt a search for (and if possible removal of) the source and consideration of an antifungal agent. Chromogenic agar plates allow rapid speciation of *Candida* colonies. Blood cultures alone are relatively insensitive and may miss cases of disseminated candidiasis (particularly deep-seated infections such as intra-abdominal candidiasis). *In vitro* susceptibility testing for *Candida* spp. is available and standardized but is less well validated than for bacteria. *Candida* spp. generally have quite well-defined susceptibility patterns and therefore accurate and rapid speciation is important.

Histopathology

If there is an amenable focal lesion (e.g. punch biopsy of a skin lesion), send tissue for histological examination, Gram stain, and culture.

Biomarkers

BD-glucan assay, though not specific for *Candida*, is a useful adjunctive test if available (positive predictive value ~70% and negative predictive value ~98%).

Treatment

All central venous catheters should be removed if possible (though not over a guidewire). Rule out a thrombus. Fundoscopy and echocardiography are important to exclude complicated infection and to guide duration of therapy. Resolution of candidaemia should be established by taking at least one blood culture per day until cultures are negative. For uncomplicated candidaemia, treatment for 14 days after resolution (i.e. first negative blood culture) is recommended. Patients with metastatic complications require prolonged therapy.

Initial therapy for candidaemia is with fluconazole or an echinocandin. If *C. glabrata* or *C. krusei* are isolated, treat with an echinocandin or liposomal amphotericin B. Micafungin or liposomal amphotericin are alternatives (these can only be given intravenously). Oral follow on is usually with fluconazole according to sensitivity.

For patients with a urinary tract infection due to a fluconazole-susceptible *Candida* spp., treatment with fluconazole is recommended. For recipients with fluconazole-resistant organisms, use liposomal amphotericin B ± oral flucytosine. Echinocandins achieve poor urinary levels and are therefore not recommended. Amphotericin B deoxycholate bladder irrigation continuously for 5–7 days may be effective. Liposomal amphotericin B may be effective as adjunctive therapy.

In non-neutropenic SOT recipients, options for treatment include echinocandins, liposomal amphotericin B (beware nephrotoxicity, especially in kidney transplant recipients), or fluconazole if sensitivities allow.

In neutropenic SOT recipients, treat with echinocandins or liposomal amphotericin, unless *C. parapsilosis* is isolated, where fluconazole can be used. Switching to oral fluconazole could be considered after 10 days of IV therapy if *Candida* spp. are susceptible, the patient is stable, can tolerate oral administration, and the drug–drug interactions (on cytochrome P450 3A4 metabolism) can be managed.

Refer to

European Society of Clinical Microbiology and Infectious Diseases (ESCMID) Fungal Infection Study Group (EFISG) and European Confederation of Medical Mycology (ECMM) guidelines ℘ https://www.escmid.org/.

Infectious Diseases Society of America (IDSA) ℘ http://www.idsociety.org/PracticeGuidelines/ for up-to-date guidelines and further information.

Cryptococcus spp.

Cryptococci are encapsulated yeasts and though long recognized as human pathogens, *C. neoformans* became prominent as a cause of meningitis during the HIV/AIDS epidemic in the 1980s. Although the genus *Cryptococcus* contains >50 species, only *C. neoformans* and *C. gattii* are considered human pathogens.

Epidemiology

C. neoformans, often found in pigeon guano, is the commonest cryptococcal species in temperate countries and serotype A is the cause of most cryptococcal infection in the immunocompromised. *C. gattii*, associated with eucalyptus trees, rarely infects the immunocompromised (for unknown reasons). Responses to infection with *C. neoformans* range from harmless airway colonization to meningitis and disseminated disease. The immune status of the host is the crucial factor; cell-mediated immunity in particular.

Transmitted via inhalation, cryptococci can infect many organ systems but show a preference for the CNS where they may cause meningitis or meningoencephalitis. The two greatest risk factors for cryptococcal disease are HIV infection and corticosteroid use (thus most transplant recipients, particularly SOT recipients, with their often prolonged high-dose steroid regimens are at risk). Though the incidence of cryptococcal meningitis is much reduced where HAART is widely available, it continues to be a major cause of mortality among the immunosuppressed and is the third most common cause of invasive fungal disease among organ transplant patients.

Other risk factors include anti-TNF therapy, lymphomas/chronic leukaemias, liver disease, and connective tissue disease.

Clinical features

Indolent fever, malaise, and headache over a week or two is the typical presentation of cryptococcal meningoencephalitis. Only about a quarter of patients present with stiff neck, photophobia, and vomiting. Lung and skin disease are also frequent manifestations of disseminated disease and present as cough/dyspnoea and a molluscum contagiosum-like rash respectively.

Diagnosis

Have a high index of suspicion for cryptococcal meningitis in patients with advanced HIV infection (CD4 cell count <100 cells/μL)) who have isolated fever and headache. BD-glucan is not helpful in the diagnosis of cryptococcal disease.

CSF examination

If lumbar puncture is possible (based on imaging and examination) send CSF for the following:

- India ink staining and microscopy (will reveal the typical round encapsulated yeast in 60–80% cases).
- CrAg can be detected in CSF by latex agglutination or lateral flow assay with sensitivities and specificities >93%.
- Cryptococcal culture (cream-coloured mucoid colonies appear in 3–7 days on agar plates).

Serum antigen testing

If lumbar puncture is not safe or possible, CrAg testing can be performed on serum.

Other methods

Diagnosis of cryptococcal disease can also be made by recovery of the organism from blood, urine, or sputum cultures.

Treatment

Initial or induction therapy for cryptococcal meningoencephalitis is with amphotericin B and flucytosine. Close laboratory monitoring is needed for renal dysfunction, electrolyte disturbances (especially hypokalaemia), and haematological problems. Second-line therapy is with fluconazole and flucytosine. Voriconazole or posaconazole can also be considered if other regimens are not possible. Oral follow on or maintenance therapy is usually with fluconazole. Repeat lumbar puncture to monitor and control raised intracranial pressure is recommended. IRIS may be a significant problem in HIV-positive patients (➔ see Chapter 5).

Refer to

British HIV Association (BHIVA) and British Infection Association (BIA) ℘ http://www.bhiva.org/Guidelines.aspx and Infectious Diseases Society of America (IDSA) ℘ http://www.idsociety.org/PracticeGuidelines/for up-to-date guidelines and further information.

Trichosporon spp.

The genus *Trichosporon* is closely related to *Cryptococcus*. These two fungi share some antigens and cross-reactivity with the cryptococcal polysaccharide latex agglutination assay can be seen in patients with trichosporonosis. *Trichosporon* spp. may be found as a constituent of normal flora but can also cause both superficial and invasive infections in humans. Invasive disease, called trichosporonosis, occurs almost exclusively in immunocompromised hosts, appears to be increasing in frequency, and is usually fatal.

Epidemiology

Widespread in the environment, predominantly in soil, humans may become colonized with *Trichosporon* spp. Rates of colonization vary from 1% to 3% in patients admitted to general hospital wards. In the immunocompetent, this fungus causes a characteristic infection of hair shafts, often in the genital region, known as 'white piedra'.

The majority of cases of invasive trichosporonosis have been seen in patients with haematological malignancies, often in the setting of neutropenia. IV catheters, burns, and heart valve surgery are other recognized risk factors.

Clinical features

Invasive trichosporonosis in a neutropenic patient most often manifests as disseminated disease and presents with an acute febrile illness progressing rapidly to multi-organ failure. Pulmonary (dyspnoea, cough, haemoptysis), renal (microscopic haematuria/proteinuria progressing to renal failure), and cutaneous (erythematous papules/bullae) involvement occur frequently in disseminated disease. Less commonly, invasive infection appears confined to a single site such as heart valves, CNS, peritoneum, or surgical wounds. Fungal endocarditis vegetations are large and prone to break off causing distal ischaemic events.

Diagnosis

Microscopy and culture

Blood, urine, sputum/BAL samples, and CSF can be examined by microscopy and cultured. Most cases of invasive trichosporonosis are diagnosed on blood culture. Cultures of *Trichosporon* spp. isolated from sputum or urine may represent colonization rather than infection.

Histopathology

If skin lesions are present, biopsy and send for staining and microscopy.

Serum antigen testing

A positive *C. neoformans* polysaccharide antigen assay (CrAg) may occasionally indicate disseminated trichosporonosis due to cross-reactivity.

Treatment

Invasive *Trichosporon* infection is treated with IV voriconazole. Several species are resistant to liposomal amphotericin B, flucytosine, and to the echinocandins.

Refer to

European Society of Clinical Microbiology and Infectious Diseases (ESCMID) Fungal Infection Study Group (EFISG) and European Confederation of Medical Mycology (ECMM) guidelines ℘ https://www.escmid.org/ for up-to-date guidelines and further information.

Dimorphic fungi/endemic mycoses

These geographically constrained fungi exhibit thermal dimorphism; they exist as a yeast at 37°C during their parasitic phase in human or animal tissue, but produce hyphae and grow as a mould in their colder saprophytic environmental phase. *In vitro* culture at different temperatures induces one form or the other.

Histoplasma capsulatum

A thermally dimorphic environmental fungus and cause of histoplasmosis, the most common endemic mycosis in HIV-infected patients.

Epidemiology

Histoplasmosis is globally distributed, but specific highly endemic areas include the St Lawrence, Ohio, and Mississippi River valleys in the United States, the Caribbean, parts of Central and South America, Southeast Asia, and Africa. The fungus is found in high concentrations in soil contaminated with bird or bat excreta and transmission occurs via inhalation of spores from the soil. Patients can acquire primary histoplasmosis infection and clinical disease when visiting areas of endemicity, or develop reactivation disease many years later, in the setting of advanced immunosuppression. In resource-rich settings, disseminated disease usually occurs in HIV-infected patients who are not taking ARV therapy at the time of diagnosis.

Clinical features

Usually presents as a febrile wasting illness, known as progressive disseminated histoplasmosis, in patients with advanced HIV infection (CD4 <150 cells/µL). Progressive disseminated histoplasmosis is also seen in transplant recipients and patients on glucocorticoid or TNFα inhibitors. Roughly half of patients will have respiratory involvement, often with cough and dyspnoea. CNS involvement (chronic meningitis, focal CNS lesions, or encephalitis) occurs in 5–20% of cases. Severely immunodeficient patients may present with overwhelming infection manifested by shock, respiratory distress, hepatic and renal failure, obtundation, and coagulopathy. Mortality rates, in spite of treatment, approach 50% in such cases. ~10% of HIV-infected patients with disseminated histoplasmosis have mucocutaneous manifestations with lesions commonly located over the face, chest, and upper extremities.

Diagnosis

Microscopy

Microscopy of stained smears (peripheral blood/buffy coat/bone marrow/lymph node or bronchial aspirates) may allow rapid visualization of the budding yeast within tissues or body fluids although the sensitivity is very low (<10%).

Serum antigen testing

Histoplasma antigen detection is the most sensitive and specific test. It can be performed on samples of urine, serum, CSF, and BAL fluid. Antigen levels decline in response to treatment and false-positive results may occur in patients with blastomycosis, coccidioidomycosis, paracoccidioidomycosis, and penicilliosis.

Culture
Culture of blood, respiratory samples, or other tissues (e.g. bone marrow) remains the gold standard for diagnosis. However, cultures of *H. capsulatum* may take up to 6 weeks to grow and sensitivity depends on disease burden.

Treatment
Patients with diffuse pulmonary or disseminated histoplasmosis are treated with IV liposomal amphotericin B initially, followed by oral itraconazole. Lifelong suppressive therapy with itraconazole may be necessary in endemic regions if immunosuppression is ongoing. Similarly, prophylaxis is recommended in patients with HIV infection with CD4 <150 cells/μL in specific areas of endemicity.

Refer to
Infectious Diseases Society of America (IDSA) ℘ http://www.idsociety.org/PracticeGuidelines/for up-to-date guidelines and further information.

Coccidioides spp.

C. immitis and C. posudasii are dimorphic fungi of the genus *Coccidioides* and cause the human infection coccidioidomycosis.

Epidemiology
Coccidioides spp. are endemic to certain desert areas in the Southwestern US, Central America, and South America. Infection may be acquired by inhalation of a single arthroconidium. There are in the region of 150,000 reported infections per year in the US. Only a small number of these will cause progressive pneumonia or disseminated disease. Altered host immunity predisposes to severe disease and coccidial pneumonia was a major opportunistic infection in patients with HIV prior to HAART. Haematological malignancy, HSCT, glucocorticoids/other immunosuppressives, and pregnancy are also recognized risk factors for coccidioidomycosis. Immunocompromised patients can develop primary coccidioidomycosis through inhalation, or previously dormant sites of infection can reactivate.

Clinical features
The diagnosis should be considered in patients who have been in an endemic area, presenting with peripheral eosinophilia, night sweats, pneumonia (usually focal but may be diffuse/bilateral in severe immunosuppression), and hilar or mediastinal lymphadenopathy. The most common sites of disseminated infection are skin, subcutaneous soft tissue, meninges, and the skeleton. Meningitis is the most lethal complication and commonly presents with persistent headache of subacute/chronic onset.

Diagnosis
The laboratory must be informed if *Coccidioides* is suspected as laboratory staff are at risk of exposure and infection.

Serology
Detection of *Coccidioides* IgM/IgG is the first-line screening test, but may not be positive for weeks/months post infection.

Microscopy
Microscopy and culture of respiratory secretions, tissue, or other specimens (e.g. CSF in suspected meningitis). Culture results are usually available
within 5 days. The fungus will occasionally be isolated from blood cultures.
Coccidioides spp. are never normal flora.

Antigen testing
Antigen testing of urine or serum is infrequently used due to its insensitivity,
but can be useful in the severely immunocompromised where serology is
negative.

Treatment
Patients with diffuse pulmonary or disseminated disease should be treated
with liposomal amphotericin and fluconazole.

Refer to
Infectious Diseases Society of America (IDSA) ℞ http://www.idsociety.
org/PracticeGuidelines/for up-to-date guidelines and further information.

Paracoccidioides spp.
P. brasiliensis and *P. lutzii* are thermally dimorpic fungi that cause
paracoccidioidomycosis.

Epidemiology
Endemic to Central and South America, *Paracoccidioides* spp. are thought to
be soil dwelling. Infection is acquired via inhalation and agricultural workers
are at particular risk. The most likely outcome of inhalation is asymptomatic pulmonary infection. However, if not contained by host immunity, the
individual may develop either acute (mostly children) or chronic disease.
Chronic disease (~90% of cases) represents reactivation of primary infection and may present months or years later.
    Paracoccidioides spp. can disseminate to any part of the body; dissemin-
ated disease is more likely in patients with HIV or other causes of T-cell-
mediated immunodeficiency.

Clinical features
Consider in any patient from (or who has visited) Central or South America
presenting with dry cough and dyspnoea. Other sites affected include the
mucosae (painful oral ulcers), skin, lymph nodes, adrenal glands (may present with Addison's disease), CNS (ring enhancing lesions in brain/spine),
or joints.

Diagnosis
Serology
Usually the first-line screen if available but is less sensitive in patients
with HIV.

Microscopy
Send accessible samples (sputum, BAL, abscess fluid, lymph node aspirates,
scrapings of skin lesions, and/or biopsy samples of affected organs) for microscopy. Direct microscopy using KOH yields a diagnosis in >90% of cases.
Culture is slow as *Paracoccidioides* spp. take 20–30 days to grow and bacteria
in the sample often inhibit fungal growth.

Histopathology
Methenamine silver or periodic acid–Schiff stain allows visualization of fungal elements in tissue samples.

Treatment
Mild or moderate paracoccidioidomycosis can be treated with oral itraconazole while more severe disease should be treated with liposomal amphotericin B.

Refer to
Consensus Brazilian guidelines for the clinical management of paracoccid ioidomycosis: ℘ http://www.scielo.br/pdf/rsbmt/2017nahead/1678-9849-rsbmt-0037868202302017.pdf.

Blastomyces dermatitidis

B. dermatitidis is a thermally dimorphic fungi and the cause of the systemic pyogranulomatous infection blastomycosis.

Epidemiology
Most cases have been reported in North America but it is also found in Africa, Asia, Central America, and South America. It is soil dwelling and infection is via inhalation into the lungs. Pulmonary disease tends to be more severe in immunocompromised hosts and dissemination is more common. Mortality is higher (up to ~40 %) in the immunocompromised.

Clinical features
Chronic pneumonia is the most common presentation. Pulmonary symptoms usually appear 3–6 weeks after exposure. As with other fungal infections and TB, there is often accompanying weight loss, night sweats, etc. The most common extrapulmonary sites involved are skin (grey/violet verrucous lesions), bone/joint (osteomyelitis), genitourinary (prostatitis/epidymo-orchitis), and CNS (single or multiple brain abscesses—seen more commonly in patients with HIV).

Diagnosis
Microscopy and histopathology
Direct examination of stained (calcofluor white or KOH) and concentrated clinical samples (sputum, urine, pleural fluid, CSF) has a low diagnostic yield (~30–50%) but if positive can provide a rapid diagnosis. Definitive diagnosis requires culturing the organism from clinical specimens. Culture of sputum or bronchoscopy samples has a diagnostic yield of ~90% and the *B. dermatitidis* mould phase grows on plates in 1–4 weeks. Colonization or contamination with *B. dermatitidis* does not occur, so identifying the organism histologically or isolation from culture confirms the diagnosis.

Antigen testing
Antigen detection in the urine or serum is ~90% sensitive but less specific due to cross-reactivity with other dimorphic fungal species.

Treatment
Liposomal amphotericin is recommended for moderate to severe pulmonary disease and extrapulmonary disease.

Refer to
Infectious Diseases Society of America (IDSA) ℘ http://www.idsociety.org/PracticeGuidelines/for up-to-date guidelines and further information.

Sporothrix schenckii

S. schenckii is a dimorphic fungus which causes the subacute/chronic infection known as sporotrichosis.

Epidemiology
While the organism is found worldwide, the disease is particularly common in parts of Peru. Most infections are through skin inoculation of soil (e.g. gardening injuries) but zoonotic transmission, mostly from cats, also occurs. In most cases, the immunocompetent host develops localized lymphocutaneous sporotrichosis (papule/ulcer at site of inoculation) but in the immunocompromised, it may cause disease in the lungs, meninges, and osteoarticular structures.

Clinical features
Lymphocutaneous disease is the most common presentation and is usually in the form of a papule or ulcer with other lesions appearing proximally along lymphatic channels. It may resemble lesions of NTM, *Nocardia*, or *Leishmania*. Pulmonary sporotrichosis (more common in COPD and alcoholism) presents like TB with fever, night sweats, and weight loss in addition to cough, dyspnoea, sputum, and haemoptysis. *S. schenckii* joint infections appear to be more common in middle-aged alcoholic males. Meningeal infection is rare, occurring mostly in patients with HIV or lymphoma and presenting with chronic fever and headache.

Diagnosis
Microscopy and histopathology
Direct microscopy of relevant samples (aspirate from a cutaneous lesion/sputum/joint aspirate/CSF) or histopathological examination of tissue is of low sensitivity as the organism is often present in very low numbers. Culture is therefore more reliable. Growth usually appears within a week (though may take longer).

Treatment
Therapy for severe disease is liposomal amphotericin followed by oral itraconazole.

Refer to
Infectious Diseases Society of America (IDSA) ℘ http://www.idsociety.org/PracticeGuidelines/for up-to-date guidelines and further information.

Penicillium (Talaromyces) marneffei

A dimorphic fungus and cause of the systemic fungal disease, penicilliosis.

Epidemiology
Penicilliosis is endemic to Southeast Asia, Taiwan, Hong Kong, Northeastern India, and Southern China. It is usually described as an opportunistic infection in patients with HIV and low CD4 counts but can cause disease in immunosuppression of any origin. The highest incidence is in Thailand where

it caused thousands of cases in association with HIV in the pre-HAART era. Humans and bamboo rats are the only known hosts. Mode of transmission is not proven but considered likely to be airborne as for other endemic fungi.

Clinical features
Consider in immunocompromised individuals from (or who have visited) endemic areas, with rash (umbilicated papules on the face, chest, and extremities) and/or cough, fever, lymphadenopathy, hepatosplenomegaly, diarrhoea, altered mentation, and mucosal lesions.

Diagnosis
Microscopy
Biopsy of lesions or blood smears may reveal oval or elongated yeast with a central septum. Culture of bone marrow/lymph node/skin lesions/blood (in descending order of sensitivity) provides definitive diagnosis. Has also been cultured from stool, urine, CSF, and joint fluid. Usually grows in 4–7 days on Sabouraud's agar at 25°C and its dimorphism can be shown by subculture at 37°C. A red pigment on the plate, though not specific for *P. marneffei*, should raise suspicion of this organism.

Treatment
Severe penicilliosis is treated with liposomal amphotericin followed by oral itraconazole.

Refer to
British HIV Association (BHIVA) and British Infection Association (BIA) http://www.bhiva.org/Guidelines.aspx for guidelines on penicilliosis in HIV.

Atypical fungi

Pneumocystis jirovecii

An atypical fungus (previously classified as a protozoan) responsible for pneumonia in the immunocompromised. Formerly known as *P. carinii*.

Epidemiology

The organism is distributed globally. It is not thought to be a zoonosis and there is no known animal reservoir of human disease, although different strains of *P. jirovecii* infect other mammals. Transmission is primarily airborne and serological studies show that the majority of people are infected by the age of 5 years. Acquisition of new infections in humans is most likely by person-to-person spread. In the immunocompetent host, it appears to cause little or no disease. It is best known as a cause of pneumonia among patients with HIV infection (CD4 cell count usually <200 cells/μL) but rates have fallen greatly where HAART and chemoprophylaxis are available. In non-HIV-infected patients, the most significant risk factors are glucocorticoid use and defective cell-mediated immunity. Other specific risk factors include haematological malignancy, organ transplantation, inflammatory conditions, and solid tumours.

Clinical features

Consider in any immunosuppressed patient with progressive dyspnoea, fever, and cough. The onset is typically over a few weeks and the cough non-productive. Patients are often tachypnoeic and desaturate markedly on exercise. The most common CXR changes are diffuse, bilateral, interstitial, or alveolar infiltrates. Prophylaxis against *P. jirovecii* with TMP–SMX is widely used and effective, though it may fail due to non-adherence and/or a very low CD4 count (<50 cells/μL). (➔ See Chapter 7.)

Diagnosis

Microscopy

Definitive diagnosis is made by visualizing the cystic or trophic forms in stained respiratory samples. The organism cannot be cultured. Induced sputum (by inhalation of hypertonic saline) has a specificity close to 100% but a lower sensitivity (60–90%) and may not be possible if the patient is too dyspnoeic or unable to cooperate. If induced sputum is not possible or non-diagnostic, proceed to BAL. This can be site directed and has a diagnostic yield approaching 100% in patients infected with HIV.

Histopathology

If neither induced sputum nor BAL are diagnostic, then occasionally biopsy of lung tissue (transbronchial or transthoracic) may be required.

Serum antigen testing

BD-glucan is usually elevated (>80 pg/mL) in PCP and is highly sensitive (~95%) in the diagnosis of PCP.

Molecular techniques

PCR of respiratory fluids is increasingly used to diagnose *P. jirovecii* in HIV-uninfected patients, but cannot distinguish between colonization and disease.

Treatment

Treatment for severe PCP is with IV TMP–SMX or IV pentamidine plus corticosteroids. Mild-to-moderate disease is treated with oral TMP–SMX or oral TMP/dapsone or clindamycin/primaquine. G6PD deficiency needs to be checked for before primaquine use. In the context of severe illness or if samples cannot be safely obtained, it is appropriate to start patients on presumptive treatment.

Refer to

European Conference on Infections in Leukaemia (ECIL) guidelines on PCP infections in leukaemia and HSCT: ℘ https://www.ebmt.org/Contents/Resources/Library/ECIL/Pages/ECIL.aspx.

British HIV Association (BHIVA) and British Infection Association (BIA): ℘ http://www.bhiva.org/Guidelines.aspx for guidelines on PCP in HIV.

Acknowledgement

This chapter was kindly reviewed by Dr Ian Bowler, Consultant in Infectious Diseases and Microbiology, Oxford University Hospitals NHS Trust.

Bacteria

Introduction

Immunocompromised patients have increased susceptibility to all the common hospital- and community-acquired bacterial infections affecting the general population. As a result, the bacterial species most frequently isolated in routine hospital inpatient blood cultures (staphylococci, streptococci, enterococci, *Escherichia coli*, *Klebsiella pneumoniae*, *Proteus mirabilis*, *Pseudomonas aeruginosa*, *Enterobacter* spp. etc.) are also the most commonly isolated in the immunocompromised.

For example, community-acquired pneumonia in both the immunocompetent and immunocompromised, is predominantly (~85%) due to *Streptococcus pneumoniae*, *Haemophilus influenza*, or *Moraxella catarrhalis*. Most of the remaining 15% is caused by *Mycoplasma pneumoniae*, *Chlamydophila pneumoniae*, or *Legionella* spp. In most circumstances, therefore, standard first-line antibiotic protocols are appropriate in the immunocompromised.

However, the immunocompromised are also more susceptible to bacterial infections that do not ordinarily cause severe disease in the immunocompetent host. Frequent hospitalization and recurrent use of antibiotics make the dangers posed by multi-resistant organisms particularly significant in this group. This chapter focuses on bacterial pathogens of particular relevance in the immunocompromised.

Mycobacteria

Mycobacteria, so named because of their fungus-like growth on culture, are aerobes with thick, waxy cell walls, rich in mycolic acid. This cell wall gives them their characteristic 'acid-fast' staining. Once stained, the mycolic acid resists de-staining by alcohol or acids. There are many species, but those causing human disease are usually divided into *Mycobacterium tuberculosis* complex (MTBC), *M. leprae*, and the free-living environmental non-tuberculous mycobacteria (NTM).

Mycobacterium tuberculosis complex

MTBC includes the genetically closely related causative pathogens of tuberculosis (TB): *M. tuberculosis, M. bovis* (including BCG), *M. africanum, M. canetti, M. microti, M. caprae,* and *M. pinipedii*. The majority of human disease is caused by the first three. They grow very slowly, with a generation time of ~20–24 hours.

Epidemiology

Approximately one-third of the global population is latently infected with *M. tuberculosis* and there are an estimated 9 million new cases of active disease and 1.5 million deaths from TB per year. Transmission is human to human by inhalation and deposition in the lungs. This leads to one of three possible outcomes: immediate clearance of the organism, primary disease, or latent infection. Latent infection may or may not lead to subsequent re-activation of disease. The most important host risk factor determining TB susceptibility is impaired immunity due to HIV co-infection. Other immunosuppressive conditions including cancer, diabetes, and medications such as glucocorticoids and TNF inhibitors also increase susceptibility to TB.

Clinical features

TB must always be considered in the immunocompromised. Of the ~9 million new cases of active TB per year, over a million of these are in patients infected with HIV. HAART greatly reduces the risk of developing TB, though incidence rates remain higher than in the general population. Presentation depends on the degree of immunosuppression. The classic presentation with fever, cough, weight loss, night sweats, and malaise with apical pulmonary cavitation is common in those with early HIV disease (CD4 count >200 cells/μL). As immunosuppression increases, pulmonary cavitation becomes less common (leading to less haemoptysis) and rates of extrapulmonary dissemination increase. The pleura and lymph nodes are the commonest site of extrapulmonary spread but any site can be involved (e.g. pericardium, meninges) Prolonged fever without respiratory symptoms should prompt a search for TB in the immunocompromised.

Rates of TB in SOT recipients are in the order of 20–80× higher than in the general population and are most frequently due to reactivation of latent disease (though nosocomially acquired and donor transmission cases have been reported). Case series of TB post SOT suggest that it manifests as pulmonary disease in ~50% of cases, extrapulmonary in ~15%, and disseminated in ~35%. Fever, night sweats, and weight loss are common symptoms.

Diagnosis
The initial laboratory workup in suspected pulmonary TB should include three sputum specimens for microscopy and culture as well as at least one specimen for NAAT. The gold standard for diagnosis remains culture and this is necessary for drug susceptibility testing. While awaiting culture results (which may take weeks), microscopy/NAAT results and clinical context will guide the decision on commencing therapy.

Microscopy
Sputum: three early morning sputum samples from different days should be collected. Nebulized hypertonic saline can be used to induce sputum if needed. Sputum smears are less sensitive then sputum cultures; >5000–10,000 bacilli/mL are needed for detection of bacteria in stained smears, whereas culture can detect as few as 10 bacilli/mL of sputum. Due to its relatively low sensitivity, sputum microscopy is considered a preliminary result that is followed up by culture. Fluorescence microscopy is more sensitive than traditional Ziehl–Neelsen or Kinyoun staining and allows much quicker detection of mycobacteria. Quantification of the bacilli seen on sputum smears, along with clinical and radiographic parameters, can be used to monitor response to treatment.

Bronchoscopy
BAL samples have improved sensitivity over induced sputum.

Fine-needle aspiration
Aspiration of enlarged lymph nodes and smear microscopy can detect AFBs in ~75% cases of extrapulmonary TB and this increases to >95% if lymph node tissue is cultured. In pleural TB, smears of pleural biopsy or aspirate give higher diagnostic yield in HIV-infected patients than sputum smears (69% vs 29%).

Culture
Is generally required for speciation and drug-susceptibility testing. The sensitivity and specificity of sputum culture are about 80% and 98% respectively. Growth in liquid media is faster (1–3 weeks) than on solid media (3–8 weeks). Culture of urine (first morning samples collected on 3 consecutive days) gives a good yield for diagnosing disseminated TB.

Molecular techniques
Allow rapid and sensitive detection of MTBC in a variety of clinical specimens including sputum and CSF, particularly when levels of mycobacteria are too low to detect by microscopy. 1–10 organisms/mL may give a positive result with NAAT and in smear-positive patients the technique has >95% positive predictive value in distinguishing MTBC from NTM. In smear-negative patients, NAATs can quickly detect MTB in 50–80% of patients (who, weeks later, would go on to be culture positive). One such assay, the Xpert® MTB/RIF assay, can rapidly amplify and detect both MTBC and rifampicin resistance with specificities approaching 99% and sensitivities of 98% in smear positive-, and ~70% in smear-negative patients.

Antigen tests

Urine antigen strip tests are cheap, quick, and easy bedside tests to detect mycobacterial lipoarabinomannan. They are useful in detecting renal TB in patients with HIV and low CD4 counts.

Treatment

Standard treatment for drug-sensitive pulmonary TB is with an intensive phase of four drugs (isoniazid, rifampin, pyrazinamide, and ethambutol) for 2 months and a continuation phase usually with isoniazid and rifampin for at least another 4 months. The exceptions are with CNS disease (12 months of therapy) and bone and joint disease (6–9 months of therapy). In cases where it is not possible to establish an immediate laboratory diagnosis, a presumptive clinical diagnosis is usually sufficient for initiating therapy.

Refer to

National Institute for Health and Care Excellence (NICE) guidelines on managing of latent and active TB: ℛ https://www.nice.org.uk/guidance/ng33.

British Infection Society (BIS) guidelines on the management of central nervous system TB: ℛ https://www.britishinfection.org.

British HIV Association (BHIVA) guidelines on HIV/TB co-infection: ℛ http://www.bhiva.org/guidelines.aspx.

World Health Organization (WHO) guidelines on management of TB: ℛ http://www.who.int/publications/guidelines/tuberculosis/en/.

Non-tuberculous mycobacteria

NTM are the non-tuberculous, non-leprae mycobacteria. They are free-living environmental organisms and globally distributed. >160 species of mycobacteria have now been classified using molecular taxonomy, but traditionally the NTMs have been organized according to their growth rate on culture.

Slow growers (>7 days to appear on in vitro culture)

Include *M. avium* complex (MAC), *M. kansasii*, *M. marinum*, *M. xenopi*, *M. simiae*, *M. malmoense*, and *M. ulcerans*.

Rapid growers (<7 days to appear on in vitro culture)

Include *M. abscessus*, *M. fortuitum*, and *M. chelonae*.

Epidemiology

NTM are free-living saprophytes found in water, soil, dust, and food worldwide. In contrast to the MTBC, NTM infection is from the environment with no known human-to human transmission. Infection usually occurs through inhalation or ingestion. They are most strongly associated with HIV infection, but are also significant pathogens in other immunocompromised groups. MAC is the most frequently found NTM in immunocompromised. Often found in drinking water and of low inherent pathogenicity, it colonizes the respiratory tract of immunocompetent. *M. kansasii* is the second commonest NTM isolate after MAC in the US. It is the only NTM not found in soil and is regularly found in tap water.

Clinical features

Patients with HIV infection

MAC disease refers to infections caused by one of two NTM species: *M. avium* or *M. intracellulare*. MAC infection is most commonly seen among patients with HIV and with CD4 counts <50 cells/μL. Latent infection does not exist with this organism, so unlike some other opportunistic infections in HIV, MAC disease always represents recent acquisition rather than reactivation. Infection is via the respiratory tract and GI tract with bacteraemia following dissemination via the lymphatics.

Presentation is with either disseminated or local disease. Disseminated MAC presents non-specifically with fever, night sweats, abdominal pain, diarrhoea, and weight loss (which often precedes the onset of fever). The diagnosis is confirmed by the isolation of MAC from the blood. Localized MAC presents as focal lymphadenitis with fever, leucocytosis, and inflammation in a lymph node (usually cervical, intra-abdominal, or mediastinal). The diagnosis is confirmed by culture of lymph node aspirate. Blood cultures are almost always been sterile. Prior to HAART, localized disease was rare in HIV.

Non-MAC disease: *M. kansasii* is the most frequently isolated NTM after MAC. Tap water is thought to be the most likely environmental source of exposure. Clinical manifestations are mostly similar to those of TB, although *M. kansasii* is a less virulent pathogen. Typical symptoms include fever, night sweats, weight loss, cough with sputum, dyspnoea, and weakness. *M. xenopi* presents with fever, wasting, and pulmonary infiltrates, similar to disseminated MAC. *M. genavense* infection has been associated with massive adenopathy and organomegaly. *M. szulgai* is associated with pulmonary disease, cutaneous lesions, osteomyelitis, and septic arthritis.

The rapidly growing mycobacteria *M. fortuitum* and *M. chelonae* can cause disseminated disease with pustular and nodular cutaneous lesions, localized pulmonary disease, multifocal osteomyelitis, and lymphadenitis.

SOT recipients

NTM are more common aetiological agents of disease in SOT recipients than MTBC in countries where TB is non-endemic. Median onset of NTM infection is usually 1 year or more after transplantation. Pleuropulmonary disease is the most common manifestation of NTM infection after transplantation and lung transplant recipients are most commonly affected. MAC species are the most common NTM species isolated and typically involve the lungs. Cutaneous and disseminated infections are the next most common presentations. *M. fortuitum* and *M. marinum* tend to cause localized skin infections and may present as purplish papules or nodules. *M. marinum* infection, known as 'fish tank granuloma', usually occurs after exposure to aquariums or marine environments. *M. abscessus* tends to be particularly virulent and can cause pulmonary, cutaneous, and/or disseminated disease. Disseminated infection caused by NTM typically presents with constitutional symptoms (weight loss, fever, night sweats).

Diagnosis

NTMs may colonize the respiratory or GI tract without causing disease, so a positive culture does not necessarily indicate infection. NTM found in sterile specimens, such as blood, are generally considered significant.

Microscopy and culture

Staining and microscopy for AFB followed by culture should be performed on all respiratory specimens. Diagnosis of NTM is made by isolation of the organism in culture usually of the blood or lymph node aspirates. When the BACTEC™ culture system is used, the cultures usually become positive in 7–10 days. Bone marrow culture often yields the organism before blood cultures turn positive. Mycobacterial blood cultures are collected in special media and the bottles must be specifically requested.

Histopathology

Biopsy of suitable lesions including skin biopsy should be performed in all patients with suspicious lesions where possible. This should be sent for microscopy and culture as well as histopathology.

Molecular techniques

Species identification using DNA probes distinguishes MAC and *M. kansasii* from *M. tuberculosis*.

Treatment

Treatment of NTM is often difficult in immunocompromised hosts due to antimicrobial resistance and often adjuvant surgery is needed. At least two active drugs should be used due to the high risk of development of resistance, but the accuracy of *in vitro* testing is variable. At least three active agents, including one injectable, are recommended for patients with severe infection. Lung disease should be treated until sputum cultures taken over 12 consecutive months are negative; skin and soft tissue infections should be treated for at least 3–6 months. Close follow-up after completion of treatment is essential.

The following treatment recommendations are supported by the British Thoracic Society guidelines (due for publication in early 2018):

- *MAC* is treated with a combination of drugs in order to reduce the risk of drug resistance. First line is clarithromycin (or azithromycin) plus ethambutol plus rifampicin. In severe disease (smear-positive/severe symptoms/cavitation), additional amikacin (IV or nebulized for up to 3 months) should be considered. In clarithromycin-resistant disease, either isoniazid or moxifloxacin should be given as a substitute for a macrolide, and amikacin should also be considered.
- *M. kansasii* is usually treated with rifampicin, ethambutol, plus one of isoniazid/clarithromycin/azithromycin.
- *M. malmoense* is usually treated with rifampicin plus ethambutol plus clarithromycin/azithromycin. Amikacin (up to 3 months) should also be considered in severe disease.
- *M. xenopi* is treated with rifampicin, ethambutol plus clarithromycin/ azithromycin, plus either moxifloxacin or isoniazid.

- *M. abscessus* is usually treated in the initial phase (≥1 month) with clarithromycin/azithromycin (if sensitive) plus amikacin plus imipenem plus tigecycline. This is followed by a continuation phase of nebulized amikacin and oral clarithromycin/azithromycin plus one to three of the following drugs: clofazimine, linezolid (and pyridoxine), minocycline, moxifloxacin, TMP–SMX. This is usually for 12 months with surgical resection if possible.
- In macrolide-resistant disease, clarithromycin should be omitted from the initial phase. The continuation phase should consist of nebulized amikacin plus two to four of the above-listed drugs.

Non-pulmonary NTM disease
- *M. fortuitum* is usually treated with amikacin plus cefoxitin for 2–6 weeks followed by TMP–SMX or doxycycline.
- *M. chelonae* is treated with clarithromycin plus either tobramycin, imipenem, or linezolid followed by clarithromycin or moxifloxacin for at least 4 months (Box 14.1).

Refer to

British Thoracic Society (BTS) guidelines on non-tuberculous mycobacteria: https://www.brit-thoracic.org.uk/standards-of-care/guidelines/.

American Thoracic Society (ATS) and the Infectious Diseases Society of America (IDSA) guidelines on non-tuberculous mycobacteria: http://www.idsociety.org/PracticeGuidelines/.

Box 14.1 *Mycobacterium chimaera* and cardiothoracic surgery

M. chimaera, an environmental NTM, has been newly recognized as a cause of severe infections in patients who have undergone cardiothoracic surgery. It is likely to be transmitted from contaminated heater cooler units used for cardiopulmonary bypass grafting (CABG) equipment or extracorporeal membrane oxygenation, where generation of a contaminated aerosol results in particles reaching the operative field. The risk is low (approximately one case per 100,000 coronary artery bypass graft procedures). The highest-risk group is patients who have undergone valve replacement or repair (approximately one case per 5000 procedures). Internationally, it has also been reported after CABG, vascular grafts, left ventricular assist device insertion, and heart/lung transplant. Only one UK patient has been reported as being immunosuppressed (due to haematological malignancy), but diabetes mellitus is a common comorbidity.

Clinical features

Include endocarditis, vascular graft infection, chronic sternal wound infection, and severe disseminated infection (liver, bone marrow, spine, lungs, lymph nodes, skin, brain, eyes). This may manifest many years after surgery on bypass (2–58 months). It has an insidious and non-specific presentation.

Diagnosis

Not always identified through conventional microbiology. Specific *M. chimaera* microbiological investigations must be undertaken in suspected cases. Mycobacterial culture is the essential investigation for all sample types. Blood cultures (three sets if suspected endocarditis or disseminated infection) and cardiac tissue/bone/pus samples (where relevant) should be sent for mycobacterial culture. Mycobacteria cannot be cultured from swabs. In addition, 16S rRNA gene sequencing may be helpful (though should not be used in isolation). Biopsies of affected sites should also be sent for histological assessment (granulomatous pathology has been described in a significant proportion of cases and sarcoidosis is also an important differential diagnosis).

Echocardiography (including transoesophageal) is supportive if abnormal but cannot alone be used to exclude current or developing infection.

Treatment

Clinical advice should be obtained from local infection and cardiology specialists. Infection teams can contact the nearest specialist National Mycobacterial Reference Service for specific treatment advice.

Mycobacteria-related bacteria

Nocardia spp.

Unusual Gram-positive aerobic bacteria of the order Actinomycetales, so called because they form branching, fungal-like filaments which break up into either coccoid or bacillary units. Other aerobic actinomycetes causing human disease include *Rhodococcus, Gordonia,* and *Tsukamurella.* They are mostly saprophytes and infection arises from environmental exposure. >30 species of *Nocardia* are known to cause human disease, but the most common are *N. asteroides, N. nova,* and *N. farcinia.*

Epidemiology

Inhalation of this globally dispersed environmental pathogen is the most common route of transmission and consequently the lung is most common site of disease. ~65% of cases are in patients with defective cell-mediated immunity and prolonged glucocorticoid use is a major risk factor.

Clinical features

Consider in any immunocompromised patient with recent or ongoing non-specific respiratory symptoms associated with CNS, skin, or soft tissue lesions. There are no pathognomonic signs and nocardiosis is commonly misdiagnosed as TB due to similar clinical and chest X-ray findings. ~50% of all lung infections disseminate, most commonly to the brain, so the brain should be imaged to look for abscess formation. Skin lesions are most commonly caused by direct inoculation and include mycetoma.

Diagnosis

Microscopy and culture

An initial presumptive diagnosis may be made if filamentous, weakly acid-fast branching rods are seen on microscopy of sputum samples or skin biopsies. Inform laboratory staff if nocardiosis is suspected so they can optimize conditions for detection. Most routine cultures are discarded at 48–72 hours, whereas *Nocardia* spp. can take between 5 and 21 days to grow and special media may be used. Precise speciation and drug sensitivity testing are essential as there is significant variability in drug susceptibility. Isolates often need to be sent to a regional/national reference laboratory for this.

Treatment

Depends on sensitivity but usually includes two out of TMP–SMX, amikacin, imipenem, and third-generation cephalosporins (ceftriaxone and cefotaxime) for severe infection. Therapy in immunocompromised patients is usually for at least 6 months with long-term suppression with oral TMP–SMX or doxycycline.

Rhodococcus equi

Like *Nocardia* spp., rhodococci are part of the diverse group of Gram-positive bacilli known as 'aerobic actinomycetes'. Of the >30 species in the genus *Rhodococcus*, only one, *R. equi*, has been frequently associated with human disease. *R. equi*, initially identified as a cause of horse pneumonia, has become increasingly recognized as a cause of pulmonary and disseminated disease in immunocompromised humans. The pathogenic potential of *R. equi* results from its ability to persist in and destroy macrophages and most cases of disease are in association with HIV infection, lymphoproliferative malignancy, organ transplant, or immunosuppressive medication.

Epidemiology

Rhodococcus spp. have a worldwide distribution and are frequently isolated from soil, particularly soil contaminated with herbivore faeces. Isolates of *R. equi* from sputum and indwelling lines point to inhalation and air contamination as primary sources of infection. Sequencing of some human isolates suggests a specific animal host and thus possible zoonotic transmission; contact with farm animals or manure has been reported in up to 50% of cases. Infection can also be acquired by traumatic inoculation or superinfection of wounds.

Clinical features

Pulmonary infections are the most common form of human disease caused by *R. equi* and most reported cases of pneumonia have occurred in immunocompromised hosts. Infection is usually subacute in onset but results in high fever, cough ($\pm$ haemoptysis), fatigue, chest pain, and weight loss. Cavitation arises in >50% of cases and pleural effusion in ~20%. Malacoplakia, a chronic granulomatous condition, can result from *R. equi* infection of the lung parenchyma.

Extrapulmonary infections, which may present weeks to years after therapy for pulmonary disease, most commonly affect the skin (subcutaneous abscesses) and brain. Brain abscesses, with associated oedema and sometimes meningitis, may present as confusion, agitation, obtundation, coma, seizures, and motor weakness. Kidney, liver, and bone involvement or isolated bacteraemia also occur. In ~25% of documented *R. equi* infections, there is no pulmonary disease; these cases include wound infections, peritoneal catheter-related peritonitis, and isolated fever with bacteraemia.

Diagnosis

Suspect *R. equi* infection in immunocompromised patients with cavitating lung disease and epidemiological risk factors.

Diagnosis is made by culturing the organism from a clinical sample and *R. equi* is easily cultivated on ordinary non-selective media when incubated aerobically at 37°C. Commercially available panels of biochemical tests (API® (RAPID) Coryne) can be employed to identify *R. equi* in cultures with the typical colony characteristics and Gram stain morphology.

The lung is the usual primary site, so send sputum $\pm$ bronchial washings, lung tissue, abscess contents, or pleural fluid.

Blood cultures are positive in >50% of immunocompromised patients with *R. equi* infection.

In suspected CNS disease, send CSF $\pm$ brain abscess aspirates.

Though easy to culture, *R. equi* may be dismissed as a contaminant, given its appearance as a diphtheroid, so the clinical team should liaise closely with the lab in suspected cases. Rhodococci may be reported as 'aerobic actinomycetes'. If available, 16S rRNA sequencing and/or mass absorption laser depolarizing ionization time-of-flight may be used to diagnose rhodococci.

Treatment

R. equi is generally susceptible *in vitro* to erythromycin and extended-spectrum macrolides, rifampin, fluoroquinolones, aminoglycosides, glycopeptides, linezolid, and imipenem.

Combination therapy, with at least two antimicrobial agents, is recommended in the immunocompromised to reduce the emergence of resistance. Initial therapy is often with a macrolide or fluoroquinolone in combination with rifampin. Survival within macrophages is a significant virulence factor in *R. equi* disease, so antibiotics with intracellular activity, such as rifampin, fluoroquinolones, and azithromycin are preferable. Once drug sensitivities are known, treatment should continue with two active agents; ideally including a macrolide or a quinolone.

In CNS involvement, the second agent must have good CNS penetration (e.g. imipenem, vancomycin, rifampin, or linezolid) since fluoroquinolones and macrolides do not penetrate CSF well.

Initial therapy in immunocompromised people should last at least 2 months and longer courses should be administered when there is persistent clinical or radiographic evidence of infection.

Secondary prophylaxis with a single oral agent with demonstrated *in vitro* activity should be administered to patients who remain immunosuppressed. Improving immune function and drainage/resection may be important adjuncts to antimicrobial therapy.

Gram-positive bacteria

Clostridium difficile

C. difficile is an anaerobic, Gram-positive, spore-forming, toxin-producing bacillus. It was so named due to the difficulties in isolating it and growing it on conventional media. First isolated from the intestinal flora of healthy newborns in the 1930s, it was not until the 1970s, when it was isolated from the stool of patients with antibiotic-associated pseudomembranous colitis, that its pathogenic role began to be appreciated. Outside the colon, it exists in a heat-, acid-, and antibiotic-resistant spore form. Inside the colon, the spores convert to their fully functional vegetative, toxin-producing forms and become susceptible to killing by antimicrobial agents. Though not invasive, certain strains release potent exotoxins (toxins A and B) which mediate diarrhoea and colitis. All known toxigenic strains contain toxin B, with or without the presence of toxin A. These toxins inactivate cellular regulatory pathways leading to cell retraction and apoptosis and disrupt intercellular tight junctions. In vivo, stool toxin levels correlate with disease severity. Up to 30% of C. difficile strains are non-toxigenic.

Antibiotic use disrupts the barrier function of normal colonic flora, allowing C. difficile to multiply and elaborate toxins.

Epidemiology

Most cases of C. difficile-associated diarrhoea (CDAD) were initially attributed to the use of clindamycin. In the last two decades, however, the emergence of C. difficile infections (CDIs) that are more severe, refractory to standard therapy, and likely to relapse has been strongly correlated with increasing fluoroquinolone use. These cases are largely caused by the fluoroquinolone-resistant and hypervirulent NAP1/BI/027 strain, which produces substantially larger quantities of toxins A and B as well as an additional toxin known as 'binary toxin'. In the last decade, a new C. difficile strain (ribotype 078) has emerged in Europe and causes infections of similar severity to type 027, though it appears to affect a younger population.

In 2011, an estimated 450,000 cases of C. difficile occurred in the US, of which approximately one-third were community acquired and two-thirds were healthcare associated. Transmission is via the faecal–oral route and the organism can be cultured from the hospital environment, including items in patients' rooms and the hands and clothing of healthcare workers.

The C. difficile carrier rate among healthy adults is in the region of 3%, but among hospitalized adults and those in long-term care facilities it reaches 20–50%. Carriers of C. difficile act as a reservoir for environmental contamination regardless of clinical infection.

Antibiotic use is the principal risk factor for CDAD; the antibiotics most frequently implicated include fluoroquinolones, clindamycin, and broad-spectrum penicillins and cephalosporins. Any antibiotic, however, can predispose to C. difficile colonization, including metronidazole and vancomycin, the primary antibiotics used to treat it. In general, increased duration of therapy, the use of broad-spectrum agents, and the use of multiple antibiotic combinations all contribute to risk of CDAD

Advanced age, hospitalization, gastric acid suppression, GI surgery, enteral feeding, obesity, cancer chemotherapy, HSCT, and inflammatory bowel disease are other known risk factors. CDAD can also occur in the absence of any identifiable risk factors.

Clinical features
CDI can range from asymptomatic carriage to fulminant disease with toxic megacolon. Symptoms usually begin during antibiotic therapy or 5–10 days following antibiotic therapy. More rarely, onset may be as late as 10 weeks after cessation of antibiotic therapy.

Asymptomatic carriage
Patients shed *C. difficile* in stool but do not have diarrhoea or other clinical symptoms.

C.difficile-associated diarrhoea
Watery diarrhoea is the cardinal symptom ± colitis.

Fulminant colitis
Diarrhoea, lower abdominal pain/distention, fever, hypovolaemia, lactic acidosis, hypoalbuminemia, elevated creatinine, and marked leucocytosis. Complications include hypotension, sepsis, renal failure, toxic megacolon, and bowel perforation with peritonitis. Occasionally, CDI presents acutely as ileus, with little or no diarrhoea.

Recurrent disease
Defined by complete cessation of CDI symptoms while on appropriate therapy, followed by recurrence of symptoms post treatment. Up to 25% of patients experience recurrent *C. difficile* within 30 days of treatment, but recurrent CDI can occur as late as 3 months after completion of treatment. One recurrence significantly increases the risk of further recurrences and a recurrence most often represents a relapse rather than a reinfection, regardless of the interval between episodes.

Diagnosis
Suspect CDI in all patients with clinically significant diarrhoea or ileus in the context of relevant risk factors.

Send liquid stool for *C. difficile* testing. This will not distinguish between CDAD and asymptomatic carriage (which does not need treatment), so only send stool for CDI testing in patients with clinically significant diarrhoea.

For patients with ileus, perirectal swabs may be sent for toxin assay or anaerobic culture; the sensitivity of rectal swab for *C. difficile* culture in the setting of ileus is high, though turnaround time is long.

Pseudomembranous colitis (seen on imaging or endoscopy) is highly suggestive and should prompt laboratory testing for CDI.

Laboratory diagnosis requires demonstration of *C. difficile* toxin(s) or detection of toxigenic *C. difficile* organisms.

Most labs now use PCR, often as part of an algorithm including initial enzyme immunoassay (EIA) screening for glutamate dehydrogenase (GDH) antigen and toxins A and B. Real-time PCR, which detects genes (usually *tcdB*) specific to toxigenic strains, is highly sensitive and specific and results can be available within hours. False negatives may occur if stool specimen collection is delayed or the patient has been treated empirically for suspected CDI.

EIA for C. difficile

GDH antigen cannot distinguish between toxigenic and non-toxigenic strains and is therefore most useful as an initial screening step in a multistep approach. GDH antigen testing has good sensitivity, and results are available quickly.

EIA for C. difficile toxins

Toxin B is the clinically important toxin, however, testing for both toxin A and B by EIA gives a higher sensitivity. The sensitivity of EIA for toxins A and B is ~75% and specificity is >95%.

Laboratory diagnostics for suspected recurrent CDI are the same as for initial infection. Repeat stool assays are *not* warranted during or following treatment in patients who are recovering or are symptom free. Up to 50% of patients have positive stool assays for as long as 6 weeks after completion of therapy. Imaging of the abdomen and pelvis is required for patients with clinical manifestations of severe illness or fulminant colitis to look for conditions needing surgical intervention, such as toxic megacolon or bowel perforation.

Treatment

Stop the contributory antibiotic(s) as soon as possible and implement infection control measures. The use of soap and water is favoured over alcohol-based hand sanitization in a CDI outbreak. Empirical antibiotic treatment is usually started on clinical suspicion of CDI (after specimens are sent) and discontinued if the laboratory tests are negative.

Antibiotic treatment of confirmed cases must follow local guidelines; a summarized example of a current protocol is found in Box 14.2.

Refer to

Public Health England (PHE) guidelines: ℘ https://www.gov.uk/government/publications/clostridium-difficile-infection-guidance-on-management-and-treatment.

European Society of Clinical Microbiology and Infectious Diseases (ESCMID) guidelines: ℘ https://www.escmid.org/escmid_publications/medical_guidelines/escmid_guidelines/.

Listeria monocytogenes

A Gram-positive rod whose natural habitat is soil and decaying vegetable matter. It may form short chains and characteristically exhibits tumbling motility on light microscopy at 25°C. It is a particularly virulent pathogen in immunocompromised groups, most notably in pregnancy, neonates, and those on corticosteroids.

Epidemiology

Most infections result from oral ingestion followed by invasion of the intestinal mucosa and systemic infection. Up to 5% of healthy adults have *listeria* detectable in the bowel. Food-borne outbreaks, usually present with fever and gastroenteritis after an incubation period of ~24 hours. Infection is most commonly associated with processed meats, soft cheeses, pâtés, and fruit. Systemic infections generally occur in those with at least one predisposing condition: pregnancy, glucocorticoid treatment, other immunocompromising condition (e.g. HIV or chemotherapy), or old

Box 14.2 Example of a protocol for antibiotic treatment of CDI

Assess severity

Mild CDI: not associated with a raised white cell count (WCC); typically associated with fewer than three loose stools per day.

Moderate CDI: associated with a raised WCC $<15 \times 10^9$/L; typically with 3–5 loose stools per day.

Severe CDI if any of the following: WCC $>15 \times 10^9$/L; acutely rising blood creatinine (e.g. >50% increase above baseline); temperature >38.5°C; evidence of severe colitis (abdominal signs, radiology).

Life-threatening CDI includes hypotension, ileus, toxic megacolon, or CT evidence of severe disease. Diarrhoea may be absent in life-threatening CDI due to ileus. Request early gastroenterology/surgical/critical care review in severe or life-threatening CDI.

Specific antibiotic therapy for CDI

First episode of mild/moderate severity: metronidazole orally (IV if nil by mouth) for 10–14 days. If clinical worsening or no improvement after 7 days, switch to vancomycin orally for 10–14 days. Do not give vancomycin IV for CDI, though the IV formulation may be given via nasogastric tube if patient is nil by mouth. Patients with mild CDI may not require any specific anti-CDI antibiotic treatment.

First episode of severe disease: vancomycin orally/nasogastrically for 10–14 days. If no improvement/worsening, add in metronidazole. Discuss with microbiology, options may include increasing the vancomycin dose, using fidaxomicin, intracolonic vancomycin, or IVIG.

Second episode of CDI: assess severity as above; if severe, treat as above. Review medication; stop gastric acid suppressants and predisposing antibiotics. If non-severe, commence vancomycin. If poor response, discuss alternatives with microbiology.

Subsequent episode of CDI, i.e. third or more episode: assess severity and review medication as above. If non-severe, commence vancomycin orally/nasogastrically and discuss options with microbiology—these may include a prolonged tapering course of oral vancomycin, the use of fidaxomicin, IVIG, or donor stool transplant.

age. Pregnant women (>20 weeks) are particularly vulnerable to *Listeria*. Infection can cross the placenta to cause fetal death, premature birth, or an infected neonate. *L. monocytogenes* is the most common cause of meningitis in patients with lymphoma, transplant recipients, and those on glucocorticoid therapy. Invasive listeriosis has a much longer incubation period (usually ~10 days).

Clinical features

Consider *Listeria* in cases of meningitis or sepsis in the immunosuppressed, elderly, or neonates. Listerial bacteraemia often leads to endocardial infection. Less common syndromes include pneumonia, arthritis, endophthalmitis, encephalitis, and CNS abscess. Most neonatal disease presents with septicaemia within 5 days of birth and has a mortality of 30–60%. In pregnancy, listerial infection is more common beyond 20 weeks and usually either asymptomatic or presents with relatively mild symptoms such as headache, sore throat, myalgia, and fever. (➲ See Chapter 9.)

Diagnosis

Microscopy and culture

Blood cultures are positive in 60–75% of patients with CNS infection and CSF cultures are positive in almost 100%. CSF microscopy with Gram staining, however, is positive in <50% of cases. Wet mounts of CSF may demonstrate the classical 'tumbling motility'. Listeria may form chains and appear Gram variable on microscopy, so can be initially misidentified as cocci or diphtheroids.

Treatment

IV ampicillin or TMX–SMT for at least 2 weeks for bacteraemia and 4 weeks for CNS infection. In severe disease, gentamicin may be added for up to 2 weeks.

Refer to

British Infection Association (BIA) UK joint specialist societies guideline on meningitis: 🕮 https://www.britishinfection.org/guidelines-resources/published-guidelines/ for guidelines on CNS infection.

European Society of Clinical Microbiology and Infectious Diseases (ESCMID) guidelines: 🕮 https://www.escmid.org/escmid_publications/medical_guidelines/escmid_guidelines/ for guidelines on CNS infection.

Gram-negative bacteria

Pseudomonas aeruginosa

P. aeruginosa is a Gram-negative, aerobic rod, commonly present in the environment, especially in water. It may act as an opportunistic pathogen causing serious infections in the immunocompromised and often has multiple inherent and acquired antibiotic resistance mechanisms.

Epidemiology

P. aeruginosa is a major pathogen worldwide and a significant cause of hospital-acquired infection; particularly ventilator-associated pneumonia, surgical site infection, catheter-related urinary infection, and nosocomial bacteraemia. It is the most common pathogen isolated from adults with cystic fibrosis and is well known as an opportunist pathogen in patients with neutropenia or burns. As well as multiple intrinsic mechanisms to avoid antibiotic killing (including AmpC beta-lactamase, efflux pumps, and biofilm formation), *P. aeruginosa* has acquired plasmids encoding both ESBLs and carbapenemases.

Clinical features

P. aeruginosa has two distinct forms of pathogenic behaviour: chronic colonization of the lungs (as in many patients with cystic fibrosis) and invasive disease (pneumonia, bacteraemia, and septic shock). Hospital-acquired *P. aeruginosa* bacteraemia can follow primary infection in the lungs, GI/biliary tract, urinary tract, skin/soft tissues, or from infected intravascular catheters. It is more common in neutropenia or other immunodeficiency states. It commonly presents, with endotoxin-induced shock, typically fever, tachycardia, tachypnoea, disorientation, and hypotension. Skin lesions, such as ecthyma gangrenosum, point towards *P. aeruginosa* as the causative organism. Mortality is higher in bacteraemia caused by *P. aeruginosa* than that caused by most other commonly isolated bacilli. Infective endocarditis due to *P. aeruginosa* is relatively rare, but strongly associated with prosthetic heart valves, pacemakers, and IV drug abuse.

Diagnosis
Culture

Send blood and/or respiratory samples for culture and follow local empirical therapy guidelines for suspected pseudomonal infection while awaiting identification and sensitivity profile. Quantitative or semi-quantitative cultures may be performed on certain respiratory specimens as an aid to diagnosing ventilator-associated pneumonia.

Molecular techniques

Molecular techniques for detection of respiratory pathogens are being developed and should allow for more rapid identification of the causes of hospital-acquired pneumonia or ventilator-associated pneumonia.

Treatment

Sensitivity patterns are crucial to treatment selection. Choices of treatment include antipseudomonal penicillins (e.g. piperacillin–tazobactam), antipseudomonal cephalosporins (e.g. ceftazidime), carbapenems (e.g. meropenem), or aminoglycosides (e.g. gentamicin). Fluoroquinolones are the only oral options, although isolates are frequently resistant. Nebulized colistin is also used in chronic respiratory infection.

Refer to

British Thoracic Society (BTS) guidelines on bronchiectasis: ℘ https://www.brit-thoracic.org.uk/standards-of-care/guidelines/.

Cystic Fibrosis Trust UK ℘ https://www.cysticfibrosis.org.uk/the-work-we-do/clinical-care/consensus-documents for guidelines related to infections in cystic fibrosis.

Burkholderia cepacia complex

The *B. cepacia* complex includes >18 phenotypically similar species of Gram-negative, non-spore-forming bacilli. When first described in the 1950s by W.H. Burkholder, they were of note for the vinegar-like stench ('sour skin') they cause in onion bulbs. In recent decades, they have been recognized as opportunistic human respiratory pathogens in individuals with weakened immune systems or chronic lung disease, especially cystic fibrosis. Molecular taxonomy has grouped the many species into nine genomovars, of which two—*B. cenocepacia* (genomovar 3) and *B. multivorans* (genomovar 2)—are the most common causes of *B. cepacia* colonization and infection in cystic fibrosis patients. Various characteristics differentiate them from other cystic fibrosis pathogens and complicate management; they are highly transmissible, more virulent, and have inherent resistance to multiple antibiotics.

Endotoxin plays an important role in their pathogenesis; lipopolysaccharide from clinical isolates of *B. cepacia* have endotoxin activity almost ten times higher than endotoxin extracted from *Pseudomonas aeruginosa*. Other virulence factors include the ability of *B. cepacia* to form biofilms, adhere to epithelial cells and mucin, invade and survive inside airway epithelial cells and macrophages, and secrete catalases, proteases, and siderophores.

Epidemiology

B. cepacia spp. are ubiquitous in nature and commonly found in soil and water. An estimated 3% of cystic fibrosis patients in the US and UK are infected with *B. cepacia* organisms and prevalence increases with age. Although transient infection occurs, the majority of infections cannot be eradicated.

Patient-to-patient spread of organisms can occur through social contact and this is particularly well described for the epidemic (ET-12) strain of *B. cenocepacia*. Recognition of this and the increased mortality rates associated with the epidemic strains, led to the policy of strict segregation in clinical units. Consequently, most new *B. cepacia* complex infections these days are with *B. multivorans*, acquired from as-yet unidentified environmental reservoirs.

B. cepacia infection is not limited to cystic fibrosis patients; other groups, such as those with chronic granulomatous disease, are vulnerable and it has occasionally caused disease in healthy individuals. It has been associated with cutaneous foot lesions in military personnel ('swamp foot') and been isolated from catheters, wounds, burns, sputum, and urine. Contamination of inhaled and IV solutions has resulted in airways infection or systemic sepsis.

Clinical features

Vary from asymptomatic carriage to accelerated decline in lung function to rapid, uncontrolled deterioration with septicaemia and necrotizing pneumonia ('cepacia syndrome'). Prognosis depends in part on the species within the *B. cepacia* complex. With *B. multivorans*, the 5-year survival is similar to *P. aeruginosa* infection; however, *B. cenocepacia* is associated with a rapid deterioration and early death in up to a third of cases.

Cystic fibrosis patients are at a significantly higher risk of post-transplant pneumonia than other lung transplant recipients and are more likely to be colonized with multidrug-resistant *B. cepacia* and *P. aeruginosa*. Individuals with *B. cenocepacia* appear to have poorer post lung transplant outcomes and colonization with this strain is viewed as a relative contraindication to transplantation. Screening of all patients with cystic fibrosis for *B. cenocepacia* is advised.

Diagnosis

The 'recA' PCR is currently the most sensitive and specific molecular identification method. More complex methods such as pulse field gel electrophoresis (PFGE) or restriction fragment length polymorphisms (RFLPs) are needed for epidemiological analysis and transmission mapping.

B. cepacia can be cultured from respiratory samples on specific media and commercial biochemical identification kits such as API™ 20NE are useful but have significant false positives. *Stenotrophomonas maltophilia, Achromobacter xyloxidans*, and occasionally *P. aeruginosa* can be erroneously diagnosed as *B. cepacia* organisms. False positives or negatives may lead to the patient being inappropriately cohorted and thereby facilitate transmission.

Treatment

There is a lack of trial evidence to guide decision-making and antimicrobial therapy should be directed by *in vitro* sensitivities where available. Most isolates show high-level resistance to antipseudomonal antibiotics, including inherent resistance to colistin. Some centres have reported pan-resistance in >80% of patient isolates. Environmental strains are generally more susceptible than clinical strains.

The most consistently active agents *in vitro* appear to be ceftazidime, piperacillin–tazobactam, meropenem, imipenem, ciprofloxacin, trimethoprim, co-trimoxazole, and tetracyclines. Various combinations of two or three antibiotics (e.g. tobramycin plus meropenem plus ceftazidime) have shown synergy against *B. cepacia* complex. Temocillin has been trialled for treating exacerbations, with modest clinical improvement observed. Anecdotal evidence suggests that eradication can be enhanced by giving aerosolized amiloride and tobramycin in combination. There is little evidence on the best therapeutic approaches for 'cepacia syndrome' but combination therapy is usually tried. Aggressive eradication therapy for all new growths should be considered.

Refer to

British Thoracic Society (BTS) guidelines on bronchiectasis: ℬ https://www.brit-thoracic.org.uk/standards-of-care/guidelines/.

Cystic Fibrosis Trust UK ℬ https://www.cysticfibrosis.org.uk/the-work-we-do/clinical-care/consensus-documents for guidelines related to infections in cystic fibrosis.

Burkholderia pseudomallei

B. pseudomallei is a facultative, intracellular, Gram-negative bacterium and a widely distributed environmental saprophyte in soil and fresh surface water in endemic regions. Infection with *B. pseudomallei* can lead to the disease melioidosis, which is associated with high case-fatality rates. Functional neutrophil defects are important in the pathogenesis of melioidosis and the disease mostly occurs in adults with an underlying predisposing condition.

Epidemiology

Melioidosis is a disease of public health importance in Southeast Asia and northern Australia, with seasonal peaks in the wet seasons. Cases may be acquired by visitors to endemic areas, with symptoms arising later.

The important risk factors for melioidosis are diabetes mellitus, alcohol abuse, and chronic renal or lung disease. B. pseudomallei can cause colonization and pulmonary infections in patients with cystic fibrosis. Children may develop infection without associated risk factors.

The major mode of transmission is thought to be percutaneous inoculation during exposure to wet season soils or contaminated water, though transmission can also occur via inhalation, aspiration, and occasionally ingestion. During severe weather events such as storms, inhalation may become the primary mode of B. pseudomallei transmission. Laboratory-acquired infections and iatrogenic infections from contaminated hospital or surgical equipment occasionally occur.

Following percutaneous inoculation the organism can disseminate via haematogenous spread. Incubation periods from inoculation range from 1 day to 3 weeks.

Clinical features

Most B. pseudomallei infections are subclinical and severe disease occurs mainly in those with risk factors.

The most common clinical manifestations are pneumonia (acute or subacute/chronic) and localized skin infection (ulcers/abscesses). >50% of all patients are bacteraemic and up to 25% present with septic shock.

Haematogenous spread of B. pseudomallei may lead to clinical manifestations in virtually any site:

- Genitourinary melioidosis (fever, suprapubic pain, dysuria, or acute retention).
- Septic arthritis or osteomyelitis.
- Encephalomyelitis—unilateral upper motor neuron limb weakness, cerebellar signs, cranial nerve palsies, or flaccid paraparesis.
- Abscesses in internal organs (spleen, kidney, prostate, and liver).
- Suppurative parotitis (particularly common in children in SE Asia).

Imaging of the chest, abdomen, pelvis, brain, and other clinically suspicious site is thus an essential part of the workup.

Diagnosis

Culture, usually on Ashdown's medium, is the mainstay of diagnosis.

Send blood, sputum, urine, ulcer swabs, abscess fluid, throat swabs, and rectal swabs. Gram stain of sputum or pus may reveal Gram-negative bacilli with a characteristic bipolar staining giving a 'safety pin' appearance.

PCR and matrix-assisted laser desorption/ionization-time of flight mass spectrometry are increasingly used for confirmation of bacterial isolates cultured from clinical samples.

Isolation of *B. pseudomallei* from any clinical specimen generally warrants treatment as residual colonization is usually associated with low-grade infection and there is a risk of subsequent invasive disease.

Treatment

All cases of melioidosis should be treated with aggressive initial antimicrobial therapy. *B. pseudomallei* is resistant to penicillin, ampicillin, first- and second-generation cephalosporins, gentamicin, tobramycin, and streptomycin. Initial therapy usually consists of at least 2 weeks of IV ceftazidime, meropenem, or imipenem.

This should be followed immediately by longer-term oral eradication therapy to prevent recrudescence or relapse. TMP–SMX for at least 3 months (longer in bone or neurological disease) is a standard regimen.

Adjunctive therapies include abscess drainage and, in septic shock, the use of recombinant human G-CSF.

Refer to

US Centers for Disease Control and Prevention (CDC) ℘ https://www.cdc.gov/melioidosis/index.html for further information.

Stenotrophomonas maltophilia

A MDR, aerobic, Gram-negative bacillus that is ubiquitous in aquatic environments. Though an organism of low virulence, it is increasingly detected as a nosocomial pathogen in the immunocompromised.

Epidemiology

Risk factors include underlying malignancy, immunosuppressant therapy, cystic fibrosis, exposure to broad-spectrum antibiotics, ICU admission, mechanical ventilation, recent surgery, HIV infection, and neutropenia. Invasive medical devices are usually the vehicle by which the organism by-passes normal host defences.

Clinical features

Consider in patients with indwelling catheters, those receiving immunosuppressant therapy or broad-spectrum antibiotics, or in patients with cystic fibrosis. *S. maltophilia* commonly colonizes the urine but is pathogenic only in those with impaired host defences. Cases of *S. maltophilia* causing a rapidly progressive haemorrhagic pneumonia have been reported in mechanically ventilated patients.

Diagnosis

Usually by culture of the organism from body fluids. However, the presence of *S. maltophilia* may represent colonization alone and not disease. Growth of *S. maltophilia* from normally sterile sites (such as blood or peritoneal fluid) should be interpreted as representing true infection.

Treatment

Empirical treatment is with TMP–SMX with the addition of ceftazidime or levofloxacin for severe infection.

Refer to

British Thoracic Society (BTS) guidelines on bronchiectasis: ℘ https://www.brit-thoracic.org.uk/standards-of-care/guidelines/.

Cystic Fibrosis Trust UK ℘ https://www.cysticfibrosis.org.uk/the-work-we-do/clinical-care/consensus-documents for guidelines related to infections in cystic fibrosis.

Bartonella spp.

Originally thought to be Rickettsiae, the bacterial genus *Bartonella* now has >20 species described. Of these, two species—*B. henselae* and *B. quintana*—are major causes of disease in patients with HIV. Transmission occurs by traumatic contact with infected animals or by insect vectors.

Epidemiology

Both *B. henselae* and *B. quintana* are globally distributed. *B. henselae* infection is associated with cat exposure, most often a scratch, whereas *B. quintana* is transmitted via lice and is most often found among the homeless. Though much less common these days, due to the wide availability of HAART, *Bartonella* infection is still seen in HIV infection with CD4 counts <100 cells/µL.

Clinical features

Suspect in patients with HIV infection presenting with violaceous skin lesions. Though the vascular lesions of bartonellosis most often affect the skin (and may resemble Kaposi's sarcoma), they also occur in lung, gut, bone, and brain. Peliosis hepatis (multiple blood-filled cavities in the liver), splenitis, and endocarditis ('culture negative') are also described in *Bartonella* co-infection with HIV. Constitutional symptoms (fever, malaise, headache, anorexia, etc.) are common.

Diagnosis

Culture

Culture from blood or tissue is difficult due to the fastidious nature of *Bartonella* spp. If informed, the laboratory can use special conditions and prolonged culture periods to maximize yield.

Histopathology

Biopsy of an accessible lesion will show vascular proliferation and silver staining often demonstrates numerous bacilli.

Serology

Can be used to support a diagnosis, but is not definitive. A significant proportion of patients with HIV will not develop detectable antibody responses to *Bartonella*.

Molecular techniques

PCR is increasingly used and if available may be the best choice. PCR of cardiac valve tissue is very sensitive and not affected by pre-surgical antibiotic treatment.

Treatment

Bacteraemia is usually treated with doxycycline and gentamicin.

Refer to

British HIV Association (BHIVA) and British Infection Association (BIA) ℘ http://www.bhiva.org/Guidelines.aspx for guidelines related to *Bartonella* spp. infections in HIV.

Capnocytophaga canimorsus

C. canimorsus are long, thin, slow-growing, Gram-negative rods which form part of the normal flora of the oral cavity of dogs and cats. They are a cause of fulminant sepsis in asplenic/hyposplenic individuals.

Epidemiology

About half of patients diagnosed with *C. canimorsus* infection report a history of dog bite and most of the rest will have had some contact with dogs or cats. As well as impaired or absent splenic function, other risk factors include prolonged corticosteroid use, alcoholism, and cirrhosis.

Clinical features

Consider *C. canimorsus* in septicaemic shock in patients with a history of dog bite/exposure, particularly in the context of impaired immunity. May also present with pneumonia, cellulitis, meningitis, or pyrexia of unknown origin.

Diagnosis

Send relevant clinical samples for culture; *C. canimorsus* is a slow-growing, fastidious bacteria, so if suspected, inform the laboratory in order that they can use appropriate media and leave the culture for a prolonged period.

Treatment

Patients with severe disease should receive a beta-lactam–beta-lactamase combination (such as piperacillin–tazobactam), a cephalosporin (such as ceftriaxone), or a carbapenem (such as imipenem-cilastatin).

Non-typhoidal *Salmonella* (NTS) spp.

NTS are motile, facultatively anaerobic, Gram-negative Enterobacteriaceae. The genus *Salmonella* consists of two species, *S. enterica* and *S. bongori*; most clinically important salmonellae are serotypes of *S. enterica*, subspecies enterica. NTS refers to all the serotypes except the human-restricted *S. typhi* and *S. paratyphi* which cause enteric fever. *S. enteritidis* and *S. typhimurium* are the pathogenic NTS serotypes most commonly isolated from blood

NTS species are associated with animal reservoirs worldwide and are a major cause of food-borne (mostly poultry, eggs, and milk) diarrhoeal outbreaks. In the context of impaired cellular immunity due to advanced HIV infection, corticosteroid use, or malignancy, NTS may cause more severe disease such as bacteraemia with metastatic foci.

Epidemiology

The greatest burden of invasive NTS disease is in Africa where NTS species are a leading cause of bacteraemia in both children and adults and can occur in epidemics with high mortality. In addition to HIV, corticosteroid use, and malignancy, other risk factors for invasive disease include extremes of age, rheumatological disease, immunomodulatory drugs, transplantation, congenital immune deficiencies, liver disease, diabetes, sickle cell disease, schistosomiasis, and chronic granulomatous disease. Prior to the widespread availability of HAART, recurrent invasive *Salmonella* infection was a relatively frequent AIDS-defining infection.

Clinical features

NTS bacteraemia can lead to suppurative foci of infection throughout the body, including long bones, joints, muscles, lung, heart, and CNS. Foci tend to occur at sites of structural abnormality, e.g. endovascular atheroma, prosthetic grafts, or bones and joints damaged by avascular necrosis from sickle crises. In immunosuppression due to malignancy or steroid use, soft tissue and lung foci are more common. Meningitis is rare and most often occurs in children <1 year old. NTS bacteraemia in HIV (usually occurring when CD4 count <200 cells/µL) most often has a non-specific febrile presentation without diarrhoea or abdominal symptoms. Hepatomegaly and/or splenomegaly occur in up to half of cases.

Diagnosis

Culture

NTS species grow vigorously in both aerobic and anaerobic culture. A 'primary bacteraemia' without preceding GI illness may be the first presentation of an underlying immune deficiency.

Laboratory isolation of salmonellae from stool usually requires a minimum of 48 hours and samples collected over several days are preferred. After stool and blood, urinary isolates are encountered next most frequently. ESBL genes are emerging in salmonellae in all areas

Treatment

Depends on sensitivity patterns but fluoroquinolones are usually first line with azithromycin where quinolone resistance has emerged.

Refer to

British HIV Association (BHIVA) and British Infection Association (BIA) ℳ http://www.bhiva.org/Guidelines.aspx for guidelines related to infections in HIV.

Emerging multidrug-resistant bacteria

The immunocompromised represent a unique group for the acquisition of antimicrobial resistant infections due to their frequent encounters with the healthcare system, need for empiric and prophylactic antimicrobials, and immune dysfunction.

Enterococci (including vancomycin-resistant enterococci)

Enterococci are normal flora in the human and animal gut. Previously known as group D streptococci, they are Gram-positive facultative anaerobes which can survive high temperatures and grow in salty conditions. The genus *Enterococcus* has >18 species described, but only a handful are known to cause disease in humans. *E. faecalis and E. faecium* are the predominant species implicated in human disease (>90% clinical isolates) and it is *E. faecium* that is the cause of most vancomycin-resistant infections. Enterococci have both intrinsic and acquired antibiotic resistance mechanisms. High-level resistance to vancomycin (defined as a minimum inhibitory concentration (MIC) >32 micrograms/mL) is encoded by different clusters of genes referred to as the vancomycin-resistance gene clusters (e.g. *vanA, vanB,* and *vanD* gene clusters). VRE, particularly *E. faecium* strains, are frequently resistant to all antibiotics effective against vancomycin-susceptible enterococci.

Epidemiology

Enterococci are among the most common causes of nosocomial infections. First reported in the 1980s, vancomycin-resistant strains are now widespread. Infecting strains of VRE most often originate from the patient's gut flora. Individuals at risk for colonization include critically ill patients on long courses of antibiotics, SOT recipients, patients with haematological malignancies, and healthcare workers. Risk factors for VRE bacteraemia include intestinal colonization, prior long-term antibiotic use, increased severity of illness, haematological malignancy, bone marrow transplant, mucositis, neutropenia, indwelling urinary catheters, corticosteroid treatment, chemotherapy, and parenteral nutrition.

Clinical features

The virulence of enterococci is generally lower than that of organisms such as *Staphylococcus aureus*, but this is counterbalanced by the fact that enterococcal infections most often occur in debilitated patients and as part of polymicrobial infections. Nosocomial infections are often in very ill patients who have been exposed to broad-spectrum antibiotics. Urinary tract infections are the most common site of VRE, followed by bacteraemia. Enterococci, predominantly *E. faecium*, cause 5–15% of all cases of endocarditis; this tends to be left-sided and subacute (often without peripheral stigmata). Other sites of enterococcal infection include the abdomen, pelvis, and rarely the meninges (often associated with neurosurgical procedures).

Diagnosis

Obtain cultures from blood, urine, and any other sites suspected to be infected (e.g. peritoneal fluid, joint fluid, CSF, pyogenic fluid collections in soft tissue). If endocarditis is suspected, obtain three sets of blood cultures over 1 hour or longer.

Send stool or perirectal cultures to screen for VRE colonization.

Treatment
Therapy depends on antibiotic sensitivities. Treatment of bacteraemia due to susceptible enterococci (in the absence of suspected endocarditis) consists of ampicillin monotherapy. Bacteraemia due to ampicillin-resistant organisms is with vancomycin. Vancomycin-resistant *E. faecium* bacteraemia may be treated with daptomycin. Endocarditis is usually treated with a combination of ampicillin and low-dose gentamicin.

Refer to
Public Health England (PHE)   https://www.gov.uk/guidance/ enterococcus-species-and-glycopeptide-resistant-enterococci-gre   for guidelines on glycopeptide-resistant enterococci.
   British Society for Antimicrobial Chemotherapy (BSAC)   https:// www.britishinfection.org/guidelines-resources/published-guidelines/   for guidelines relating to enterococcal endocarditis.

Staphylococcus aureus (MRSA/VRSA)
In the early 1960s, just a couple of years after the introduction of methicillin, resistant *S. aureus* isolates were first described. Resistance is defined as an oxacillin MIC >4 micrograms/mL and results from the PBP-2a encoding *mecA* gene. Studies suggest that the *mec* gene was acquired from closely related coagulase-negative staphylococci (CoNS) species. MRSA is now globally distributed and a common pathogen, both in hospitals and the community. The ability of *S. aureus* to form biofilms on invasive devices (such as endovascular catheters) partly accounts for its ubiquity as a nosocomial pathogen. Immunosuppression is associated with an increased risk of *S. aureus* colonization and therefore an increased risk of infection and morbidity. Mortality appears to be higher with bacteraemia due to MRSA than with methicillin-sensitive *S. aureus* (MSSA) organisms.
   Vancomycin-intermediate and vancomycin-resistant (VISA/VRSA MIC 4–8 micrograms/mL and MIC ≥16 micrograms/mL respectively) *S. aureus*, were first described in 1997 and 2002 respectively. These have arisen via different mechanisms. VISA are thought to have resulted from mutations of MRSA strains exposed to vancomycin, whereas VRSA arose from transfer of genetic material from VRE.

Epidemiology
Based on differences in clinical and molecular epidemiology, MRSA has traditionally been divided into healthcare-associated (HA-MRSA) and community-associated (CA-MRSA).
   HA-MRSA is defined as infection occurring >48 hours after hospital admission or within 1 year of healthcare exposure. It is classically associated with severe disease such as pneumonia and bloodstream infection. Antibiotic use, long hospital stays, ICU admission, haemodialysis, MRSA colonization, and proximity to others with MRSA are all risk factors for HA-MRSA infection. By contrast, CA-MRSA has been most associated with skin and soft tissue infections in otherwise healthy individuals. Over recent years, however, the boundaries between CA- and HA-MRSA have blurred. HIV infection is a risk factor for MRSA colonization and infection, with skin and soft tissue infections being the predominant manifestation. Antibiotic use (particularly cephalosporin and fluoroquinolone use) strongly correlates

with the risk of MRSA colonization and infection. MRSA transmission occurs via contact with a colonized individual or a contaminated fomite.

There have been globally scattered case reports of VRSA, with over a dozen cases reported in the US since 2002.

Clinical features

Immunocompetent

While skin and soft tissue infections are the most common presentations, *S. aureus* also is responsible for a wide spectrum of invasive infections including musculoskeletal infections, complicated pneumonia, and endocarditis. *S. aureus* is a leading cause of community- and hospital-acquired bacteraemia. Vascular catheters are a common source of infection and cardiac devices such as pacemakers often become colonized. The incidence of infective endocarditis in the setting of *S. aureus* bacteraemia is 10–15% and can be more aggressive than endocarditis due to other organisms. Osteomyelitis (most frequently vertebral) commonly occurs due to either haematogenous or direct spread from a contiguous focus of infection. Back or joint pain in a patient with *S. aureus* should prompt imaging to look for an osteomyelitic lesion. Among hospital inpatients, *S. aureus* pneumonia is associated with intubation or other respiratory tract instrumentation.

Immunocompromised

HIV-positive adults are known to have more frequent invasive *S. aureus* infections, notably bacteraemia, than HIV-negative controls and these infections are more often with drug-resistant strains.

S. aureus accounted for 10% of total cases of bacteraemia in a series of adults with malignancy with mortality rates ranging from 15% to 25%. The mortality rate for *S. aureus* pneumonia in adult cancer patients is particularly high (almost 50%).

Diagnosis

Cultures

Blood cultures and other sterile site sampling are the mainstay of diagnosis. Failure to clear bacteraemia on repeat culture (taken ~48 hours after initiation of therapy) should prompt evaluation of susceptibility data to ensure appropriate antibiotic selection and dosing, as well as clinical evaluation for occult focus of infection that may require drainage or surgery.

Repeated isolation of *S. aureus* despite seemingly appropriate therapy should prompt consideration of MRSA, VISA, or VRSA. VISA may emerge during treatment even if the MIC of the original isolate was within the susceptible range. Alternatively, persistent bacteraemia may reflect abscess or metastatic infection rather than reduced antibiotic susceptibility.

Disc diffusion or automated methods are insufficient for detection of *S. aureus* with reduced susceptibility to vancomycin; a MIC susceptibility testing method (such as broth microdilution or agar-gradient diffusion) should be used.

Treatment

Eliminate potential sources of ongoing infection (e.g. implanted medical material, vascular catheter, abscess, etc.) Vancomycin or daptomycin are the agents of choice for treatment of invasive MRSA infections. Alternatives, if available, include teicoplanin, ceftaroline, linezolid, and telavancin. If the vancomycin MIC nears the limit of the susceptible range (2 micrograms/mL) and initial clinical response is poor, vancomycin should be discontinued and replaced with daptomycin.

Optimal regimens for infection due to VISA or VRSA are uncertain.

In the context of bacteraemia but with proven absence of deep-seated infection, monotherapy may be considered and options include ceftaroline, linezolid, and telavancin. In cases of bacteraemia and concomitant deep-seated infection, combination therapy is warranted to minimize the risk of resistance emerging during therapy. Possible combinations include daptomycin plus ceftaroline (or other beta-lactams); vancomycin plus ceftaroline (or other beta-lactams); daptomycin plus TMP–SMX; or ceftaroline plus TMP–SMX.

Refer to

British Society for Antimicrobial Chemotherapy (BSAC) ℘ https://www.ncbi.nlm.nih.gov/pubmed/19282331 for guidelines on prophylaxis and treatment of MRSA.

Infectious Diseases Society of America (IDSA) guidelines on MRSA infection: ℘ http://www.idsociety.org/PracticeGuidelines/.

Enterobacteriaceae: extended-spectrum beta-lactamases and carbapenemases

Extended-spectrum beta-lactamases (ESBL) are enzymes which open the beta-lactam ring and inactivate most beta-lactam antibiotics. ESBL have so far been found exclusively in Gram-negative organisms, primarily *Escherichia coli*, *Klebsiella pneumoniae*, and *Klebsiella oxytoca*, but also in *Acinetobacter, Burkholderia, Citrobacter, Enterobacter, Morganella, Proteus, Pseudomonas, Salmonella, Serratia*, and *Shigella* spp. First reported in Gram-negative bacteria in the 1960s, plasmids encoding ESBL are now prevalent in Enterobacteriaceae worldwide. The most common ESBL currently described are CTX-M, TEM, and SHV beta-lactamases. The proportion of *Enterobacter* isolates producing ESBL is increasing and recent estimates from some centres are in the region of 15% of *K. pneumoniae*, 12% of *E. coli*, 10% of *K. oxytoca*, and 5% of *P. mirabilis*.

Carbapenemases are carbapenem-hydrolysing beta-lactamases which confer resistance to carbapenems as well as penicillins, cephalosporins, and other antibiotics. The widespread use of carbapenems to treat suspected cases of ESBL-producing bacteria has now led to the development and increasing prevalence of carbapenem resistance in these same bacterial species. They have been organized into four classes (A–D) based on their amino acid sequences; class A contains the best known and most prevalent carbapenemase, *K. pneumonia* carbapenemase (KPC).

Epidemiology

GI colonization with ESBL/carbapenemase producing Enterobacteriaceae is a strong risk factor for subsequent infection and colonization and is often driven by the use of broad-spectrum antibiotics. Prolonged hospitalization, mechanical ventilation, haemodialysis, malignancy, organ transplantation, and intravascular catheters are all associated with an increased risk of infection with resistant Gram-negative bacilli. Travelling to, and particularly receiving medical treatment in, regions with high rates of ESBL/carbapenemases, such as parts of Asia and Latin America, is also a well-described risk factor. Environmental, animal, and food contamination with ESBL-producing Gram-negative organisms have been extensively documented.

Clinical features

Gram-negative bacilli were once the predominant organisms associated with hospital-onset bloodstream infections, but over the last few decades, Gram-positive aerobes (e.g. coagulase-negative staphylococci, *S. aureus*, and entero-cocci), and *Candida* spp. have increased in relative importance. Gram negatives still account for a higher proportion of community-onset bacteraemias as these are more likely related to primary infections of the urinary tract, abdomen, and respiratory tract as opposed to device-related infections.

Fever and rigors are the most common presentation of Gram-negative bacteraemia, with hypotension, mental state changes, and respiratory failure suggestive of developing shock. Most hospitalized patients with Gram-negative bacteraemia will have at least one immunocompromising comorbidity and Gram-negative bacillary sepsis with shock has a high mortality rate (~10–40%).

Drug-resistant Enterobacteriaceae may cause infection at diverse sites but are most commonly encountered in bloodstream infections, ventilator-associated pneumonia, urinary tract infections, and catheter-related infections. Clusters and outbreaks have occurred due to hospital-based clonal spread.

Diagnosis

Cultures of blood, urine, CSF, respiratory secretions, or any other clinically relevant and accessible sample should be taken prior to initiation of antimicrobial therapy. At least two sets of blood cultures taken from separate venepuncture sites should be obtained. Most clinically significant bacteraemias are detected within 48 hours with the use of instrument-based, continuous monitoring blood culture systems.

Recent technologies for organism identification, such as matrix-assisted laser desorption/ionization time-of-flight mass spectrometry and next-generation gene sequencing may increase the speed of diagnosis and detection of known resistant strains.

The isolation of a drug-resistant strain should be discussed with the local microbiology team to consider antimicrobial options, infection control, and contact tracing/screening. Follow-up blood cultures are normally recommended when MDR strains are detected.

Treatment

Optimal treatment should be guided by location and severity of infection as well as the sensitivity profile of the isolate. The only current proven therapeutic options for serious infections caused by ESBL producers are the carbapenems (meropenem, ertapenem, imipenem, and doripenem).

Carbapenem-resistant Enterobacteriaceae (CRE) causing an uncomplicated urinary tract infection can often be effectively treated with fosfomycin or an aminoglycoside (assuming they remain susceptible). Combination therapy with at least two drugs is used for more serious infections (including bacteraemia). The optimal combination is uncertain, but a polymyxin-based (colistin or polymyxin B) regimen should be used unless there is documented resistance. Meropenem, especially if the isolate has a MIC to meropenem ≤8 micrograms/mL, can be added as a second agent. For infections involving the GI tract and lungs, consider tigecycline as the second agent as it penetrates well into these tissues. Ceftazidime–avibactam is an alternative agent to use as part of a combination regimen if the isolate is susceptible. Aztreonam may be a useful additional agent for patients whose isolates carry a metallo-beta-lactamase and demonstrate *in vitro* susceptibility to this drug.

Refer to

European Society of Clinical Microbiology and Infectious Diseases (ESCMID) ℘ https://www.escmid.org/escmid_publications/medical_guidelines/escmid_guidelines/for guidelines on treatment of hospital-associated MDR Gram-negative bacteria.

Public Health England (PHE) ℘ https://www.gov.uk/government/publications/carbapenemase-producing-enterobacteriaceae-early-detection-management-and-control-toolkit-for-acute-trusts for guidelines on carbapenemase-producing Enterobacteriaceae.

Acinetobacter spp.

Aerobic, Gram-negative, motile coccobacilli which naturally inhabit soil and water. >30 species have been described in the *Acinetobacter* genus, but *A. baumannii* is the most frequently isolated and clinically important species. It colonizes skin, wounds, the GI and respiratory tracts, and is associated with hospital outbreaks, particularly among ICU patients. *A. baumannii* has acquired many different antibiotic resistance mechanisms and MDR strains are an increasing threat.

Epidemiology

A. baumannii is a significant cause of hospital-acquired infection worldwide and tends to occur in debilitated ICU patients—accounting for up to 10% of Gram-negative isolates in ventilator-associated pneumonia. Outbreaks have been linked to contaminated ventilator equipment as well as cross-infection from the contaminated hands of healthcare workers. Some *Acinetobacter* strains can survive desiccation for weeks.

Clinical features

Consider in all ventilator-associated pneumonia and hospital-acquired sepsis. Bloodstream infection usually results from pneumonia and vascular catheters, though wounds and the urinary tract are other possible primary sites. Risk factors for *A. baumanni* bacteraemia include immunosuppression, prior use of broad-spectrum antibiotics, mechanical ventilation, trauma, burns, malignancy, and prolonged hospitalization. *Acinetobacter* are also rare causes of infective endocarditis and nosocomial meningitis. Traumatic wound infections (notably war-related blast injuries) with MDR *Acinetobacter* are increasingly reported.

Diagnosis

Culture: send clinically relevant samples (blood, respiratory samples, CSF) for culture and sensitivity. Distinction between colonization and infection can often be difficult and depends crucially on the clinical context and site of sampling. As with *Pseudomonas* spp., quantitative or semi-quantitative culture of respiratory samples may be helpful.

Treatment
Treatment of severe disease depends on sensitivity but empirical treatment should be with a carbapenem ± a quinolone.

Refer to
Public Health England (PHE) guidelines on multi-resistant *Acinetobacter* infections: ℘ https://www.gov.uk/government/publications/acinetobacter-working-party-guidance-on-the-control-of-multi-resistant-acinetobacter-outbreaks/working-party-guidance-on-the-control-of-multi-resistant-acinetobacter-outbreaks.

Acknowledgement

This chapter was kindly reviewed by Dr Ian Bowler, Consultant in Infectious Diseases and Microbiology, Oxford University Hospitals NHS Trust.

Index